PHARMACOLOGY
SECRETS

PHARMACOLOGY SECRETS

PATRICIA K. ANTHONY, Ph.D.

Chair, Department of Pharmacology
Medical University of the Americas
Nevis, West Indies

HANLEY & BELFUS, INC./Philadelphia

Publisher: HANLEY & BELFUS, INC.
              Medical Publishers
              210 South 13th Street
              Philadelphia, PA 19107
              (215) 546-7293; 800-962-1892
              FAX (215) 790-9330
              Web site: http://www.hanleyandbelfus.com

Note to the reader: Although the information in this book has been carefully reviewed for correctness of dosage and indications, neither the authors nor the editor nor the publisher can accept any legal responsibility for any errors or omissions that may be made. Neither the publisher nor the editor makes any warranty, expressed or implied, with respect to the material contained herein. Before prescribing any drug, the reader must review the manufacturer's current product information (package inserts) for accepted indications, absolute dosage recommendations, and other information pertinent to the safe and effective use of the product described.

Library of Congress Cataloging-in-Publication Data

Pharmacology secrets / edited by Patricia K. Anthony.
    p. ; cm.—(The Secrets Series®)
  Includes index.
  ISBN 1-56053-470-2 (alk. paper)
   1. Pharmacology—Miscellanea. I. Anthony, Patricia K. II. Series.
  |DNLM: 1. Pharmaceutical Preparations—Examination Questions. 2. Drug
Therapy—Examination Questions. 3. Pharmaceutical Services—Examination Questions.
QV 18.2 P5357 2001|
RM301.P475 2002
615'.1—dc21

                        2001026398

PHARMACOLOGY SECRETS   ISBN 1-56053-470-2

Last digit is the print number: 9 8 7 6 5 4 3 2 1

DEDICATION

To my father, who inspired me to aspire, and to my family
To physicians and medical professionals everywhere,
    and to their patients
To my professors, and their students
To my students, past and present

    (and to Mary—the smartest turnip to fall off of the truck)

CONTENTS

XI. CANCER CHEMOTHERAPY
Patricia K. Anthony, Ph.D., and Dal Yoo, M.D.

XII. HERBAL AND OVER-THE-COUNTER PREPARATIONS AND TOXICOLOGY
Patricia K. Anthony, Ph.D., and Donald Kautz, Ph.D.

PREFACE

In writing *Pharmacology Secrets*, we have attempted to promote a better understanding of pharmacology by integrating the basic sciences with the practice of clinical pharmacology. Pharmacology is a truly "multidisciplinary" field and is based on the integration of disciplines such as physiology and biochemistry in the study of the actions of drugs. Thus, we have reviewed basic principles from these disciplines within the context of pharmacologic therapy.

In order to differentiate *Pharmacology Secrets* from the plethora of pharmacology texts in the market, an attempt has been made to orient the text to the needs of students and medical professionals, and to enhance the *understanding* of the basic principles of pharmacologic intervention. Most notably, we have presented ideas and concepts in a manner that promotes *thought*, as well as understanding, presenting clear discussions of pharmacologic mechanisms and the physiologic bases of drug action. In this way, we hope to have presented some of the true "secrets" of pharmacology.

In writing and editing this book, I have drawn on over nineteen years of collective teaching and research experience in pharmacology to reveal to the reader the collective cellular, subcellular, and physiologic mechanisms underlying drug action and the ultimate actions of therapy on the "whole" patient, rather than simply looking at the therapeutic goal and related drug action. I hope that this book will stimulate independent thought and understanding in the reader, and ultimately foster an integrated, novel approach to pharmacologic therapy.

Many thanks to my contributors, who took the time and effort to "broaden the Secrets palette" and added much to the text.

Patricia K. Anthony Ph.D.

I. General Pharmacology

Patricia K. Anthony, Ph.D.

1. PHARMACOKINETICS

1. Define the term *pharmacokinetics*.
The movement of drugs within the body from dosage to elimination. Pharmacokinetics encompasses the absorption, distribution, metabolism, and excretion of drugs.

2. State the Henderson-Hasselbalch equation and describe its use in pharmacology.
The equation:

$$pK_a \text{ (of drug)} = pH - \log \frac{\text{protonated drug particles}}{\text{nonprotonated drug particles}}$$

This equation is used to predict the degree of ionization of a drug or substance at a particular pH range, in order to predict the movement of the drug across cell membranes. This information allows a more accurate prediction of the potency and efficacy of a drug.

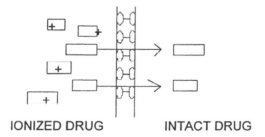

IONIZED DRUG   INTACT DRUG

3. What is the role of the cell membrane in drug absorption?
The cell membrane is lipophilic in nature, and therefore acts as a barrier to drugs that are water-soluble. Those drugs that are dissociated (charged) at physiologic pH for a particular compartment will not cross the lipophilic cell membrane, and will therefore not be absorbed, or will be absorbed in lesser quantities, which are predicted by the Henderson-Hasselbalch equation.

4. State the role of the cell membrane in relation to drug potency.
Drug potency is a measure of the amount of drug necessary to achieve a desired result. The potency of a drug may be reduced if the drug is ionized at physiologic pH, as the ionized fraction will not cross cell membranes. A higher dose (resulting in a higher concentration of nonionized drug) will thus be necessary to achieve the desired result. Thus, potency is decreased

5. Discuss drugs as weak bases.
Most drugs are weak bases, that is, they exist in a neutral state within a basic environment. Upon exposure to an acidic environment, however, the neutral molecule accepts a proton [H⁺], forming a charged (protonated, ionized) molecule that will not cross cell membranes. The neutral (nonionized) form is thus the intact (and more lipophilic) form. Only in this form will the drug cross cell membranes. Thus, a drug that is a weak base will only cross cell membranes from a basic environment as shown in the figure on the next page.

Weak Acid		Weak Base	
R-COOH	RCOO⁻ H⁺	RC-NH₂	RC-NH₃⁺
protenated	non-protenated	non-protenated	protenated
form	form	form	form
(non-ionized)	*(ionized)*	*(non-ionized)*	*(ionized)*

6. Discuss drugs as weak acids.

Drugs that are weak acids exist in a protonated state within an acid environment, but when exposed to a basic environment, the proton dissociates, forming an anion and a cation (the molecule ionizes). The protonated (non-dissociated, non-ionized) state is thus the more lipophilic for a drug that is a weak acid. This becomes important when utilizing the Henderson-Hasselbalch equation to predict the degree of absorption across cell membranes.

7. Acetaminophen has a pK_a of 9.5. Is it a weak acid or a weak base?

The consideration of the pK_a value is irrelevant to the question. The classification of drugs as weak acids or bases is independent of the pK_a of the drug; rather, it is a function of the protonation of the drug molecule. Acetaminophen is actually a weak acid, as it ionizes in a basic environment.

8. Define *drug absorption*.

Drug absorption refers to the entrance of the drug into the bloodstream. Thus, the term is only applicable to drugs administered by an enteral or topical route. As injectable drugs are administered directly into the blood stream, they are not absorbed.

9. What is the relevance of pH to drug absorption?

The pH of a physiologic compartment in relation to the pK_a of a particular drug and the classification of the drug as a weak acid or weak base determines the amount of drug that will be absorbed in that compartment. Because drugs can only pass through cell membranes in nonionized (neutral) form, optimizing the pH of the compartment to the pK_a of the drug will result in more drug particles existing in nonionized form (as calculated using the Henderson-Hasselbalch equation). This will result in a greater absorption of drug in that compartment. For example, codeine, a weak base with a pK_a of 8.2, will be 61.4 percent absorbed in the basic milieu of the duodenum (pH = 8), but less than 0.0002 percent of the drug will be absorbed in the acid milieu of the stomach (pH = 2.5).

10. Discuss the effect of concurrent administration of antacids and aspirin.

Ingestion of an antacid (alternatively an H_2 blocker or proton pump inhibitor) results in an increase in the pH of the gastric milieu. Because the pK_a of aspirin (a weak acid) is 3.5, and therefore exists mainly in nonionized form in the gastric milieu, an increase in gastric pH would shift the equilibrium to the right, resulting in an increase in the ionized form and decreased absorption of the drug.

11. What is the partition coefficient for a drug?

It is a measure of how lipophilic a drug is. The more lipophilic a drug is, the higher is its partition coefficient.

12. State the significance of the partition coefficient.

Drugs with low partition coefficients are likely to distribute in the plasma and thus are more likely to have peripheral effects. They are also more likely to be eliminated by renal filtration. In contrast, those with high partition coefficients will distribute in adipose tissue and are more likely to cross the blood-brain barrier and distribute into the central nervous system (CNS), with CNS effects. These drugs are likely to undergo hepatic metabolism and be eliminated in the bile.

13. Describe the role of the partition coefficient in the rapidity of onset of a CNS drug.

In general, lipid-soluble drugs have a higher partition coefficient. Because the brain and spinal cord contain a large amount of fatty tissue (e.g., myelin) and are protected by the blood-brain barrier, the more lipophilic a drug is, the better it will cross into the CNS. This will also result in a faster onset and faster withdrawal of effects as well, because the drug will cross very rapidly into (and out of) the lipophilic environment of the CNS.

14. To what does the term *drug distribution* refer?
After a drug is absorbed into the bloodstream, it is distributed among the bodily compartments such as plasma and adipose tissue. Where the drug is distributed depends on the degree of ionization at physiologic pH and on the partition coefficient. More water-soluble drugs distribute into plasma and may bind to plasma proteins. The type of proteins to which a drug binds is specific to that drug; it may bind to albumin, or it may preferentially bind to more specialized proteins in the plasma (e.g., thyroid-binding protein, IGF-binding protein), or to other types of plasma proteins. More lipophilic drugs distribute into the CNS and into adipose tissue. Drugs that are less hydrophilic may also bind to tissue proteins.

15. Which types of drugs extensively bind to plasma albumin?
Drugs such as phenytoin, prednisolone, and aspirin extensively bind to plasma albumin.

16. In addition to albumin, which other plasma proteins may serve as drug-binding sites?
Plasma globulins and α_1-acid glycoprotein.

17. State the pharmacologic ramifications of the type of plasma protein to which a drug binds.
The protein type can determine how stable the plasma levels of drug will be. For example, albumin is in relatively high concentrations in the plasma (barring genetic abnormalities), providing plentiful and relatively constant binding sites for drugs, under a variety of conditions. Drugs that bind to plasma globulins and to α_1-acid glycoproteins, however, may fluctuate in level under inflammatory conditions, as the amounts of these proteins may increase when inflammation is present and decrease at other times. Thus, the concentration of free drug in the plasma (and the pharmacologic effect) is more difficult to predict.

18. Define *volume of distribution*.
Volume of distribution is the amount of space available in the body in which drugs may be stored. Theoretically, it refers to a homogenous distribution of drug.

19. What effect does a large volume of distribution have on drug dosage?
In general, it means that a higher dose can be tolerated. A drug with a large volume of distribution allows a correspondingly higher therapeutic dose.

20. Describe the effect of concurrent administration of drugs that are highly protein bound (e.g., warfarin and carbamazepine).
When two drugs that both bind with high affinity to plasma proteins are administered concurrently, a competition exists between the two drugs for plasma protein-binding sites. Because protein-binding sites are not unlimited, the drug that has the greatest affinity will occupy more sites. This results in increased levels of the second drug existing as free drug in the plasma. Recalling that the pharmacologically active drug is not that which is in the bound form, but that which is free in the plasma, the increase in free drug may result in an apparent increased effect, with a potential increase in toxicity.

21. Does concurrent administration of drugs that are highly protein bound necessarily result in toxicity?
Toxicity depends on the individual patient. If clearance rates increase, which correlate with the increased plasma drug levels, theoretically no toxicity would result. However, while it is true that clearance rate for the free drug could increase with an increase in plasma level, which might eventually stabilize plasma levels, continued concurrent administration would exacerbate the problem by continually replacing the cleared drug. Thus, elevated plasma

levels of free drug might continue to be maintained, regardless of an increase in clearance, resulting in potential toxicity. A dosage adjustment would need to be made, particularly in the elderly.

22. How are drugs eliminated from the system?

Drugs are normally eliminated by liver metabolism, by renal filtration, and by redistribution.
Metabolism within major organs, such as the lung, intestine, cardiac myocytes, and the
blood/vascular system, may also occur. For example, drugs such as acetylcholine are metabolized
by plasma esterases. Still other drugs, such as prostaglandin analogs, are metabolized by the lung
and eliminated, and still others are so poorly absorbed (e.g., sulfasalazine) as to pass through the
feces to be metabolized by intestinal flora.

23. Explain the phenomenon of redistribution.

Redistribution is the process whereby drugs that are concentrated and have activity in a particular tissue or organ may be eliminated by removal of the drug from the target tissue to other
storage sites in the body. This may occur, for example, with drugs that are active in the central
nervous system, such as general anesthetics. These drugs rapidly concentrate in the central nervous system, resulting in a rapid onset of drug effects. An equally rapid redistribution to sites in
the periphery terminates the drug action.

24. What is meant by drug clearance?

Drug clearance is the rate of elimination of the drug as a function of drug concentration.
Depending on the properties of the drug, clearance may be a function of concentration in the
plasma or blood, that is:

$$\text{Clearance} = \frac{\text{Rate of elimination}}{\text{Plasma concentration}}$$

25. What kinds of drugs are eliminated by renal filtration?

Drugs that are small in molecular size and highly soluble in water may be eliminated unchanged through renal filtration. The degree of elimination is dependent upon urine pH. Drugs
that are less soluble in water (less polar) are first metabolized by enzymes in the liver (e.g., cytochrome P_{450}), and made more polar by the subsequent attachment of a polar group, such as an
organic acid (e.g., glucuronic acid or acetic acid (acetate)). This metabolic transformation allows
the molecule to be excreted by the kidney as shown in the figure below.

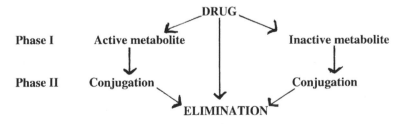

26. Discuss the elimination of drugs by hepatic metabolism.

Drugs that are lipid soluble, such as CNS drugs, may be excreted unchanged through the
bile, or enzymatically converted to metabolites, which are then excreted through the bile. This
metabolism may require several enzymatic steps, some of which may generate active metabolites
or metabolites that are toxic.

27. What is zero order enzymatic metabolism?

Under zero order metabolism (zero order kinetics), drugs are metabolized at a constant rate
per time. This occurs when the enzymes involved become saturated.

28. Describe first-order enzymatic metabolism.

First-order kinetics are followed when a drug is eliminated as a constant percent of the plasma concentration per time. In this instance, the metabolizing enzymes are not saturated, with therapeutic dose. The majority of drugs follow first-order kinetics in their metabolism.

29. What are phase I and phase II biotransformations?

Both phase I and phase II biotransformations are enzymatic reactions that normally take place in the liver. The type of phase I and phase II biotransformations, and the order and number in which they occur, are a function of the drug structure and available liver enzymes. A drug may undergo only phase I metabolism, or a phase I reaction with a subsequent phase II reaction. It is also possible for a drug to undergo the phase II reaction before undergoing the phase I and possibly a second phase II reaction, as well (e.g., the antituberculin drug isoniazid).

30. How are phase I and phase II biotransformations generally accomplished?

In phase I biotransformations the parent drug molecule is enzymatically converted to a polar metabolite by the conjugation of a functional group to the drug molecule (or removal of a functional group, depending on the structure), making the molecule more polar in character. If the metabolite produced is not readily excreted, a subsequent phase II reaction occurs.

Phase II biotransformation involves the enzymatic conjugation of a polar molecule to the drug molecule or to the phase I metabolite. These reactions include glucuronidation, acetylation, sulfation, or amidation.

31. List some examples of drugs that are metabolized by phase II glucuronidation.

Glucuronidated drugs include aspirin, barbiturates, opiates, diazepam, meprobamate, mescaline, acetaminophen, and digitalis glycosides.

32. What role do genetic factors play in drug metabolism?

Genetic expression of enzymes and their cofactors may influence the metabolism of drugs and therefore play a role in determining dosage and dosage frequency. An example is acetylation—patients may be classified into "fast" and "slow" acetylators, depending on the level of expression and activity of acetylases. This influences the rate of metabolism and must be considered when prescribing a drug such as isoniazid. The same is true for persons expressing decreased levels or defective pseudocholinesterases, which would affect the clearance of drugs such as succinylcholine.

33. Describe the "first-pass" effect and its significance.

Drugs taken orally are absorbed and subsequently pass through the hepatic portal system into the liver. Many drugs are quickly metabolized on this initial pass through the liver (hence, the "first-pass" effect). Depending on the drug, this may result in complete inactivation or an alteration of activity. Examples of drugs with a high hepatic first-pass effect are catecholamines, morphine, verapamil, isoniazid, and aspirin. Other drugs, such as clonazepam, may also be metabolized by intestinal flora, contributing to the first-pass effect.

34. What is *enterohepatic recycling*?

Enterohepatic recycling refers to the reabsorption of an excreted drug or an active metabolite from the gut. This occurs with drugs that are excreted unchanged by the liver or that generate active metabolites, which are then excreted in the bile. As the bile is reabsorbed in the course of digestion, the drug or active metabolite is also reabsorbed, or "recycled." Clinically, this results in an increased duration of action of the drug.

35. How do drugs induce metabolic enzymes?

Some drugs act on the enzymes that metabolize them to increase the activity or the number of enzyme molecules present. This is termed *induction of the metabolic enzymes*. Ethanol and carbamazepine are examples of this type of drug.

36. What is the half-life ($T\frac{1}{2}$) of a drug?

The half-life is the amount of time that is required for half of the absorbed dose of drug to be cleared from the body.

37. Assume that a drug has a $T\frac{1}{2}$ of 8 hours. How long will it take for 75 percent of the drug to be cleared from the body?

By definition, in 8 hours, 50 percent of the drug will be cleared from the body; 50 percent of the remaining drug will be cleared in another 8 hours, leaving 25 percent of the original plasma concentration. Thus, 75 percent of the drug has been cleared in two half-lives, or 16 hours.

38. A drug (e.g., carbamazepine or ethanol) induces enzymes required for its metabolism. How does induction affect the half-life of the drug?

Chronic use of the drug will increase the amount and/or activity of metabolic enzymes, which will result in faster metabolism and a decrease in drug half-life. This leads to drug tolerance, and the dosage may need to be adjusted over time.

39. Does the age of a patient have an effect on drug half-life?

In a very young patient, particularly a neonate, the kidney and liver are still continuing to develop, and renal and hepatic clearance are decreased, as compared to an adult. In a geriatric patient, renal function and glomerular filtration rate are decreased, as well as hepatic metabolism. Thus, both increased and decreased age could result in an increase in the half-life of a drug.

40. Describe the effect of urine pH on renal excretion and drug half-life.

Drugs that are ionized in the tubular fluid are eliminated in the urine, as drugs in ionized form are not reabsorbed across the tubular membrane. Drug molecules that do not ionize, however, may be reabsorbed, extending the half-life of the drug. Thus, a basic drug is more quickly eliminated in acid urine, whereas an acidic drug remains in the intact form in an acidic environment, and is reabsorbed. The degree of reabsorption is predicted by the Henderson-Hasselbalch equation.

41. Predict the effect of concurrent acetazolamide administration on the half-life of an acidic drug such as ampicillin ($pK_a = 2.5$).

Acetazolamide increases the concentration of bicarbonate in renal tubular fluid, resulting in basic urine. An acidic drug such as ampicillin would be primarily in ionized form at basic pH, resulting in increased excretion and a decrease in the half-life of the drug.

42. Discuss the relationship between drug half-life and dosage interval.

The objective of therapy is to achieve and maintain a therapeutic level of drug in the plasma. This level should remain constant throughout therapy, avoiding fluctuations in levels that may result in toxic symptoms (peaks) or subtherapeutic levels (troughs). Correlating the dosage interval with the drug half-life enables a more constant level to be maintained (ideally the drug should be replaced as it is cleared).

BIBLIOGRAPHY

1. Bearden DT, Rodvold KA: Dosage adjustments for antibacterials in obese patients: Applying clinical pharmacokinetics. Clin Pharmacokinet 38(5):415–426, 2000.
2. Fauvelle F, Petitjean O, Tod M, Guillevin L: Clinical pharmacokinetics during plasma exchange. Therapie 55(2):269–275, 2000.
3. Fuhr U: Induction of drug metabolising enzymes: Pharmacokinetic and toxicological consequences in humans. Clin Pharmacokinet 38(6):493–504, 2000.
4. Miners JO, Birkett DJ: Cytochrome P4502C9: An enzyme of major importance in human drug metabolism. Br J Clin Pharmacol 45(6):525–538, 1998.
5. Park K, Verotta D, Blaschke TF, Sheiner LB: A simiparametric method for describing noisy population pharmacokinetic data. J Pharmacokinet Biopharm 25(5):615–642, 1997.

2. PHARMACODYNAMICS

1. Define *pharmacodynamics*.

Pharmacodynamics refers to the action of the drug at the cellular level. This term encompasses the binding of a drug to its receptor or binding site, the relationship of dose and therapeutic level to the physiologic response, and the relationship of drug action and efficacy to dosage interval.

2. Distinguish between drug potency and drug efficacy.

Drug *potency* refers to the dose (amount of drug required) to produce a particular effect. The higher the dose that is required to produce the desired physiologic effect, the less potent the drug. Drug *efficacy* refers to the maximum effect that can be produced by a drug. It is independent of dose.

3. Refer to the figure below and discuss the relative potency of the three drugs (A, B, and C).

Drug A produces an equal response to that of drugs B and C, but with a lower dose. It is therefore the most potent drug of the three. Drug C is the least potent, as the greatest dose is required to produce a therapeutic effect.

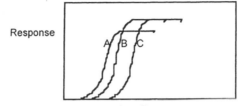

4. Refer to the above figure and explain the relative efficacy of the three drugs.

Drugs B and C are equally efficacious—the two drugs produce the same maximum effect, albeit at different doses (recall that efficacy is independent of dose). Drug A, on the other hand, never produces the amount of response seen with drugs B and C, regardless of how much drug is administered. The maximum therapeutic effect produced by drug A is seen at a relatively low dose, so further increases in dose would only produce toxicity, not increased therapeutic benefit. It is therefore the least efficacious of the three drugs.

5. What is the ED_{50}?

The ED_{50}, or effective dose 50, is the dose that produces the desired therapeutic response in 50 percent of patients.

6. What is the EC_{50}?

The EC_{50}, or effective concentration 50, is the plasma concentration of drug at which 50 percent of the maximum response for the drug is seen. It can be calculated using the plasma concentration-response curve as follows:

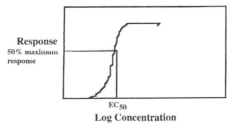

7. Discuss the significance of the LD$_{50}$.

This number represents the lethal dose in 50 percent of animal test subjects. The higher the value of the LD$_{50}$ for a drug, the safer it is, because a higher dose is required to produce toxic effects and death.

8. What is the clinical significance of prescribing a drug with a low LD$_{50}$?

A drug with a low LD$_{50}$ would produce toxic symptoms and death with a lower dose. Such a drug can easily result in a fatal overdose simply by inappropriate dosing.

9. What is the therapeutic index (TI)?

The therapeutic index is a measure of the relative safety of a drug. Mathematically, it is a ratio of the value of the LD$_{50}$ and ED$_{50}$ of a drug:

$$TI = \frac{LD_{50}}{ED_{50}}$$

10. What is the significance of the therapeutic index?

Recall that a high LD$_{50}$ gives a wide safety margin in case of inappropriate dosing, while a low ED$_{50}$ means that only a small amount is required for therapeutic effect. Therefore, because the TI is a ratio of the two, the higher the therapeutic index, the safer the drug.

11. Define *therapeutic level*.

For a drug to be therapeutically active, an optimum ratio of drug to storage sites and sites of activity must be maintained. Thus, there is a minimum concentration of drug per unit of plasma that must be maintained for therapeutic efficacy. This is called the therapeutic level, and is usually expressed in milligrams per deciliter (mg/dl).

The particular numeric plasma concentration necessary for therapeutic action is dependent on the particular drug and on the individual patient.

12. Define *therapeutic window*.

The area between the minimum efficacious dose and the maximum allowable dose is the therapeutic window. It may also be thought of as a range of acceptable plasma levels in which positive therapeutic results are seen. The smallest plasma drug level that produces a positive response is the lower limit of the therapeutic window, and the upper boundary of the window is the level at which undesirable effects or toxic responses are seen.

13. What is the clinical significance of the therapeutic window?

It is extremely important in light of patient compliance: a patient who is lax in adherence to a dosing regimen may not maintain therapeutic levels, while the patient who is dosing too frequently (as happens with lapses of memory, or adherence to the concept of "if a little is good, more is better") will build plasma levels at or above the upper boundary, producing toxicity.

14. Which physiologic conditions might alter a drug's potency?

The pH of the surrounding tissue: The drug may become ionized and thus be less capable of crossing cell membranes, requiring a higher dose. (Recall that the Henderson-Hasselbalch equation predicts a ratio of ionized drug to nonionized drug. An increased dose will increase the amount of nonionized drug available in an ionizing environment.) An example of a case in which this is an issue is the use of a weak, basic local anesthetic (e.g., lidocaine, prilocaine) when an infection or inflammation is present.

Altered gastric pH: An acidic drug may be incompletely absorbed if gastric pH is increased. This may occur through the use of antacids, H$_2$-receptor antagonists, or the use of proton pump inhibitors, or in conditions where vomiting is present. This may result in systemic alkalosis, which further lowers drug potency.

Drug metabolism: Production of active metabolites or saturation of metabolic enzymes may result in higher level of drug availability, resulting in a lower therapeutic dosage.

15. Define *loading dose*.

A loading dose is the amount initially given to bring plasma concentration to approximate therapeutic levels. If a loading dose is not given, the patient must build to therapeutic levels using the prescribed dosage regimen. This may take time, depending on the drug and rate of clearance, and therapeutic benefit is decreased during this interval.

16. Define *maintenance dose*.

Once therapeutic levels are reached, the optimum amount of drug necessary to be administered is equal to the amount of drug cleared per time. The maintenance dose is therefore calculated based on the drug half-life and clearance rate, in order to maintain a constant therapeutic level.

17. How do tolerance and tachyphylaxis differ?

When a drug is given over time, the effects may decrease accordingly. This may be the consequence of, for example, desensitization of receptors or depletion of neurotransmitter stores. This effect is termed *tolerance*. If a drug is administered and produces a response that diminishes with subsequent doses, the effect is termed *tachyphylaxis*. This phenomenon is a rapid decrease in drug effect with subsequent dosing.

RECEPTOR PHARMACOLOGY

18. Which types of molecules may serve as drug receptors?

The majority of drug receptors are classified as regulatory proteins. Molecules such as enzymes, transport proteins, or structural proteins (e.g., histone, tubulin) may also be classified as drug receptors.

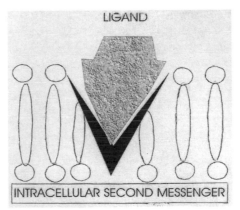

The "lock and key" model.

19. Describe the two general classifications of receptors and how they differ.

The first classification is extracellular receptors, which work through a second messenger, and the second is intracellular receptors, which alter gene expression by altering the configuration of structural proteins regulating DNA transcription.

20. What is the role of the receptor in the selectivity of drug action?

The molecular size, shape, and charge of a drug in relation to that of the receptor determines the degree of binding of the drug to that receptor. This has been referred to as the "lock and key" effect. Thus, specific changes in the structure of a drug may dramatically influence the type of receptor to which it binds, subsequently altering the potency of the drug and its physiologic effects, as well as the degree of toxic effects.

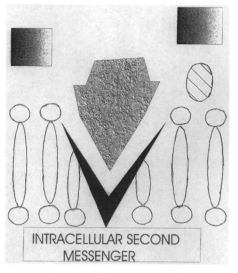

The extracellular receptor model.

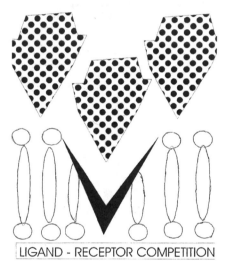

21. Describe the relationship of dose and therapeutic levels to the role of the drug receptor.

A drug's potency is a function of the degree of drug-receptor complexes formed. Drug-receptor complexes are dynamic—drugs and their receptors are constantly dissociating and reassociating, in accordance with the binding affinity of the drug for the receptor, and the stability of the drug-receptor complex. Thus, the drug which is bound to the receptors is in equilibrium with drug that is free. A larger dose results in more free drug available (a greater plasma drug level) which forces the equilibrium to the right, resulting in a greater number of drug-receptor complexes and greater therapeutic effect, up to the maximum effect of the drug.

22. What factors may limit the maximum effect of a drug?
- The number and affinity of receptors present in a particular tissue or organ.
- The number and affinity of receptors present which may mediate adverse effects associated with the drug.

- The ability of a drug to reach the target site.
- Endogenous factors or other drugs which may compete with the drug for binding.
- The maximum ability of the target tissue to respond to the drug.

23. How do drugs mediate physiologic effects by binding receptors?

Most drugs bind to receptors on the cell membrane. These receptors are proteins that are coupled to **second messengers** such as enzymes (e.g., adenlyate cyclase, guanylate cyclase, protein kinase C, or tyrosine kinase), or calcium. The activation of the receptor results in the activation and release of the second messenger, which initiates a **cascade response** within the cell, ending in a specific cellular response (e.g., smooth muscle contraction, increased heart rate, energy storage, etc.).

24. Define *"drug receptor agonist"*.

A drug receptor agonist is a substance that binds to an endogenous receptor and elicits a stimulatory response.

25. How does a direct receptor agonist work?

A drug binds to the receptor and elicits one response—the receptor is activated only upon binding of the drug (or ligand). The process is dynamic—in order to continue receptor stimulation, the drug must then dissociate and reattach to the receptor site.

26. What problems are associated with chronic or high dose therapy with a receptor agonist?

The more drug molecules which are present (up to a point), the more consistently the receptor may be stimulated. Constant stimulation of a receptor may result in desensitization of the receptor, or in receptor "down regulation," and a lower number of available receptors. This is a tolerance effect, and may necessitate a drug holiday.

27. How does an indirect receptor agonist work?

Simply stated, an indirect agonist is a substance which increases levels of an endogenous agonist. Normally, an indirect agonist inhibits the degradation of the endogenous agonist (e.g., acetylcholine esterase inhibitors, monoamine oxidase inhibitors), or increases its rate of release (e.g., amphetamines). In this way, the concentrations of the endogenous (direct) agonist are increased, which increases the pharmacologic effect. The drug itself plays no direct agonistic role.

28. Describe the relationship between receptor affinity and drug potency.

The drug must bind repeatedly to the receptor in order to mediate maximal stimulation of the receptor. If the affinity of the drug for the receptor is too high, the drug remains on the receptor, essentially acting as an antagonist.

29. Contrast a weak and strong receptor agonist.

To be an effective agonist, a drug must have at least the potency of the endogenous ligand—the object of a therapeutically useful agonist is to mediate an increase in receptor activity. If the drug has decreased potency relative to the endogenous agonist, it may actually act as an antagonist (see the discussion of partial agonists). A strong agonist may have several times the potency of the endogenous ligand, while a weak agonist may have a potency and affinity for the receptor similar to the endogenous ligand.

30. Describe a drug receptor antagonist.

A drug receptor antagonist binds to an endogenous receptor and does not elicit a response. Since receptors by definition have an endogenous ligand, the binding of the antagonistic drug prevents the binding of the endogenous agonist, resulting in decreased activation of the receptor.

31. Describe a competitive antagonist.

A competitive antagonist binds and dissociates from the receptor, in accordance with the binding affinity of the drug for the receptor.

32. What is the relationship between drug concentration and receptor stimulation?

Once a drug molecule binds to the receptor, produces activation, and dissociates, the opportunity exists for a second drug molecule to occupy the binding site on the receptor. If this molecule is a receptor agonist, continued stimulation occurs. If, however, the molecule is an antagonist, or is decreased in potency with regard to the endogenous agonist, stimulation decreases and pharmacologic effect is impaired.

33. Describe a noncompetitive antagonist.

A noncompetitive antagonist has a strong affinity for the receptor binding site. This type of drug may bind covalently to the site, resulting in a relatively permanent association. Thus, because the drug does not dissociate, it blocks the receptor permanently. (Recall that receptors are fairly short-lived, and are endocytosed and recycled frequently, so the term "permanent" is relative.)

34. Is a competitive antagonist safer than a noncompetitive antagonist?

Yes. A competitive antagonist dissociates and re-attaches to the receptor site. Thus, it competes with the endogenous ligand. Should an accidental overdose of a competitive antagonist be administered, it can be countered by the administration of a compensatory amount of receptor agonist. Should an overdose of the noncompetitive drug be administered, however, this safeguard would not apply, and supportive measures would need to be instituted until receptor recycling could take place. The competitive antagonist therefore has a wider margin of safety.

36. Describe a partial agonist.

A partial agonist (e.g., pindolol, pentazocine) is that which has the ability to stimulate the receptor, but has less potency at the receptor than the endogenous ligand.

37. What is the physiologic action of a partial agonist?

The endogenous ligand is always in the body and competes with the drug for receptor binding sites. When concentrations of the endogenous ligand are low, the partial agonist acts as an agonist, because it binds to and stimulates unbound receptors, albeit with decreased potency. However, when endogenous ligand concentrations are high, the drug competes for binding sites on the receptors, and, because of the drug's decreased activity at the receptor, effectively blocks the binding sites for the more potent endogenous ligand. In this case, the drug is effectively acting as an antagonist.

38. Describe the pharmacologic use of a partial agonist.

The use of a partial agonist helps to promote a constant level of receptor stimulation when secretion of the endogenous ligand is erratic. For example, patients with inappropriate secretion of norepinephrine (where levels are increased at rest and decreased during exercise), benefit from pindolol therapy, and those involved in the recovery of opiate addiction benefit from pentazocine therapy to prevent reintroduction of the opiate narcotic.

39. Describe nonreceptor mediated drug antagonism.

Drug antagonism may occur when a drug is inactivated by an antagonizing drug or substance. Rather than blocking a receptor site, the substance acts directly on the drug, or antagonizes its actions. An example would be the chelation of tetracylines by divalent ions, which prevents its absorption, the chemical inactivation of heparin by protamine sulfate, or the inhibition of the actions of methotrexate by folinic acid.

40. Refer to the figure below and discuss which two of the three drugs (A, B, or C) are antagonistic?

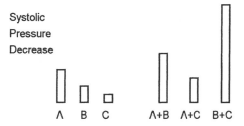

The response of drug A alone is greater than the combination with drug C. Drug C is therefore antagonistic to the actions of drug A.

41. Which of the drugs in the above figure have additive effects in lowering blood pressure?
The amount of response produced by drug A plus the amount of response produced by drug B equals the response produced by the combination of drugs A and B. The effects are therefore additive.

42. Mechanistically, what does the additive effect of drugs A and B tell you about them?
Since the effects are additive, the two drugs are most likely working by the same mechanism.

43. Discuss which drugs in the figure above are synergistic?
Drugs that are synergistic produce a far greater effect when used together than the total effect of the two drugs put together (i.e., much more than an additive effect). This occurs with the combination of drugs B and C. These drugs are probably working by different mechanisms.

BIBLIOGRAPHY

1. Bos JD, Meinardi MM: The 500 Dalton rule for the skin penetration of chemical compounds and drugs. Exper Dermatol 9(3):165–169, 2000.
2. Hardman J, Limbird L, Gilman A: Goodman & Gilman's The Pharmacological Basis of Therapeutics, 10th ed. McGraw-Hill Publishers, 2001.
3. Katzung B: Basic and Clinical Pharmacology, 8th ed. Appleton & Lange, 2001.
4. Olson SC, Bockbrader H, Boyd RA, Cook J, et al: Impact of population pharmacokinetic-pharmacodynamic analyses on the drug development process: Experience at Parke-Davis. Clin Pharmacokinet 38(5):449–459, 2000.

II. *Drugs that Affect the Central Nervous System*

Patricia K. Anthony, Ph.D., and C. Andrew Powers, Ph.D.

3. SEDATIVE-HYPNOTIC DRUGS

1. Compare sedation and hypnosis.
   Sedation is an anxiolytic effect. A sedative drug depresses the central nervous system enough to exert a calming effect, but the higher brain centers and motor functions are not affected. Hypnosis occurs with further depression of the central nervous system, where a normal sleep cycle is induced. In the state of hypnosis, cognitive functions and motor skills are impaired.

2. Describe the clinical uses of sedative-hypnotic drugs.
   The depressant actions of these drugs are useful in the treatment of anxiety, insomnia, or as an adjunct to general anesthesia. They are also useful in the therapy of stimulant overdose (e.g., amphetamines).

3. What physical manifestations are seen with increasing central nervous system (CNS) depression (increasing dose of sedative-hypnotic drugs)?
   Sedation generally results with a low dose of a sedative-hypnotic drug. As the dosage is increased (see figure), one sees hypnosis, progressing to anesthesia. With increasing dose, medullary respiratory centers and vagomotor centers are depressed, the patient becomes comatose, and finally, death ensues. These effects are dose dependent. However, the dosage required and the final result depends on the drug.

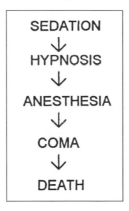

4. Do sedative-hypnotic drugs cross the fetal-placental barrier?
   Yes. These drugs tend to be highly lipophilic and therefore will easily cross into the fetal circulation. They will also be released into breast milk.

5. Discuss the general mechanism of action of benzodiazepines.
   The action of these drugs is mediated through the inhibitory neurotransmitter gamma-aminobutyric acid (GABA), which governs the activation of the chloride channel within the membrane

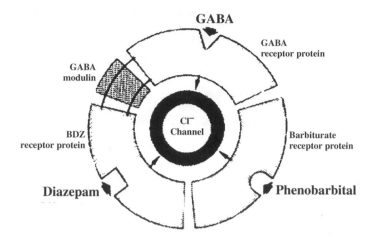

of excitable cells. Central benzodiazepine receptors interact allosterically with GABA receptors, potentiating the effects of GABA, which increases chloride flux across the neuronal cell membrane. This tends to partially repolarize (stabilize) the membrane and decrease conduction.

6. What accounts for the differences in activity of various drugs which mimic the actions of GABA (e.g., increase chloride conductance)?

Evidence suggests that GABA receptors are heterogeneous with many different subtypes. This may account for the differential effects of the various GABA receptor agonists.

7. Describe the general therapeutic uses of benzodiazepines.

These drugs may be used as sedatives, anxiolytics, muscle relaxants, or hypnotics, depending on the individual drug.

8. What paradoxical effects may be seen with benzodiazepine therapy?

Irritability, excitability, and hallucinations are known to occur with the use of benzodiazepines.

9. Do specific benzodiazepine class drugs have activity in only one area?

Older drugs of the class (e.g., diazepam) have sedative, hypnotic, and muscle relaxant properties. This may be due primarily to the formation of active metabolites with various actions. Newer drugs, however, have been engineered to have increased activity in a specific area (e.g., triazolam as a hypnotic and alprazolam as an anxiolytic).

10. Discuss the contraindications to benzodiazepine therapy.

Benzodiazepines are contraindicated in a patient who is pregnant or lactating, due to the ability of the drug to pass into breast milk and to cross the fetal placental barrier. These drugs also are contraindicated in a patient diagnosed with myasthenia gravis (due to muscle relaxant activity), acute depression, or psychosis (due to general CNS depression). Because of the anticholinergic effects of drugs of this class, therapy in patients with narrow angle glaucoma also is contraindicated.

11. Describe the actions of benzodiazepines on the cardiovascular system.

These drugs stabilize excitable membranes, primarily in the CNS. Similarly, they stabilize excitable membranes in cardiac tissue and vascular smooth muscle. In susceptible individuals (e.g., the elderly, patients with existing cardiac dysfunction or hepatic dysfunction), this may lead to hypotension and abnormal cardiac activity.

12. Which benzodiazepine class drug has a pronounced muscle relaxant activity?

Diazepam, in particular, has a very pronounced depressant activity on skeletal muscle. While all drugs of this class have some activity in this regard, due to the stabilization of excitable tissue in skeletal muscle, certain older drugs of the class (e.g., diazepam) may have a direct muscle relaxant effect.

13. Describe the metabolism of benzodiazepines.

Most benzodiazepines first undergo microsomal oxidation through cytochrome P_{450} mixed function oxidases (phase I). The metabolites then undergo phase II glucuronide conjugation and are eliminated in the urine. Metabolites produced through phase I oxidation may have pharmacologic activity, depending on the parent drug. Secondary metabolites may also be pharmacologically active.

14. Which benzodiazepine is inactive as the parent drug and must undergo phase I metabolism?

Chlorazepate is a pharmacologically inactive "pro-drug." It is metabolically converted to desmethyldiazepam, which is pharmacologically active. Desmethyldiazepam is in turn metabolized to oxazepam, which is also pharmacologically active.

15. Which of the benzodiazepines have active metabolites?

Chlordiazepoxide, desmethyldiazepam, diazepam, and flurazepam have active metabolites that are subject to enterohepatic recycling, which accounts for their relatively long half lives. Alprazolam and triazolam also have active metabolites. However, these are rapidly inactivated by glucuronidation, which accounts for their relatively short half-lives.

16. Why is flurazepam useful in treating the "premature awakening" type of insomnia?

Flurazepam is rapidly metabolized into hydroxyethylflurazepam (the major metabolite) and N-desalkyl flurazepam. These metabolites are pharmacologically active, resulting in a relatively long duration of drug action.

17. Describe the clinical use of lorazepam.

Lorazepam has been used as a hypnotic.It is useful in the "premature awakening" type of insomnia, due to its long half-life. It is also used as an anxiolytic and skeletal muscle relaxant.

18. Discuss the pharmacokinetics of lorazepam.

As with most benzodiazepines, lorazepam is highly bound to plasma proteins (over 85 percent). The serum half-life of lorazepam is approximately 12 to 15 hours. The drug undergoes hepatic metabolism and is rapidly conjugated to an inactive glucuronide. Excretion of the metabolite is primarily renal, with a small percentage excreted through the bile.

19. What is the major adverse effect of benzodiazepine therapy?

A dose-related anterograde amnesia.

20. Why is triazolam useful in inducing sleep?

Triazolam has a rapid onset (30–60 minutes) and short duration (2–4 hours). It is therefore useful in sleep induction, but not in the "premature awakening" type of insomnia.

21. Describe the adverse effects of triazolam therapy.

Patients may develop a tolerance to drug effects with chronic use, and a rebound anxiety is also seen in waking hours. Impaired cognitive and motor functions also may occur, particularly in the elderly.

22. What is the major clinical use of alprazolam?

It is used in the therapy of chronic anxiety or panic disorder, in the absence of a behavioral disorder.

23. Discuss diazepam's therapeutic window.

Diazepam has a flatter dose-response curve than the other benzodiazepines. However, the drug's margin of safety is still very large.

24. What dose-related effects may be seen with diazepam?

Diazepam initially may produce a disinhibitory effect, followed by sedation, dose-related anticonvulsant, muscle relaxant, ataxic, and hypnotic effects.

25. Does diazepam decrease amphetamine-induced excitation?

No. Diazepam is relatively devoid of autonomic effects.

26. What are the indications of use for diazepam?

Diazepam is useful in the short-term therapy of anxiety, and in the relief of skeletal muscle spasm as seen with upper motor neuron disorders (e.g., cerebral palsy, athetosis). It may also be of use in alcohol withdrawal, in the symptomatic relief of acute agitation, tremor, and impending acute delirium tremens.

27. Is diazepam useful in the therapy of psychosis or depression?

No. Because of the paradoxical reactions and potential induction of suicidal tendencies, diazepam is not indicated in these states.

28. Describe the symptoms of diazepam overdosage.

Confusion, ataxia, and reduced reflex activity are seen. Decreased respiration, pulse and blood pressure may be seen with a large overdose, and coma may be seen with extreme overdose.

29. Why are benzodiazepines used in uncomfortable procedures such as endoscopy?

These agents tend to calm the patient, which is conducive to the procedure. In addition, benzodiazepines tend to produce anterograde amnesia, which inhibits the patient's memory of the procedure.

30. Do benzodiazepines cause difficulties in learning?

Yes. They can inhibit short-term memory (anterograde amnesia), while leaving long-term memory intact.

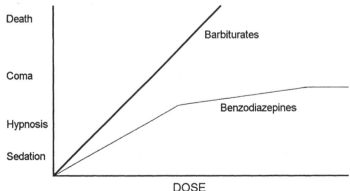

31. Explain why benzodiazepines have a much safer dose-response curve than other sedative hypnotic drugs (e.g., barbiturates).

Among the reasons for increased safety is a benzodiazepine receptor that, when stimulated, produces effects **opposite** to those of the benzodiazepines—effectively turning the drug into an **inverse agonist**. Because of the relative lack of sensitivity of these receptors, they are stimulated only with high doses of drug. Thus, as plasma levels increase, and the patient progresses from sedation through anesthesia, the drug activates these less sensitive receptors and further dose-related progression to respiratory depression and coma is opposed (see Figure on previous page).

32. Is flumazenil useful in reversing the respiratory depression caused by benzodiazepine overdose?

No. Flumazenil antagonizes central benzodiazepine receptors and is primarily useful in reversing CNS depression in benzodiazepine overdose. It is also used to speed recovery from drugs of this class, when used for diagnostic procedures or in anesthesia.

33. Does flumazenil reverse the CNS effects of nonbenzodiazepine sedative hypnotics?

No. The antagonism is specific for benzodiazepines.

34. Describe the pharmacokinetics and administration of flumazenil.

Flumazenil, when given intravenously, has a rapid onset, and is rapidly metabolized and cleared by the liver ($T\frac{1}{2}$ = 50–70 minutes). Because the duration of most benzodiazepines is very long, by comparison, the drug must be administered frequently over the course of treatment.

35. Describe the classification and use of zolpidem.

Zolpidem is of the imidazopyridine class, and is used as a hypnotic agent. It is not considered a benzodiazepine.

36. What is the mechanism of action of zolpidem?

Zolpidem acts at the omega-1 subtype of the benzodiazepine receptor on the chloride channel. Like the benzodiazepines, it potentiates the actions of GABA.

37. Does zolpidem exhibit anticonvulsant activity or promote muscle relaxation?

No.

38. What is the primary clinical use of zolpidem?

Due to its rapid onset and short duration of action (approximately 4 hours) zolpidem is useful only in the types of insomnia which exhibit delayed sleep onset. It is not useful in the "premature awakening" types of insomnia.

39. What would be the result of combining zolpidem with other CNS depressants (e.g., ethanol)?

Particularly in large doses, these drugs may synergize to cause respiratory depression.

40. Does zolpidem cause altered sleep patterns?

In doses recommended for hypnosis, the drug does not affect REM sleep. However, in larger doses, REM sleep may be shortened.

41. Describe the metabolism of zolpidem.

It is rapidly metabolized in the liver by oxidation and hydroxylation. The metabolites are inactive.

42. What is the clinical use of buspirone?

Buspirone is used as an anxiolytic in the short-term therapy of psychoneurosis.

43. Describe the drug classification of buspirone.

It is classified as an azaspirodecanedione.

44. What is the mechanism of action of buspirone?

The mechanism of action is not fully elucidated. However, the drug acts as a mixed agonist-antagonist at the D_2 receptor and an agonist at the $5HT_{1A}$ receptor, the combination of which produces a state of well-being.

45. Does buspirone activate the benzodiazepine receptor/GABA complex?

No. It is devoid of benzodiazepine-like activity.

46. Describe the pharmacokinetics of buspirone.

Buspirone undergoes an extensive first pass metabolism upon oral absorption. It is metabolized primarily by microsomal oxidation and produces a pharmacologically active metabolite. Multiple-dose studies suggest that steady-state plasma levels are achieved within 2 to 3 days.

BARBITURATES

47. Describe the mechanism of action of barbiturates.

Barbiturates bind to barbiturate receptors on the chloride channel (see Figure, question 5). Activation of the receptor potentiates the effects of GABA, and increases chloride flux across the neuronal membrane, causing partial hyperpolarization of the neuronal membrane, and decreased conduction. Because the barbiturate receptor is adjacent to both the benzodiazepine receptor and GABA receptor on the channel, the action of barbiturates enhances not only the binding of GABA to its receptor, but the receptor binding of benzodiazepines as well.

48. Describe the general actions of barbiturates in the CNS.

They exhibit a non-selective CNS depression.

49. Describe the metabolism of barbiturates.

Barbiturates are metabolized by hepatic cytochrome P_{450}. Most intermediates are then glucuronidated and excreted through the urine.

50. Which of the commercially available barbiturates is the longest acting?

Phenobarbital, which has a half-life of 72 hours. CNS effects such as impaired motor skills, impaired thought processes, and impaired judgment may persist for several days after treatment.

51. Describe the effects of systemic acidosis on phenobarbital therapy.

Systemic acidosis increases the potency of phenobarbital by shifting the ionization equilibrium to the left. Because the drug is a weak acid, a lowering of physiologic pH results in an increase in the amount of nonionized drug and an increase in the amount of drug which enters the CNS. (Recall that a drug may only cross the blood-brain barrier in nonionized form.)

52. Describe the distribution of phenobarbital.

The distribution of phenobarbital is slow, due to its relative lack of lipid solubility. It disseminates into all tissues of the body and is moderately plasma protein bound (20–40 percent).

53. Which of the barbiturates is shortest acting?

Methohexital and thiopental are ultra short-acting agents. Pentobarbital and secobarbital have a longer duration and are considered short-acting agents.

54. Which barbiturate has the fastest onset?

Secobarbital, as it is the most lipid-soluble of the barbiturates.

55. Describe the clinical uses of secobarbital.

Secobarbital is useful in the short-term therapy of insomnia, and in the control of status epilepticus. It is also useful in the therapy of preoperative anxiety and the therapy of psychosis, as an agent to control agitation.

56. Describe the use of barbiturates in lowering serum bilirubin.

Barbiturates such as phenobarbital, amobarbital, and butabarbital induce glucuronyl transferase, an enzyme obligatory in bilirubin metabolism. Thus, they may be used in patients with chronic cholestasis. Phenobarbital is also used for lowering serum bilirubin in the neonate.

57. What is the result of rapid bolus injection of amobarbital or butabarbital?

Rapid administration of these drugs precipitates a rapid and severe respiratory depression, possibly resulting in coma and death.

58. Describe the major clinical uses of butabarbital.

Butabarbital is used clinically for daytime sedation, to relieve preoperative anxiety, to provide sedation, and in the short-term treatment of insomnia.

59. Discuss the pharmacokinetics of butabarbital.

Butabarbital has an onset of action of 60 minutes and a duration of 6 to 8 hours. Distribution is rapid to all body fluids and tissues, and plasma protein binding is low. Hepatic metabolism produces an inactive metabolite, which is excreted in the urine. Only a very small portion of the drug is excreted unchanged.

60. What are the clinical uses of methohexital?

Methohexital can be used alone as an anesthetic for short procedures. It may also be used as an inducing agent or adjunct to regional anesthesia.

61. Compare the thiobarbiturates methohexital and thiopental.

Methohexital is more lipophilic than thiopental, and thus has a faster onset of action. It exhibits minimal accumulation in fatty tissues and thus has a shorter duration of action, leading to a faster recovery time. The potency of methohexital is approximately twice that of thiopental.

62. Discuss the clinical ramifications of the muscle relaxant effects of methohexital.

Methohexital has no muscle relaxant properties. Thus, it may be safely used in conjunction with skeletal muscle relaxant agents. However, unlike thiopental, methohexital does not prevent postanesthesia excitatory phenomena.

63. Does toxicity develop with repeated dosing of methohexital?

No. The drug does not accumulate in fatty tissues, making repeated dosing relatively safe.

64. Describe the anticonvulsant properties of barbiturates.

In general, barbiturates produce a generalized depression of synaptic function. The threshold for electrical stimulation in the motor cortex is increased by barbiturates, resulting in a decreased propensity for motor seizures.

65. Which sedative hypnotic drugs may be useful in the prevention of withdrawal symptoms in a severe alcoholic who has stopped drinking?

Both barbiturates and benzodiazepines are useful.

66. Which sedative hypnotics are of the piperidinedione class?

The older sedative hypnotics such as glutethimide and methyprylon belong to this class.

67. Explain the dangers of nightly administration of chloral hydrate.

Chloral hydrate is metabolized into two major metabolites—one which is pharmacologically active and relatively non-toxic (trichloroethanol) and the other which is toxic (trichloroacetic acid). Trichloroethanol is cleared fairly rapidly, with a half-life of less than ten hours. Trichloroacetic acid is cleared much more slowly, and will accumulate with nightly administration.

ETHANOL

68. What are the pharmacologic uses of ethanol administration?
Clinically, ethanol is used in the therapy of poisoning from ingestion of methanol or ethylene glycol ("antifreeze").

69. Describe the actions of ethanol in the therapy of alcohol poisoning (e.g., methanol or ethylene glycol).
These chemicals are metabolized by alcohol dehydrogenase, which is also the enzyme responsible for the first step in the metabolism of ethanol. The metabolites produced by the dehydration of these chemicals produce toxicity rather than the parent chemicals. Pharmacologically administered ethanol competes with the ingested chemicals for sites on the enzyme, decreasing production of toxic metabolites, and allowing more of the ingested alcohols to be excreted unchanged in the urine.

70. Describe the mechanism of action of ethanol in the depression of the CNS.
Ethanol acts to increase the fluidity of neuronal cell membranes, potentiate the conformational changes of the GABA receptor, and increase chloride flux across the membrane. This results in decreased excitability of the membrane.

71. Does ethanol exhibit a tolerance effect?
Yes. Ethanol induces the enzymes that metabolize it, and thus, chronic use will result in an increase in metabolism and tolerance.

72. Describe the metabolism of ethanol.
Ethanol is metabolized in a two step process (see figure below), according to zero order kinetics. As the drug passes through the liver, it is first dehydrated by alcohol dehydrogenase, forming acetaldehyde (which dissociates into methanol and formaldehyde, should the next metabolic step be inhibited). Acetaldehyde is then metabolized by aldehyde dehydrogenase into acetate, which may then enter the citric acid cycle.

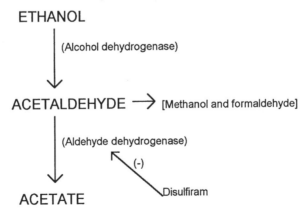

73. Is there cross-tolerance between ethanol and other CNS depressants?
Yes. Benzodiazepines, barbiturates, and ethanol all exhibit cross-tolerance. Thus, prolonged use of any of these drugs will result in tolerance, not only to the effects of that drug, but to those of the other drugs as well.

74. Explain the mechanism of action of disulfiram.
Disulfiram inhibits aldehyde dehydrogenase. Thus, consumption of ethanol will produce increased levels of acetaldehyde which will form the toxic intermediates methanol and formaldehyde

(see Figure above). As the levels of these products increase, the patient feels nauseous and experiences unpleasant symptoms such as dyspnea and a decrease in blood pressure (secondary to a drop in total peripheral resistance), which precipitates tachycardia.

75. Discuss the actions of disulfiram on the sympathetic nervous system.

Disulfiram inhibits the actions of dopamine β-hydroxylase in the adrenergic neuron. Thus, sympathetic nervous system activity is decreased in a dose-dependent manner.

BIBLIOGRAPHY

1. Akk G, Steinbach JH: Activation and block of recombinant GABA(A) receptors by pentobarbitone: A single-channel study. Br J Pharmacol 130(2):249–258, 2000.
2. Bowery NG, Enna SJ: Gamma-aminobutyric acid (B) receptors: First of the functional metabotropic heterodimers [review] [published erratum appears in J Pharmacol Exp Ther 293(1):following 312, 2000]. J Pharmacol Exp Ther 292(1):2–7, 2000.
3. Hardman J, Limbird L, Gilman A: Goodman & Gilman's The Pharmacological Basis of Therapeutics, 10th ed. New York, McGraw-Hill Publishers, 2001.
4. Jentsch TJ, Gunther W: Chloride channels: an emerging molecular picture. Bioessays 19(2):117–126, 1997.
5. Katzung, B: Basic and Clinical Pharmacology, 8th ed. Appleton & Lange, 2001.
6. Krogsgaard-Larsen P, Frolund B, Frydenvang K: GABA uptake inhibitors: Design, molecular pharmacology and therapeutic aspects [review]. Curr Pharm Des 6(12):1193–1209, 2000.
7. Pages KP, Ries RK: Use of anticonvulsants in benzodiazepine withdrawal. Am J Addicts 7(3):198–204, 1998.
8. Rudolph U, Crestani F, Benke D, et al: Benzodiazepine actions mediated by specific gamma-aminobutyric acid (A) receptor subtypes. Nature 401(6755):796–800, 1999.
9. Teuber L, Watjens F, Jensen LH: Ligands for the benzodiazepine binding site—A survey [review]. Curr Pharm Des 5(5):317–343, 1999 .
10. Zeidenberg P, Orrenius S, Ernster L: Increase in levels of glucuronylating enzymes and associated rise in activities of mitochondrial oxidative enzymes upon phenobarbital administration in the rat. J Cell Biol 32(2):528–531, 1967.

4. ANTICONVULSANT DRUGS

GENERAL PRINCIPLES

1. Explain the general mechanism of action of anticonvulsant drugs.

Seizures are due to abnormalities in conduction and conduction pathways. Thus, anticonvulsant drugs tend to make the neuron less excitable and more refractory to stimuli.

2. What are mechanisms of the therapeutic actions of an anticonvulsant drug?

- Potentiation of the effects or levels of the inhibitory neurotransmitter gamma-aminobutyric acid (GABA). The actions of GABA result in increased chloride flux across the neuronal membrane, causing the inner surface of the membrane to become more negative with respect to the outer surface. This results in an increased threshold for stimulation. The neuron is thus less excitable.
- Decreased membrane permeability to sodium, which decreases the degree of potential membrane excitation.
- Increased membrane permeability to potassium. This makes the membrane more refractory to stimulation.
- Modulation of excitatory neurotransmitters.
- Decreased calcium release, which is necessary for neurotransmission.

3. Why is systemic administration of GABA not useful in the control of seizures?

GABA is charged at physiologic pH and does not cross the blood brain barrier.

4. Is the clinical efficacy of anticonvulsant drugs manifested immediately upon initiation of therapy?

No. Therapeutic levels must be attained before clinical efficacy is seen. Maximal clinical efficacy is seen at steady-state level, which is attained in approximately five drug half-lives.

5. May anticonvulsant drugs be withdrawn immediately upon the cessation of therapy?

No. Abrupt withdrawal may precipitate status epilepticus.

6. Describe the events associated with a change in anticonvulsant therapy.

Normally, the new drug should be started concurrently with the drug to be replaced. Dosage of the first drug should be gradually reduced, as the plasma levels of the replacement drug increase. Once steady-state levels of the replacement drug are reached, the first drug may be withdrawn.

7. Discuss the use of anticonvulsants during pregnancy.

The risk of seizures may increase during pregnancy, due to changes in general physiology and acid-base balance. Anticonvulsant therapy should not be discontinued during pregnancy. However, many anticonvulsants (e.g., trimethadione, valproic acid, phenytoin) have been shown to cause fetal malformations and are contraindicated in pregnancy.

8. Which anticonvulsant medications are effective in the treatment of status epilepticus?

Intravenous lorazepam or diazepam. The use of intravenous secobarbital or phenytoin may also be effective in the therapy of status epilepticus, depending on the origin.

PHENYTOIN

9. What is the mechanism of action of phenytoin?
Phenytoin alters the conductance of sodium, potassium, and calcium channels within the membrane of excitable cells. At therapeutic levels, the effects of the drug are mainly due to a decrease in sodium conduction.

10. Describe the effects of phenytoin on neurotransmitter release.
Phenytoin affects the release of norepinephrine, acetylcholine, and serotonin. It also affects the levels of excitatory amino acids.

11. State the adverse effects of phenytoin.
A common adverse effect is a "measles-like" rash, which persists for initial therapy and disappears. In some patients, urticaria may be seen, which may signify a hypersensitivity to the drug. Other adverse effects include morning depression (probably due to the effects of the drug on serotonin levels), gingival hyperplasia, and hirsutism.

12. Discuss the distribution of phenytoin.
Phenytoin is highly bound to plasma proteins. It is lipophilic and so is widely distributed into cerebral spinal fluid, as well as muscle, fat, and brain tissue, where it has been shown to bind to and accumulate in cellular endoplasmic reticulum.

13. Describe the metabolism of phenytoin.
Phenytoin undergoes phase I parahydroxylation. The resulting intermediate (5-OH-phenyl-5-phenylhydantion, or HPPH) undergoes phase II glucuronidation and is excreted in the urine.

14. How is phenytoin eliminated?
A small amount of the drug is eliminated unchanged. The majority is eliminated as the glucuronide. Elimination of the drug is dose-dependent.

15. Describe the kinetics of phenytoin elimination.
The enzymatic pathways are saturable. Thus, with very low plasma levels of drug, the elimination follows first order kinetics. However, as plasma levels increase to therapeutic range, the enzymatic pathways begin to saturate, and a progressively smaller proportion of the plasma concentration of drug is metabolized. In the upper therapeutic range, plasma concentrations increase markedly with only a very small dosage increase, and the half-life of the drug increases markedly, producing toxicity.

16. What is the half-life of phenytoin?
The half-life in the low to mid therapeutic range is approximately 12 to 24 hours. As dosage increases, the half-life increases to 36 hours or longer.

17. Explain the action of phenytoin in prevention of grand mal seizures.
Phenytoin inhibits the tonic phase of the grand mal seizure by stabilizing excitable tissue in the brain stem.

18. What are the clinical uses of phenytoin in the prevention of seizures?
It is useful in the therapy of chronic epilepsy. It is particularly useful in tonic-clonic and psychomotor seizures.

19. Is phenytoin useful in the therapy of absence seizures?
No. It is possible that the drug increases the frequency of absence seizures.

CARBAMAZEPINE

20. What are the clinical uses of carbamazepine?
Carbamazepine is useful in the prophylaxis and therapy of partial seizures and psychomotor seizures. It is also useful in the therapy of trigeminal neuralgia, and as adjunct therapy in the treatment of manic-depressive disorders.

21. Describe the mechanism of action of carbamazepine.
Carbamazepine decreases the excitability of nervous tissue by decreasing membrane conductance to sodium.

22. Discuss the use of carbamazepine in manic-depressive disorder.
The carbamazepine molecule shares structural homology with that of the tricyclic antidepressants, and has weak antidepressant activity. The depression of cortical excitability, due to sodium blockade, also makes it useful as adjunct therapy in the treatment of acute mania.

23. Explain the actions of carbamazepine on the heart.
Carbamazepine suppresses ventricular automaticity, decreases the rate of conduction of the AV node, and suppresses phase 4 depolarization. These effects may be partially offset by the drug's anticholinergic action.

24. Is carbamazepine bound to plasma proteins?
Yes. The drug is heavily plasma protein bound (70–80 percent).

25. What is the relationship between saliva concentration and plasma concentration of unbound carbamazepine?
The concentrations are equal.

26. State the half-life of carbamazepine.
The serum half-life is 36 hours with initial dosing. Carbamazepine does, however, autoinduce metabolizing enzymes, so, with increased duration of therapy, the half-life decreases to approximately 16 hours (24 hours with the extended release form). The half-life of the drug varies slightly with each patient and decreases with concomitant anticonvulsant therapy.

27. Describe the metabolism of carbamazepine.
Carbamazepine is metabolized primarily by oxidation by the CYP 3A4 isozyme of hepatic cytochrome P_{450}. The primary metabolite is a pharmacologically active 10,10 epoxide, which undergoes phase II glucuronidation. Carbamazepine is a potent enzyme inducer, and increases its own rate of metabolism throughout the induction of cytochrome P_{450}.

28. What are the adverse effects of carbamazepine?
Carbamazepine has a moderate anticholinergic action that may cause symptoms of dry mouth and constipation. CNS effects include somnolence, ataxia, diplopia, loss of accommodation, dizziness, and headache, which are most prominent with overdosage. Erythroderma, photosensitivity, and skin rashes may also be seen, and, rarely, Stevens-Johnson syndrome or systemic lupus-like syndrome also occur. The drug also has other serious adverse effects, such as suppression of ventricular automaticity, and, rarely, blood dyscrasias (e.g., agranulocytosis, leukopenia, thrombocytopenia, and aplastic anemia). Due to hepatic metabolism, hepatocellular and cholestatic jaundice may also be seen.

29. Why is caution advised in the administration of carbamazepine to patients with a hypersensitivity to tricyclic antidepressants (e.g., amitriptyline, nortriptyline)?
Carbamazepine has a similar tricyclic structure to these drugs and may precipitate a hypersensitivity reaction.

30. Is carbamazepine useful in the treatment of petit mal or myoclonic seizures?
No. It is most useful in temporal lobe epilepsy (generalized seizures).

31. Describe the use of carbamazepine during pregnancy.
Carbamazepine should, if at all possible, not be administered, particularly during the first three months of pregnancy. Regardless of a change in therapy, administration of folic acid before and during the gestational period, and of vitamin K in the last trimester, may be useful in protecting the mother and fetus.

32. Does carbamazepine pass into breast milk?
Yes. Somnolence and hypersensitivity reactions have been observed in nursing infants.

33. State the toxicities that should be monitored during long-term carbamazepine therapy.
Complete blood work should be done on a regular basis to monitor for bone marrow depression. In addition, liver function tests, particularly in the elderly, should be performed. Carbamazepine also causes pathologic changes in the eye, so regular ophthalmic evaluations should be performed.

34. Describe the efficacy of contraceptive drugs in patients under carbamazepine therapy.
As carbamazepine induces hepatic enzymes, including those that metabolize contraceptive drugs, the efficacy of these drugs may be reduced.

35. Why should concurrent therapy with carbamazepine and isoniazid be monitored closely?
Carbamazepine potentiates isoniazid, the use of which may induce hepatotoxicity.

36. Describe the effects of carbamazepine therapy concurrent with diuretics.
The use of diuretics which promote heavy potassium loss (e.g., loop diuretics and thiazide diuretics) with carbamazepine therapy may precipitate a marked hyponatremia.

CLONAZEPAM

37. What is the clinical use of clonazepam?
Clonazepam is useful in myoclonic and akinetic seizures, and in the management of petit mal seizures. It may also be of use in the therapy of absence seizures.

38. What is the half-life of clonazepam?
It is 18 to 50 hours.

39. Describe the metabolism and elimination of clonazepam.
Clonazepam is primarily metabolized in the liver to inactive metabolites. These metabolites are excreted in the urine. A very small percentage of the drug (up to 0.5 percent) may be excreted unchanged in the urine. Up to 25 to 27 percent may be excreted unchanged in the bile.

40. Is clonazepam indicated in patients with narrow-angle glaucoma?
No. The drug may exacerbate the condition.

41. Why is clonazepam contraindicated in patients experiencing more than one type of seizure?
In such patients, clonazepam may increase the incidence of tonic-clonic (grand mal) seizures.

42. Describe the result of concomitant administration of clonazepam and valproic acid.
The combination of these drugs may induce absence status epilepticus.

43. What problems may be encountered in the administration of clonazepam to patients with chronic respiratory diseases?

Clonazepam has been shown to cause hypersecretion in upper respiratory tracts and may exacerbate existing respiratory conditions. Dyspnea and respiratory depression may also be seen, which may be due in part to the actions of the benzodiazepine on the skeletal muscle of the diaphragm.

44. What are the most frequently seen adverse effects to clonazepam therapy?

The major adverse effects are due to CNS depression, such as sedation and ataxia. Behavioral changes may also be seen.

45. Describe the behavioral changes that may result from clonazepam therapy.

Alterations in behavior may include aggressiveness, argumentative behavior, hyperactivity, agitation, depression, euphoria, irritability, forgetfulness, and confusion. These effects are most common in patients with chronic seizure disorders, or those with prior psychiatric disorders.

46. Does clonazepam administration result in dermatological abnormalities?

Yes. Clonazepam administration may result in non-specific rashes, urticaria, pruritus, and swelling of the face or eyelids.

BARBITURATES

47. Describe the usage of butabarbital.

Butabarbital is primarily used as a sedative hypnotic drug, but may also be useful in the suppression of the spread of seizure activity in the cortex, thalamus, and limbic systems.

48. Explain the use of phenobarbital in the control of seizure disorders.

Phenobarbital is a nonspecific CNS depressant that is useful in suppressing various types of seizures. It may be used as monotherapy in children, but is usually combined with other drugs in the therapy of adults.

49. Describe the administration of phenobarbital.

It is administered both orally and parenterally.

50. Discuss the relative absorption of phenobarbital.

Phenobarbital is well absorbed from the gut (70–90 percent) after oral dosage, but its absorption is delayed by the presence of food. Peak plasma concentrations are achieved 12–18 hours after oral dosage.

51. Why does the attainment of a steady-state plasma concentration take several weeks with phenobarbital administration?

Daily oral dosing over several weeks is required due to the exceptionally long half-life of the drug (72 hours).

52. Describe the onset of action of intravenous phenobarbital.

Onset of action of IV phenobarbital is less than 5 minutes, reaching peak concentration in approximately 30 minutes.

53. Does phenobarbital produce sedation at anticonvulsant doses?

Yes. The lowest plasma concentration that is therapeutically effective as an anticonvulsant is 10 µg/ml, ranging to 40 µg/ml; sedation occurs at 10 µg/ml.

54. What is the plasma concentration of phenobarbital necessary to induce coma?

Plasma concentrations of 50 µg/ml or above will result in coma.

55. How can phenobarbital's rate of elimination be increased, in case of poisoning?
An increase in urinary flow rate (i.e., using mannitol), and decreasing urinary acidity (i.e., using acetazolamide).

56. Is pentobarbital useful in chronic seizure disorders in adults?
No. It is primarily useful in the control of seizures due to isolated events, such as seizures resulting from meningitis, tetanus, alcohol withdrawal, poisons, chorea, or eclampsia.

57. Describe the use of pentobarbital in head trauma or stroke.
Pentobarbital administration is effective in the management of the induction of coma in cases involving cerebral ischemia. It is also useful in the management of increased intracranial pressure following stroke or head trauma.

58. How is pentobarbital administered?
Orally, parenterally, and rectally.

59. Compare the rate of absorption of pentobarbital through its routes of administration.
Absorption is faster from rectal or parenteral administration than from an oral dose. Sodium salts of the drug are more rapidly absorbed orally than are other forms of the drug. Oral absorption is also increased if the drug is well-diluted or taken on an empty stomach.

60. Does tolerance develop to the hypnotic effects of pentobarbital?
Yes. Tolerance occurs after about 2 weeks of continuous dosing.

61. Describe the mechanism of action of secobarbital in the prophylaxis of seizures.
Secobarbital depresses the sensory cortex; decreases motor activity; depresses cerebral function; and produces drowsiness, sedation, and hypnosis. In the motor cortex, secobarbital increases the threshold for electrical stimulation, which contributes to its anticonvulsant properties.

62. Why would secobarbital administration be useful in stroke or head injury?
Secobarbital, in high doses, exerts a protective effect on the brain, decreasing the effects of ischemia and increased intracranial pressure.

63. What is primidone?
Primidone is an anticonvulsant drug that is structurally related to phenobarbital.

64. Describe the major metabolites of primidone.
Primidone is metabolized by the liver into two metabolites, both of which have pharmacological activity. These are phenobarbital and phenylethylmalonamide (PEMA).

65. What are the clinical uses of primidone?
Primidone is effective in all types of seizure disorders except absence seizures.

VALPROIC ACID AND DERIVATIVES

66. What are the clinical uses of valproic acid?
Valproic acid is effective in the control of simple or complex absence seizures and partial seizures. It is also useful as adjunct therapy in patients who exhibit multiple seizure types, including absence or tonic-clonic seizures.

67. Explain the mechanism of action of valproic acid.
Valproic acid is thought to increase concentrations of GABA, which decreases the frequency of neuronal firing. It may also have a direct effect on the neuronal membrane by the inhibition of voltage-gated sodium channels and the resulting decrease in sodium influx.

90. How is lamotrigine eliminated?

Elimination of lamotrigine is renal, with the majority of the drug eliminated as the glucuronide conjugate. Less than 10 percent of the dose is eliminated unchanged in the urine.

91. What effect does concurrent administration of valproic acid have on lamotrigine levels?

Valproic acid significantly decreases the clearance of lamotrigine, due to competition for hepatic glucuronidases. Elimination half-life is more than doubled if valproate is administered concurrently.

GABAPENTIN (NEURONTIN)

92. Discuss the mechanism of action of gabapentin.

Gabapentin binds to proteins in the CNS which are associated with the release of glutamate. Thus, it appears to decrease the release of glutamic acid, resulting in decreased neuronal excitation and reduced rate of firing.

93. Describe the structure-activity relationships of gabapentin.

Gabapentin is an analog of GABA, and was originally thought to act by GABAergic mechanism.

94. Does gabapentin act by mimicking the effects of GABA, or by increasing its levels?

No. Gabapentin does not interact with GABA receptors, nor does it interfere with GABA metabolism.

95. Compare the actions of gabapentin with those of other anticonvulsant agents.

Unlike other agents, which alter sodium or chloride flux, and which may have cross-reactivity with receptors for various neurotransmitters, gabapentin does not interact with sodium channels, nor does it influence receptors for benzodiazepines, opioids, catecholamines, or acetylcholine.

96. What is the advantage of using gabapentin concurrently with other anticonvulsant drugs?

Since gabapentin does not act by conventional mechanisms and has little or no cross-reactivity with neurotransmitter receptors, concurrent use with other agents produces a synergistic effect. This allows less of the anticonvulsant agent to be used, minimizing side effects, and increasing patient compliance.

97. Describe the absorption of gabapentin.

Gabapentin is rapidly absorbed from the GI tract, irrespective of the presence of food.

98. Describe the pharmacokinetics of gabapentin.

Gabapentin has a wide volume of distribution, is lipid soluble, and does not bind plasma proteins. It is not metabolized. Kinetics are linear at therapeutic doses.

99. What is the half-life of gabapentin?

It is 5 to 7 hours, so dosage three times a day may be necessary.

100. State the side effects reported with gabapentin.

Somnolence, dizziness, ataxia, fatigue, nystagmus, headache, and nausea.

101. Is routine blood work required with gabapentin therapy?

No. Gabapentin does not appear to alter hematologic or biochemical variables, so routine testing is not necessary.

VIGABATRIN (SABRIL)

102. Describe the mechanism of action of vigabatrin.
Vigabatrin inhibits the metabolism of GABA, by irreversible inhibition of GABA transaminase. This appears to increase the concentrations of GABA in the midbrain. The drug does not affect GABA receptors or neuronal reuptake of GABA.

103. What are the clinical uses for vigabatrin?
Vigabatrin is useful as adjunct therapy in the therapy of refractive partial seizures. It also may be effective in the therapy of infantile spasm syndrome and GABA-mediated muscle spasticity.

104. Describe the pharmacokinetics of vigabatrin.
The half-life of vigabatrin ranges from 6 to 8 hours. The drug has a narrow volume of distribution and is not significantly protein bound. It is not metabolized but is excreted unchanged in the urine.

105. What are the major adverse reactions of vigabatrin?
The most common adverse reaction is somnolescence (although agitation and hyperactivity may be seen in pediatric patients), followed by sedation depression and, infrequently, psychosis. Nausea and vomiting may also occur.

TIAGABINE (GABATRIL)

106. Describe the mechanism of action of tiagabine.
Tiagabine inhibits the neuronal reuptake of GABA, resulting in increased levels of available neurotransmitter, which precipitates a subsequent increase in chloride conductance.

107. What is the primary clinical use of tiagabine?
Tiagabine is used as adjunct therapy in the control refractive partial seizures. When added to other antiepileptic drug regimens, tiagabine significantly decreases seizure frequency (by 50 percent or more) in about 25 percent of patients with refractory complex partial seizures and in roughly 32 percent of patients with simple complex seizures.

108. Describe the pharmacokinetics of tiagabine.
Tiagabine is almost completely absorbed from the stomach and extensively bound to plasma proteins (96 percent)—primarily serum albumin and alpha$_1$-acid glycoprotein. The metabolism of tiagabine appears to involve oxidation by the 3A isoform subfamiliy of cytochrome P_{450}, with subsequent glucuronidation. Excretion of the drug is both hepatic and renal. Serum half-life is 7 to 9 hours in an adult patient but varies under concurrent therapy with drugs that alter levels of cytochrome P_{450}.

BIBLIOGRAPHY

1. Beydoun A, Sachdeo RC, Rosenfeld WE, et al: Oxcarbazepine monotherapy for partial-onset seizures: a multicenter, double-blind, clinical trial. Neurology 54(12):2245–2251, 2000.
2. Borusiak P, Bettendorf U, Karenfort M, et al: Seizure-inducing paradoxical reaction to antiepileptic drugs. Brain Dev 22(4):243–245, 2000.
3. Cereghino JJ, Biton V, Abou-Khalil B, et al:Levetiracetam for partial seizures: results of a double-blind, randomized clinical trial. Neurology 55(2):236–242, 2000.
4. Cleton A, Altorf BA, Voskuyl RA, et al: Effect of amygdala kindling on the central nervous system effects of tiagabine: EEG effects versus brain GABA levels. Br J Pharmacol 130(5):1037–1044, 2000.
5. Collins TL, Petroff OA, Mattson RH: A comparison of four new antiepileptic medications. Seizure 9(4):291–293, 2000.
6. Cuttle L, Munns AJ, Hogg NA, et al: Phenytoin metabolism by human cytochrome P_{450}: involvement of P_{450} 3A and 2C forms in secondary metabolism and drug-protein adduct formation. Drug Metab Dispos 28(8):945–950, 2000.

7. Hardman J, Limbird L, Gilman A: Goodman & Gilman's The Pharmacological Basis of Therapeutics, 10th ed. New York, McGraw-Hill Publishers, 2001.
8. Johannessen CU: Mechanisms of action of valproate: A commentary [review]. Neurochemistry International. 37(2-3):103–110, 2000.
9. Katzung B: Basic and Clinical Pharmacology, 8th ed. Appleton & Lange, 2001.
10. Lamusuo S, Pitkanen A, Jutila L, et al: [^{11}C]Flumazenil binding in the medial temporal lobe in patients with temporal lobe epilepsy: Correlation with hippocampal MR volumetry, T2 relaxometry, and neuropathology. Neurology 54(12):2252–2260, 2000.
11. Main MJ, Cryan JE, Dupere JR,et al: Modulation of KCNQ2/3 potassium channels by the novel anticonvulsant retigabine. Mol Pharmacol 58(2):253–262, 2000.
12. Morrell MJ, McLean MJ, Willmore LJ, et al: Efficacy of gabapentin as adjunctive therapy in a large, multicenter study. The Steps Study Group. Seizure 9(4):241–248, 2000.
13. Moshe SL: Mechanisms of action of anticonvulsant agents [review]. Neurology 55(5 Suppl 1):S32–S40; discussion, S54–S58, 2000.
14. Musshoff U, Kohling R, Lucke A, et al: Vigabatrin reduces epileptiform activity in brain slices from pharmacoresistent epilepsy patients. Eur J Pharmacol 401(2):167–172, 2000.
15. Schmidt D, Gram L, Brodie M, et al: Tiagabine in the treatment of epilepsy—a clinical review with a guide for the prescribing physician [review]. Epilepsy Res 41(3):245–251, 2000.
16. Ross EL: The evolving role of antiepileptic drugs in treating neuropathic pain [review]. Neurology 55(5 Suppl 1):S41–S46; discussion, S54–S58, 2000.
17. Shorvon S: Oxcarbazepine: A review [editorial; review]. Seizure 9(2):75–79, 2000.
18. Starreveld E, Starreveld AA: Status epilepticus. Current concepts and management [review]. Can Fam Physician 46:1817–1823, 2000.
19. Wickenden AD, Yu W, Zou A, et al: Retigabine, a novel anti-convulsant, enhances activation of KCNQ2/Q3 potassium channels. Mol Pharmacol 58(3):591–600, 2000.

5. DRUGS USED IN THE THERAPY OF DEPRESSION

1. Describe the physiologic objectives of antidepressant drugs.

Antidepressant drugs elevate levels of key neurotransmitters in the central nervous system (CNS), such as norepinephrine and serotonin, which have been shown to have effects in mood elevation. Alternatively, these drugs may also act as agonists at the receptor level.

2. What are the major adverse effects of antidepressant drugs?

Adverse effects include insomnia, sedation, and cardiovascular abnormalities due to anticholinergic activity and a direct quinidine-like effect on the heart.

3. What prominent adverse effect is seen with antidepressants affecting adrenergic nerve terminals?

Orthostatic hypotension.

4. Describe the general duration of action of antidepressant drugs.

These drugs tend to have long durations of action, due to their lipophilic nature and extensive metabolism.

5. Explain the limited abuse potential of antidepressant drugs.

Antidepressant drugs do not elevate mood in patients who are not clinically depressed. Adverse effects, however, will manifest almost immediately, making these drugs a poor choice as drugs of abuse.

TRICYCLIC ANTIDEPRESSANTS

6. What is the general mechanism of action of tricyclic antidepressant drugs?

Tricyclics inhibit the reuptake of catecholamines and indolamines from the synaptic cleft, thus increasing the amount of transmitter available for postsynaptic stimulation (see Figure below). The neurotransmitters affected and the degree to which they are affected varies with the individual drug.

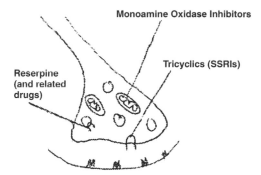

7. Discuss the secondary mechanisms of action of tricyclic antidepressants.

Due to the lag time in therapeutic effect, it is thought that tricyclics manifest their true clinical effects by down regulation of beta receptors in the limbic system. With increased concentrations in synaptic norepinephrine, over a period of time the receptors desensitize and down regulate.

8. Do therapeutic effects of tricyclic antidepressants present immediately upon institution of therapy?

No. Although inhibition of neurotransmitter reuptake is immediate, therapeutic effects take 3 to 5 weeks to be manifested. However, adverse effects are immediate.

9. State the general side effects of tricyclic antidepressants.

These drugs are sedating, and have a variety of untoward effects. The most commonly seen major adverse effect is postural hypotension. Other adverse effects include anticholinergic effects (e.g., dry mouth, constipation, urinary retention, paralytic ileus, and tachycardia), blurred vision, increased intraocular pressure, gynecomastia, galactorrhea, and changes in libido. Glucose tolerance may also be affected.

10. Describe the general pharmacokinetics and pharmacodynamics of tricyclic antidepressants.

Tricyclics are highly lipophilic and heavily protein-bound, both in plasma and tissues. These drugs have a very large volume of distribution, and are extensively metabolized. Active metabolites are subject to enterohepatic recycling.

11. Discuss the metabolism and elimination of tricyclic antidepressants.

Tricyclics undergo phase I metabolism by the cytochrome P_{450} mixed function oxidase system, resulting in either hydroxylation of the aromatic ring, or N-demethylation of the side chain amino group. These intermediates are pharmacologically active, and may be excreted through the bile and recycled. Hydroxylated intermediates may be further subjected to phase II glucuronidation and excreted through the urine.

12. In general, what is the duration of action of tricyclic antidepressants?

These drugs tend to have a long duration of action due to the formation of active metabolites. The half-life of imipramaine, for example, may exceed 20 hours.

13. Would protein binding interactions with other drugs (e.g., warfarin) be likely to occur with tricyclic antidepressants?

No. The preferential binding protein for these drugs is α_1-glycoprotein, rather than albumin.

14. Describe the cardiac effects of tricyclic antidepressants.

These drugs decrease conduction rate through a direct, quinidine-like effect on myocardial tissue. This may be offset by the strong anticholinergic effect of the drugs, and the increase in sympathetic activity.

15. What is the mechanism of the anticholinergic effects seen with tricyclics?

Anticholinergic effects are produced by a direct blockade of the muscarinic receptor. These effects are potentiated by an increase in adrenergic activity.

16. Discuss the ramifications of administering a monoamine oxidase inhibitor and a tricyclic antidepressant concurrently.

Monoamine oxidase inhibitors decrease the rate of metabolism of norepinephrine, and tricyclics increase the amount of circulating norepinephrine by decreasing the rate of neuronal uptake. Thus, concurrent therapy could synergize to cause a hypertensive crisis.

17. Describe the effects of alcohol consumption on the patient on tricyclic therapy.

The sedation and related CNS effects produced by the alcohol would synergize with the effects of the tricyclic antidepressant (e.g., sedation, ataxia, and diplopia).

18. Compare the relative potencies of nortriptyline, desipramine, and imipramine on serotonergic neurons and adrenergic neurons.

Nortriptyline has a more potent activity at the serotonergic neuron than at noradrenergic neurons. Imipramine has potent activity at both adrenergic and serotonergic neurons, but is a parent drug which is metabolized to desipramine. Desipramine selectively inhibits the reuptake of norepinephrine.

19. How are tricyclic antidepressants classified?
According to ring structure and by side chains attached to the three-ring nucleus.

20. Describe the clinical relevance of side chains on the three-ring nucleus of tricyclics.
The clinically relevant side chains are the number of amine groups attached to the tricyclic nucleus. Parent drugs tend to be tertiary amines, while their metabolites are secondary amines.

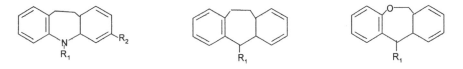

Dibenzazepine nucleus   Dibenzocycloheptadiene nucleus   Dibenzoxepin nucleus

21. What are the three classes of tricyclic antidepressants, based on ring structure, and their respective prototypes?
The three types of tricyclics (see Figure above) are the dibenzazepine type (e.g., imipramine), the dibenzocycloheptadiene type (e.g., amitriptyline), and the dibenzoxepin type (e.g., doxepin). Drugs are further classified by the type of side chain attached to the tricyclic nucleus.

22. Which tricyclic antidepressants are classified as tertiary amines?
Amitriptyline, clomipramine, doxepin, imipramine, and trimipramine are tertiary amines.

23. What are the distinguishing clinical features of tertiary amines?
These drugs tend to be more sedating and have more anticholinergic effects. They are also parent drugs and are metabolized to secondary amines.

24. What are the distinguishing clinical features of secondary amines?
These drugs have less effect on serotonergic neurons than the tertiary amines, and tend to be more selective for adrenergic neurons. In general, these drugs are better tolerated than the tertiary amines.

25. What are the clinical uses of tricyclic antidepressants?
These drugs are used to alleviate depression, and are also used in the therapy of diabetic neuropathy. They may also be effective in the treatment of obsessive compulsive disorder (OCD) and attention-deficit hyperactivity disorder. Certain drugs of this class have also been therapeutically useful in the treatment of childhood enuresis (e.g., imipramine), fibromyalgia (e.g., amitriptyline), and chronic obstructive pulmonary disease (COPD) (e.g., protriptyline).

26. Compare the degree of sedation of imipramine and doxepin.
Imipramine has a moderate degree of sedation, due to a correspondingly moderate binding affinity for histamine receptors. The degree of sedation seen with doxepin is high, due to a strong affinity for histamine receptors.

27. Should imipramine be used in the prescience of prostatic hypertrophy?
No. This drug causes urinary retention.

28. Explain the ramifications of tricyclic therapy in a hyperthyroid patient.
Tricyclics, especially secondary amines, should be administered with caution to a hyperthyroid patient, or avoided altogether. Thyroid hormone sensitizes the myocardium to catecholamines, and, because tricyclics raise the circulating level of catecholamines by decreasing

adrenergic reuptake, there is a synergistic effect that could result in ventricular arrhythmias and, in the worst case, ventricular fibrillation.

29. Explain the ramifications of using tricyclics in patients with adrenal tumors.
    Use of tricyclics in the presence of catecholamine-secreting tumors of the adrenal medulla (e.g., pheochromocytoma, neuroblastoma), may precipitate a hypertensive crisis, due to the increase in catecholamine production in the face of decreased adrenergic reuptake.

30. Why is the use of tricyclics contraindicated in seizure patients?
    Tricyclics lower seizure threshold.

31. What are the effects of tricyclic therapy on psychiatric patients?
    Tricyclic antidepressants may aggravate latent or existing psychoses, and will increase the level of agitation in hyperactive or manic-depressive patients.

32. Which tricyclic antidepressants are useful in the therapy of diabetic neuropathy?
    Those which have activity at noradrenergic nerve terminals, including doxepin, amitriptyline, and desipramine.

33. Are tricyclics a good choice for therapy in a diabetic patient?
    No, as increased sympathetic activity may result in an increase in blood glucose.

34. Explain the mechanism of action of heterocyclic antidepressants.
    Heterocyclic antidepressants antagonize α_2 receptors ("heterocyclic" receptors) located on serotonergic neurons. This results in an increase in serotonergic outflow. In addition, antagonism of presynaptic α_2-adrenergic receptors in the CNS increases norepinephrine outflow, further contributing to mood elevation.

35. Do heterocyclic drugs affect α_1 receptors?
    Yes. These drugs potently antagonize α_2 receptors. However, as like-receptor agonist or antagonist activity is never truly selective, some antagonist activity for the α_1 receptor exists, as well. The degree of this effect varies with the individual drug.

36. Discuss the effects of alpha-receptor blockade by heterocyclic drugs.
    Blockade of the α_2 receptors mediates the major therapeutic effect of these drugs. Adverse effects (e.g., sedation and hypotension) are mediated by α_1 receptor blockade.

37. Are heterocyclic antidepressants considered first-line therapeutic agents?
    No. These drugs are used as third- or fourth-line agents.

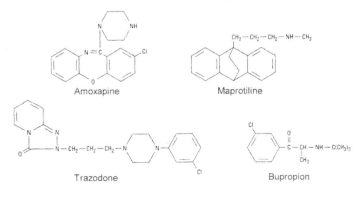

Amoxapine   Maprotiline

Trazodone   Bupropion

38. Do all heterocyclic antidepressant drugs have similar chemical structures?

No. Some are tricyclic in nature, some tetracyclic, and others unrelated in structure (see Figure at bottom of p. 40).

39. Discuss the pharmacokinetics of heterocyclic antidepressants.

These drugs tend to be highly protein-bound, with large volumes of distribution. They are erratically absorbed, extensively metabolized, and excreted as conjugates through the bile and urine. Some drugs of the class have active metabolites, which are subject to enterohepatic recycling.

40. What is the mechanism of action of amoxapine?

Amoxapine is considered a heterocyclic drug even though it blocks the reuptake of norepinephrine in the CNS.

41. Discuss the actions of amoxapine on dopamine receptors.

Amoxapine is a heterocyclic antidepressant. It is a metabolite of the antipsychotic drug, loxapine, and thus has the additional action of dopaminergic blockade. This action makes it a potentially useful therapy in depressed psychotic patients.

42. What adverse effects are seen with amoxapine?

Adverse effects are similar to those seen with tricyclic antidepressants. Additionally, dopamine-related effects, such as akathisia, galactorrhea/amenorrhea, and Parkinson-like symptoms are seen.

43. Describe the effects of amoxapine overdose.

Severe neurotoxicity results, often manifested by seizures which are unresponsive to therapy.

44. Does amoxapine cause orthostatic hypotension?

Yes. Though classified as moderate, dosage is limited to 400 mg per dose for that reason.

45. Describe the pharmacokinetics of amoxapine.

Amoxapine is rapidly absorbed and widely distributed. It is metabolized in the liver and subsequently excreted through the urine in conjugated form.

46. Does amoxipine have active metabolites?

Yes. 8-hydroxyamoxapine ($T\frac{1}{2}$ = 30 hours), and 7-hydroxyamoxapine ($T\frac{1}{2}$ = 6.5 hours).

47. Describe the mechanism of action of mirtazapine.

Mirtazapine blocks central α_2-adrenergic receptors, interrupting the negative feedback loop and increasing circulating norepinephrine. In addition, it acts at α_2 receptors on central serotonergic neurons, increasing the amount of circulating serotonin.

48. Why are adverse cardiovascular effects not prominent with mirtazapine?

The drug is ten times more potent at central receptors than peripheral receptors, so cardiac effects are not prominent at therapeutic doses.

49. Describe the pharmacokinetics of mirtazapine.

Mirtazapine is rapidly absorbed from the gut, is highly protein-bound, and extensively metabolized by cytochrome P_{450}. The metabolites, which are active, are excreted in the urine, following glucuronidation.

50. Describe the metabolites of mirtazapine and the cytochrome P_{450} isozymes involved.

The three active metabolites formed from mirtazapine metabolism are 8-hydroxymirtazapine, N-oxidomirtazapine, and N-desmethylmirtazapine. Cytochrome P_{450} isozymes 2D6 and 1A2 are involved in the formation of the 8-hydroxy metabolite, whereas isozyme 3A is responsible for the formation of the N-desmethyl and N-oxide metabolites.

51. What is the elimination half-life of mirtazapine?
It is 20–40 hours, depending on age and gender.

52. What is the mechanism of action of nefazodone?
Nefazodone antagonizes α_2 receptors (heteroreceptors), which mediates an increase in serotonin outflow. In addition, the drug is a potent antagonist at 5-HT_2 receptors, and, additionally, inhibits presynaptic reuptake of serotonin. Thus, the actions of serotonin in mood elevation are maximally potentiated.

53. Describe the cardiovascular toxicity seen with nefazodone.
Unlike tricyclic drugs, nefazodone lacks the potential for major cardiotoxicity, as the drug has comparatively less anticholinergic effect than tricyclics and only moderate quinidine-like depression of cardiac function.

54. What similarities exist between nefazodone and antipsychotic drugs?
Nefazodone is a synthetically derived piperazine drug.

55. What is the relationship between nefazodone and trazodone?
Trazodone is a metabolite of nefazodone, and shares many drug properties.

56. Describe the mechanism of action of trazodone.
Trazodone inhibits the reuptake of serotonin at the presynaptic nerve terminal. In addition, it acts as an α_2-receptor antagonist, causing an increase in serotonin outflow.

57. Discuss the dose-response relationship of trazodone.
Trazodone acts as a serotonin agonist at high therapeutic doses (6–8 mg/kg), but at low doses (< 1 mg/kg) acts as an antagonist.

58. What are the effects of long-term trazodone therapy?
Postsynaptic serotonin receptors may become desensitized.

59. Compare the adverse effects of trazodone and those of tricyclic antidepressants.
Trazodone has substantially less anticholinergic activity than tricyclics, and no cardiodepressant actions. It thus has less of an adverse cardiovascular effect. In addition, trazodone is sedating but does not interfere with phase 4 sleep.

60. Does trazodone have active metabolites?
No.

61. Discuss the elimination of trazodone.
Elimination is biphasic. The first phase occurs approximately 3 hours after absorption, followed by another phase at approximately 6 to 9 hours. This is due to a high degree of plasma protein binding. The first phase occurs with plasma concentrations of free drug; the second phase occurs after bound drug has dissociated and equilibrium has been reestablished.

62. What is the major route of elimination of trazodone?
Elimination is renal, with approximately 75 to 80 percent of the drug being cleared in the urine (mainly as water-soluble metabolites), and the remainder cleared through the bile.

63. What is the mechanism of action of maprotiline?
Maprotiline selectively inhibits the reuptake of norepinephrine at the neuronal membrane.

64. Describe the pharmacokinetics of maprotiline

Absorption from the digestive tract is slow but complete, and the drug has a very large volume of distribution. It is highly protein-bound (> 88 percent), and is metabolized to active metabolites that undergo enterohepatic recycling. Excretion is primarily via the urine.

65. How does vomiting affect maprotiline elimination?

Vomiting increases the rate of elimination, because both parent drug and active metabolites are secreted into gastric fluids and normally reabsorbed.

66. What is the half-life of maprotiline?

Plasma half-life ranges between 28 to 58 hours.

67. Describe the toxicity of maprotiline

Maprotiline may precipitate seizures in toxic doses, as well as cardiotoxicity.

SELECTIVE SEROTONIN REUPTAKE INHIBITORS (SSRIs)

68. Which of the SSRIs has the longest half-life?

Fluoxetine, with a half-life of 2 to 3 days for the parent drug, and 7 to 9 days for the active metabolite.

69. Compare the adverse effects of SSRIs to those of tricyclic antidepressants.

SSRIs have less sedative, anticholinergic, and cardiovascular effects than do the tricyclic antidepressants, due to dramatically decreased binding to receptors of histamine, acetylcholine, and norepinephrine.

70. Do SSRIs have significant cardiovascular toxicity?

No. Quinidine-like effects are absent, and there is little anticholinergic activity.

71. Describe the metabolism of fluoxetine.

Fluoxetine is demethylated in the liver to inactive metabolites and a pharmacologically active metabolite, norfluoxetine.

72. Describe the duration of action of fluoxetine.

The duration of action is long, due to a long half-life, both in the parent drug and metabolite. The $T\frac{1}{2}$ of fluoxetine is 2 to 3 days, while that of norfluoxetine is 7 to 9 days.

73. What is the pharmacologic potency of norfluoxetine?

Norfluoxetine is approximately equal to fluoxetine in potency.

74. Describe the metabolites of citalopram.

Citalopram is metabolized by cytochrome P_{450} (CYP 3A4 and CYP 2C19 isozymes) into two major metabolites—demethylcitalopram (DCT) and didemethylcitalopram (DDCT). These metabolites have pharmacologic activity, but are much less potent than the parent drug.

75. Does reboxitine have anticholinergic effects?

Yes. Typical manifestations include: dry mouth, constipation, insomnia, increased sweating, tachycardia, vertigo, urinary hesitance/retention, and impotence.

76. Describe the interactions of reboxitine and ketoconazole.

Concurrent therapy with ketoconazole has been shown to substantially increase plasma levels of reboxitine. This is due to the fact that reboxitine is primarily metabolized by the CYP 3A4 isozyme of cytochrome P_{450} and ketoconazole is a potent inhibitor of this isozyme.

77. What is the effect of sertraline on platelets?

At doses therapeutic for depression, sertraline inhibits the uptake of serotonin into platelets.

78. Is there a tolerance effect to sertraline administration?

Yes. Chronic use leads to down regulation of receptors.

79. Does sertraline undergo first-pass metabolism?

Yes. It undergoes significant hepatic first-pass metabolism.

80. Does sertraline bind significantly to proteins?

Yes. The drug is approximately 98 percent protein-bound.

81. Does sertraline interfere significantly with drugs which are highly protein-bound (e.g., warfarin)?

No. These drugs bind primarily to albumin, whereas sertraline binds primarily to α_1 glycoprotein.

82. Describe the metabolism of sertraline.

Sertraline is metabolized by N-demethylation to N-desmethylsertraline. Both parent drug and metabolite undergo oxidative deamination and subsequent reduction, hydroxylation, and glucuronide conjugation.

83. Describe the elimination of sertraline.

Conjugated drug and metabolites are eliminated through the urine. Unchanged drug is released into bile and eliminated though the feces.

84. What is the half-life of sertraline?

The elimination half-life is approximately 24 hours.

85. Describe the effect of renal or hepatic impairment on sertraline clearance.

Renal impairment does not significantly impact on drug clearance. However, serum half-life, as well as plasma drug levels, can increase by as much as 150 percent in the presence of hepatic impairment.

86. Which of the SSRIs has the highest specificity for serotonin receptors?

Paroxetine.

87. Compare the relative potencies of paroxetine, sertraline, and fluoxetine.

In-vivo studies show paroxetine to be significantly more potent than either fluoxetine or sertraline in the inhibition of serotonin reuptake.

88. Does paroxetine have active metabolites?

No.

89. Describe the metabolism of paroxetine.

Paroxetine is metabolized primarily by the CYP 2D6 isozyme of cytochrome P_{450}. This enzyme is readily saturable, and, with increased dosage, a nonlinear relationship between dose and plasma concentration is seen. Thus, steady-state concentrations in ongoing therapy are several times greater than would be predicted with a single dose.

90. Compare the pharmacokinetics of paroxetine therapy with the controlled release dosage form and the immediate release form.

Controlled release tablets are designed for a 4 to 5 hour dissolution rate. This is reflected in an increase in T_{max} as compared to the immediate release form. Nonlinear kinetics are present with ongoing therapy, regardless of dosage form.

91. Describe the role of the kidney in paroxetine elimination.

Sixty percent of serum paroxetine is eliminated through renal filtration. Mild to moderate renal impairment may cause a two-fold increase in peak serum concentrations. Severe renal impairment (creatinine clearance < 30 ml/min) may increase the half-life of the drug by over 150 percent.

92. What is the serum half-life of paroxetine?

Approximately 21 hours.

MONOAMINE OXIDASE INHIBITORS (MAOIs)

93. Describe the mechanism of action of MAOIs in the treatment of depression.

These agents bind to and inhibit the actions of the "A" type of the mitochondrial enzyme monoamine oxidase (MAO_A). As this enzyme is of major importance in the degradation of catecholamines, particularly norepinephrine and epinephrine, its inhibition results in elevated levels of both norepinephrine and epinephrine. As most of these agents are non-selective agents, binding and inactivation of MAO_B also occurs, resulting in increased levels of dopamine and serotonin. These agents are thought to have a role in mood elevation.

94. Are the therapeutic effects of MAOIs immediate?

No. It may take up to 4 weeks for antidepressant effects to be manifested.

95. Describe the effects of MAOIs on receptor sensitivity.

This class of drugs desensitizes serotonergic receptors, as well as adrenergic receptors. This may account for the delayed onset of therapeutic effects, as upregulation of receptors may result.

96. How does tranylcypromine differ from other MAOIs?

Tranylcypromine binds reversibly to MAO, while binding of the other agents is irreversible.

97. Is isocarboxazid first-line therapy for depression?

No. Due to its adverse effects, it is considered second-line therapy for refractory depression.

98. Describe the actions of MAOIs on blood pressure.

Blood pressure effects are unpredictable. The action of these drugs increases circulating levels of norepinephrine and epinephrine, which tend to raise pressure. At the same time, they stimulate the inhibition of central vasoregulatory centers that tend to decrease sympathetic activity.

99. Describe the effects of interactions of foods containing tyramine with MAOIs.

Many foods and beverages (e.g., wine, cheese, and chocolate) contain tyramine. This chemical is normally degraded by MAO_A, before systemic absorption. When the inhibition of MAO_A occurs, due to the administration of these drugs, tyramine from ingested food is absorbed. It is then taken up into adrenergic neurons, where it enters the synthetic pathway and is converted to octopamine, a "false transmitter." This results in a massive release of norepinephrine, and may result in a hypertensive crisis.

100. Explain the interaction between MAOIs and alpha-receptor agonists.

Administration of a MAOI for therapy of depression results in elevated levels of circulating norepinephrine and epinephrine. Concurrent administration of an alpha-receptor agonist results in elevated vascular tension.

101. Describe the result of concurrent administration of a MAOI and a tricyclic antidepressant.

Inhibition of MAO results in higher levels of epinephrine and norepinephrine, due to decreased catabolism. Administration of a tricyclic results in a decrease in reuptake of norepinephrine into the nerve terminus. Concurrent administration of these drugs thus results in elevated levels of norepinephrine and hypertensive crisis.

102. Upon withdrawal of an MAOI, is cessation of effects immediate?

That depends on the drug. Effects of drugs that reversibly bind to MAO (e.g., tranyl-cypromine) immediately cease upon withdrawal. Effects of drugs that bind irreversibly (e.g., phenelzine) continue until new enzyme is formed, which may take as long as several weeks.

103. What might be the result of concurrent administration of phenelzine and phenylephrine?

Concurrent administration of an α_1-receptor antagonist and a MAOI could result in postural hypotension.

104. Explain the possible result of coadministration of fluoxetine and tranylcypromine.

Tranylcypromine is a nonselective MAOI. Thus, it not only inhibits MAO_A, which is responsible for norepinephrine degradation, but also MAO_B, which results in increased levels of serotonin. Thus, coadministration of a SSRI and a nonselective MAOI would result in dramatic increases in serotonin levels, leading to serotonin syndrome.

105. How would the change in therapy between a MAOI and a SSRI be accomplished?

In general, a two-week waiting period is required between therapy with a MAOI and subsequent therapy with a SSRI. The exception is with fluoxetine, as it has a delayed onset of action. A change in therapy from fluoxetine to a MOAI requires a five-week interval, due to fluoxetine's long duration of action.

106. Describe the interactions of doxapram or levodopa with MAOIs.

These drugs cause pressor effects, which are exacerbated by the increased catecholamine levels produced by a MAOI.

107. Describe the interactions of MAOIs with local anesthetic preparations or over-the-counter (OTC) cold medications.

Local anesthetic preparations often contain a sympathomimetic drug. Cold medications contain pseudoephedrine or ephedrine-type drugs. All of these would synergize with the increased levels of catecholamines produced by a MAOI.

108. What would be the effect of concurrent administration of tolcapone with a MAOI?

Administration of a catechol-*O*-methyltransferase (COMT) inhibitor in conjunction with a drug that increases catecholamine levels would dramatically increase levels of catecholamines, leading to a hypertensive crisis, cardiac insufficiency, and possibly death.

109. Describe the interaction between MAOIs and antihistamines.

H_1 receptor blockade produces sedation, which would synergize with sedation produced by the MAOI. In addition, drugs that block H_1 receptors produce anticholinergic effects as well, which would synergize with increased catecholamine levels to produce a marked increase in sympathetic activity.

110. What might be the result of concomitant therapy with opiates and MAOIs?

The anticholinergic effect of opiates (including OTC cough preparations containing dextromethorphan) would synergize with the actions of catecholamines produced by the MAOI. This could result in heart failure.

111. Describe the use of MAOIs in a seizure patient.

MAOIs alter the concentrations of neurotransmitters that may be involved in regulatory feedback of neuronal activity. Thus, these drugs may alter seizure activity.

112. Describe the interaction of MAOIs with spinal anesthetics.

Concomitant use of these drugs (i.e., surgical procedures, labor and delivery) may cause marked hypotension, due to blockade of alpha receptors in the face of increased levels of circulating catecholamines.

113. Discuss the interaction of MAOIs with psychostimulant drugs (e.g., methylphenidate).

Psychostimulant drugs increase the amounts of available norepinephrine and/or dopamine in the CNS. The effects of MAOIs may synergize with the effects of these drugs. Thus, psychostimulant drugs should be used cautiously in conjunction with MAOIs.

114. Describe the elimination half-life and time to maximal efficacy of MAOI's.

These drugs have a half-life of about 2.5 hours. Maximum binding of MAO (maximal efficacy) is seen approximately 14 hours post absorption.

115. Should MAOIs be given to a patient with hepatic insufficiency?

No. The liver heavily metabolizes these drugs and toxicity may occur.

MISCELLANEOUS DRUGS USED FOR DEPRESSION

116. What is the mechanism of action of lithium in the adjunctive therapy of depression?

Lithium enhances the uptake of tryptophan and increases the synthesis of serotonin. It is also thought to decrease the reuptake of monamine neurotransmitters (e.g., catecholamines and serotonin). Reactions can be idiosyncratic, however, as lithium also decreases the conversion of thyroxine to triiodothyronine in the CNS.

117. Discuss the mechanism of action and use of methylphenidate in depression therapy.

Methylphenidate increases dopamine levels in the CNS, which then may be converted to norepinephrine in adrenergic terminals. This may result in mood elevation. The use of this drug, however, is limited to treatment-refractory cases or when standard medical therapies are not tolerated, as CNS stimulants may aggravate coexisting anxiety or agitation in depressed patients.

118. What is the use of liothyronine in the therapy of depression?

Liothyronine is T_4, which is selectively taken up in the CNS and converted to T_3 by 5' deiodinase. It is thought that the newly converted T_3 mediates an increase in receptor number in the CNS—primarily in the hippocampus. This may then increase the activity of mood-elevating neurotransmitters.

119. Is the use of liothyronine gender-specific?

Yes. Thyroid hormone levels in depressed patients seem to be lowered more in females than in males.

120. Is liothyronine useful as monotherapy?

No. It appears to further increase mood primarily in patients on antidepressive therapy. This, at least in part, is due to the fact that many antidepressant drugs (e.g., imipramine) decrease levels of T_3 in the CNS.

121. What are the potential systemic effects of liothyronine therapy in depression?

Potential systemic effects are minimal. In the periphery, most T_4 is in the bound state, and, when dissociation occurs, conversion relies on the activity of the kidney and liver. T_3, as well as T_4 (in the bound state), will not cross the blood-brain barrier. Thus, uptake of unbound T_4, and its subsequent conversion, is preferential in the CNS (as opposed to the periphery), and, because feedback mechanisms to the pituitary are based on T_3, thyroid function is not disrupted.

122. Which "natural" products are used in the therapy of depression?

Natural products currently sold over the counter and currently under investigation are SAM-e and St. John's Wort.

BIBLIOGRAPHY

1. Ashford JW, Ford CV: Use of MAO inhibitors in elderly patients. Am J Psychiatry 136:1466–1467, 1979.
2. Balon R, Mufti R, Arfken, CL: A survey of prescribing practices for monoamine oxidase inhibitors. Psychiatr Serv 50:945–947, 1999.
3. Beaubrun G, Gray GE: A review of herbal medicines for psychiatric disorders. Psychiatr Serv 51:1130–1134, 2000.
4. Bonomo V, Fogliani AM: Citalopram and haloperidol for psychotic depression. Am J Psychiatry 157:1706-a–1707-a, 2000.
5. Fava M, Mulroy R, Alpert J, et al: Emergence of adverse events following discontinuation of treatment with extended-release venlafaxine. Am J Psychiatry 154:1760–1762, 1997.
6. Golwin D, Seville C: Fluoxetine versus phenelzine in obsessive-compulsive disorder. Am J Psychiatry 156:159, 1999.
7. Hardman J, Limbird L, Gilman A: Goodman & Gilman's The Pharmacological Basis of Therapeutics, 10th ed. McGraw-Hill Publishers, 2001.
8. Hollister LE: Current antidepressants. Annu Rev Pharmacol Toxicol 26:23–37, 1986.
9. Janicak PG, Pandey GN, Davis, JM, et al:Response of psychotic and nonpsychotic depression to phenelzine. Am J Psychiatry 145:93–95, 1988.
10. Katzung B: Basic and Clinical Pharmacology, 8th ed. Appleton & Lange, 2001.
11. Kornstein SG, Schatzberg AF, Thase ME, et al: Gender differences in treatment response to sertraline versus imipramine in chronic depression. Am J Psychiatry 157:1445–1452, 2000.
12. Magai C, Kennedy G, Cohen CI, et al: A controlled clinical trial of sertraline in the treatment of depression in nursing home patients with late-stage alzheimer's disease. Am J Geriatr Psychiatry 8:66–74, 2000.
13. Meyer JH, Kapur S, Eisfeld B, et al: The effect of paroxetine on 5-HT2A receptors in depression: An [18F]setoperone PET imaging study. Am J Psychiatry 158:78–85, 2001.
14. Peroutka SJ, Sleight AJ, McCarthy BG, et al: The clinical utility of pharmacological agents that act at serotonin receptors. J Neuropsychiatry Clin Neurosci 1:253–262, 1989.
15. Rihmer Z, Szanto K, Arato M, et al: Response of phobic disorders with obsessive symptoms to MAO inhibitors. Am J Psychiatry 139:1374b, 1982.
16. Rothschild A, Phillips K: Selective serotonin reuptake inhibitors and delusional depression. Am J Psychiatry 156:977a–978a, 1999.
17. Sanford I. Finkel, Sanford I, Richter EM, Clary CM, et al: Comparative efficacy of sertraline vs. fluoxetine in patients age 70 or over with major depression. Am J Geriatr Psychiatry 7:221–227, 1999.
18. Trappler B, Cohen CI: Use of SSRIs in "very old" depressed nursing home residents. Am J Geriatr Psychiatry 6:83–89, 1998.
19. Zesiewicz TA, Gold M, Chari, G, et al: Current issues in depression in Parkinson's disease. Am J Geriatr Psychiatry 7:110–118, 1999.

6. ANTIPSYCHOTICS AND DRUGS USED IN THE THERAPY OF PSYCHIATRIC DISORDERS

DRUGS USED IN THE THERAPY OF SCHIZOPHRENIA

1. What is the general mechanism of action of antipsychotic drugs?

Antipsychotic drugs block dopaminergic receptors, specifically the D_2 receptors. Neuroleptic potency does not appear to correlate absolutely with the degree of receptor binding, so a secondary mechanism is also postulated.

2. What adverse effects can be expected with antipsychotics?

Depending on the class of drugs, varying degrees of extrapyramidal effects may be expected, as well as anticholinergic, antihistaminic (including sedation) and autonomic effects. Cardiovascular effects such as hypotension may be due to the autonomic effects, but direct cardiodepressant effects also occur with these drugs.

3. What are the endocrine effects of antipsychotic drugs?

Dopamine is an inhibitor of prolactin release. Thus, a patient on antipsychotics may experience (depending on gender) galactorrhea, amenorrhea, gynecomastia, and changes in libido.

4. Are the therapeutic effects of antipsychotic drugs immediate?

No. Therapeutic effects may take as long as several weeks to be manifested.

5. Discuss the phenomenon known as neuroleptic malignant syndrome.

This syndrome is a combination of symptomatic effects produced by antipsychotic drug therapy. Symptoms and signs include hyperpyrexia, muscle rigidity, altered mental status (e.g., catatonia) and cardiovascular instability (e.g., unstable heart rate and blood pressure). Acute renal failure may ultimately occur. Diagnostic signs include elevated creatine phosphokinase (CPK) and myoglobinuria.

6. What is the therapy of neuroleptic malignant syndrome?

Accepted therapies include the administration of dantrolene to reduce muscle rigidity, and antiparkinson drugs such as bromocriptine and amantadine to mediate extrapyramidal symptoms. Supportive therapy is also instituted. Withdrawal of the neuroleptic drug is mandatory.

7. Describe the symptoms of neuroleptic overdose.

Parkinson-like effects and acute dystonias may be seen. Central nervous system (CNS) effects include somnolence and seizure activity, as well as a lack of core temperature regulation due to hypothalamic effects. Autonomic effects include dry mouth, blurred vision, and urinary retention, coupled with cardiovascular effects such as tachycardia, cardiac arrhythmias, and hypotension.

8. What is the limiting effect of antipsychotic therapy?

Tardive dyskinesia, which, once established, is irreversible.

9. Which drugs are more likely to cause tardive dyskinesia?

The occurrence of tardive dyskinesia appears to be related to the degree of potency of the drug on the D_2 receptor and tends to increase with the total cumulative dose.

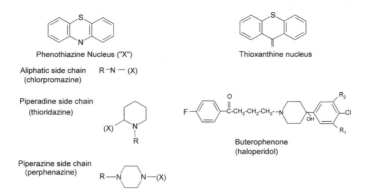

10. How are antipsychotic drugs classified?

By ring structure. They may be further classified by structural side chain group. The various ring structures and their associated side chain groups give an indication of both antipsychotic potency and the type and degree of adverse effects (see Table).

DRUG CLASS	PROTOTYPE(S)	POTENCY	DEGREE OF ADVERSE EFFECTS
Phenothiazines			
Aliphatic side chain	promazine, chlorpromazine	low	autonomic effects, sedation, cardiovascular, extrapyramidal
Piperidine side chain	thioridazine, mesoridazine	low	Cardiotoxicity, less extrapyramidal effect
Piperazine side chain	fluphenazine	intermediate	low sedation, decreased hypotensive effects
Thioxanthenes	thiothixene chlorprothixene	intermediate	less sedation, extrapyramidal effects, decreased risk of TD
Butyrophenones	haloperidol	high	less autonomic effects, low sedation, severe extrapyramidal effects
Dibenzoxazapines	loxapine clozapine	low low	agranulocytosis, seizures extrapyramidal effects low sedation/hypotension
Benzisoxazoles	risperidone	high	low extrapyramidal effects low sedation/hypotension
Thienobenzodiazepines	olanzapine	high	sedation, low hypotension low extrapyramidal effects
Floourophenylindoles	sertindole	high	low extrapyramidal effects low sedation/hypotension

11. Discuss the structure-function relationships in the phenothiazine class of antipsychotics.

Phenothiazines have a ring structure that contains both nitrogen and sulfur. The phenothiazine three-ring nucleus may have one of three types of side chains—aliphatic, piperidine, or piperazine. The type of side chain dictates the potency and degree of adverse effects of the drug.

12. Describe the pharmacokinetics of phenothiazines, thioxanthenes, and butyrophenones.

These drugs are incompletely absorbed, have a high first-pass effect, and are completely metabolized by the liver. Excretion is via the kidney and through the bile.

13. Compare the first pass effect of phenothiazines and thioxanthenes with those of butyrophenones.

The phenothiazines and thioxanthenes are 65–75 percent removed by the liver on the first pass through the portal system. Butyrophenones, in contrast, have less of a first-pass effect and are less than 35 percent metabolized before reaching the systemic circulation.

14. Describe the distribution of antipsychotic drugs.

These drugs, particularly the older drugs, have a large volume of distribution (> 7 l/kg), and are highly protein-bound (92–99 percent). They are highly lipid soluble, cross easily into the CNS, and accumulate in fatty tissues.

15. What are the cardiovascular effects seen with the phenothiazine class of antipsychotics?

These agents have significant alpha-receptor blockade, which produces acute postural hypotension, particularly after intravenous administration. Blockade of α_1 receptors may also precipitate systemic hypotension and reflex tachycardia.

16. Do phenothiazines have a direct effect on the myocardium?

Yes. These drugs have a "quinidine-like" effect and depress myocardial function.

17. Discuss the properties of phenothiazine-type drugs with aliphatic side chains (e.g., chlorpromazine).

These drugs have decreased potency as neuroleptics, and a high degree of crossreactivity between receptor types, resulting in the blockade of muscarinic, H_1, α_1, and 5-HT_2 receptors. They also have a high degree of extrapyramidal effects, and a propensity to cause tardive dyskinesia.

18. What are the general adverse effects of the aliphatic-phenothiazine class of antipsychotics (e.g., chlorpromazine)?

Members of the aliphatic group of phenothiazines tend to have strong sedative, hypotensive and anticholinergic properties. Extrapyramidal effects are mild to moderate.

19. Why might epinephrine therapy not be appropriate for a patient on antipsychotic drugs?

Epinephrine stimulates both adrenergic α_1 and β_2 receptors, providing a balance of vasoconstrictor and vasodilator actions. With antipsychotic therapy, the α_1 receptors are blocked in a dose-dependent manner. Thus, the effects of epinephrine on the vasodilatory β_2 receptors would predominate, resulting in hypotension.

20. Is therapy with chlorpromazine appropriate for a patient taking antiarrhythmic drugs?

This depends largely on the antiarrhythmic drug. Phenothiazines in particular produce a quinidine-like depression of the myocardium. Thus, the use of phenothiazines in conjunction with antiarrhythmic drugs that depress myocardial excitability such as quinidine, disopyramide, or digitalis glycosides could produce marked depression of the myocardium.

21. What might be the effect of antipsychotic therapy on a patient under antihypertensive therapy?

The α receptor blockade produced by antipsychotics would produce vasodilatation and lower systemic pressure. This effect must be considered in the dosing regimens of the drugs.

22. Contrast the properties of thioridazine and fluphenazine

Thioridazine, a piperidine phenothiazine derivative, is much less potent and less selective for dopamine (D_2) receptors than is fluphenazine, a piperazine derivative. Thus, thioridazine is likely to have more autonomic effects, more unpleasant adverse effects, and will also require a higher therapeutic dosage than fluphenazine. Because of the increased dosage required for effect, thioridazine will also be more likely to lead to tardive dyskinesia.

23. State the advantages of therapy with haloperidol over thiothixene.
Haloperidol is a member of the butyrophenone class of drugs. It thus has greater potency and less autonomic effects than thiothixene, a member of the thioxanthene class of antipsychotics.

24. Which antipsychotic of the phenothiazine class has a piperazine side chain and is considered a typical antipsychotic with "high specificity" in its pharmacological effects?
Trifluoperazine.

25. Which antipsychotic has little antimuscarinic activity and is unlikely to produce adverse effects on the extrapyramidal system at low to moderate doses?
Risperidone.

26. Which antipsychotic drug is most likely to produce a therapeutic response in schizophrenia patients who do not respond to "typical" antipsychotics?
Clozapine.

27. Why is clozapine not used as first line therapy?
Clozapine has decreased potency as an antipsychotic, and is likely to produce marked sedation and symptoms of altered autonomic function.

28. Describe the receptor selectivity of clozapine.
Clozapine has more affinity for the D_4 receptor than the D_1 or D_2 receptors. This drug also has a higher affinity for non-dopaminergic receptors (e.g., $5HT_2$, H_1, α_1) than for dopaminergic receptors. This accounts for the marked sedation and autonomic effects seen with the drug.

29. Describe the beneficial effects of clozapine in the therapy of schizophrenia.
Clozapine may improve "negative" symptoms related to lack of motivation, asocial behavior, and poverty of speech often seen in schizophrenia.

30. Which mechanism is believed to contribute to the beneficial effects of 'atypical' antipsychotics on the 'negative' symptoms of schizophrenia?
A high degree of blockade of $5HT_{2\alpha}$ receptors.

31. Which effects of clozapine limit therapy?
Agranulocytosis in a small proportion of patients. This drug may also cause seizures.

32. Which antipsychotic drugs are relatively selective for the D_2 receptor?
Pimozide is a selective D_2 receptor antagonist. In addition, perphenazine and haloperidol also have a high degree of selectivity for this receptor.

33. Which antipsychotic drugs are used as antiemetics?
Prochlorperazine and promethazine. Droperidol also may be used.

34. Which antipsychotic drug is used in neuroleptanesthesia?
Droperidol, a short-acting neuroleptic.

DRUGS USED IN THE THERAPY OF OTHER PSYCHIATRIC DISORDERS

35. Which neurotransmitter does methylphenidate affect to produce benefits for attention-deficit hyperactivity disorder (ADHD)?
Dopamine.

36. Describe the mechanism of action of methylphenidate.

Methylphenidate blocks the transport of dopamine, resulting in a dose-dependent decrease in dopamine reuptake by adrenergic neurons. The result is an increase in available dopamine in the cerebral cortex.

37. Compare the actions of methylphenidate and amphetamines.

The peripheral pharmacologic actions of methylphenidate are milder than those of the amphetamines. In addition, methylphenidate has preferential effects on mental stimulation, rather than motor function.

38. Describe the major sites of action of methylphenidate in the CNS.

The main sites of CNS activity appear to be the brain stem arousal system and the cerebral cortex.

39. Are addiction and tolerance seen with methylphenidate?

Not in normal clinical doses. These effects may occur with abuse, particularly if administered intravenously.

40. Describe the metabolism and elimination of methylphenidate.

Metabolism takes place in the liver, via hydroxylation. Metabolites are eliminated through the urine.

41. Which antidepressants are useful in the therapy of obsessive-compulsive disorder (OCD) and panic disorder?

It has been well documented that tricyclic antidepressants or SSRIs (e.g., fluoxetine) produce therapeutic responses significantly greater than placebo in the therapy of these conditions.

42. Which anticonvulsant drugs are useful in the therapy of manic depression, for the prevention of mood swings?

Valproic acid is first line therapy for this condition. Gabapentin and carbamazepine may also be useful. (See chapter 4 for a discussion of these drugs.)

43. Describe the cellular actions of lithium carbonate.

Lithium decreases production of adenosine 3c,5c-cyclic monophosphate (cAMP), and inhibits the recycling of phosphatidyl inositol phosphate to inositol, resulting in a decrease in inositol triphosphate (IP_3). Lithium also affects the permeability of membranes to sodium and potassium.

44. State the actions of lithium on neurotransmitter function.

Lithium decreases the release of serotonin and norepinephrine. In addition, it facilitates the reuptake of these neurotransmitters into neuronal endings.

45. What are the effects of lithium on potassium distribution?

Lithium causes a shift in potassium distribution from intracellular to extracellular potassium.

46. Describe the cellular mechanism of action of lithium, and relate it to it anti-manic effects.

Lithium readily enters excitable cells via sodium channels. It is not, however, removed well by the sodium/potassium ATPase exchange mechanism. It therefore accumulates within the cell. Thus, the intracellular concentration of potassium is decreased as the influx of potassium is reduced, both through inhibition of active transport (by Na^+/K^+ ATPase) and the decrease in the electrical gradient for potassium. Extracellular potassium therefore increases. The reversal in potassium levels results in a decrease in neuronal excitability, producing a therapeutic calming effect.

47. Discuss the effects of lithium carbonate on white blood cell count.

Lithium enhances granulocyte production via stimulation of monocyte colony stimulating factor production. Neutrophil count is also increased.

48. Are effects of lithium on bone marrow reversible?

Yes. White blood cell counts will decrease within 7 to 10 days after withdrawal of therapy.

49. Describe the effects of lithium on heart function.

Lithium causes disturbances in electrical conduction (i.e., flattening of T-wave). The shift in potassium distribution caused by the drug also causes supersensitivity to potassium, and may lead to cardiac arrest.

50. What is the distribution of lithium?

Lithium is not appreciably bound to serum proteins, and is distributed throughout the body. The drug appears to concentrate in fatty tissues such as bone, thyroid and brain.

51. Discuss the half-life and elimination of lithium.

Lithium is eliminated through the urine. About 80 percent of the lithium presented is reabsorbed through the renal tubules. The half-life is approximately 24 hours, which is substantially increased in the geriatric or renally compromised patient.

52. Is lithium a drug of first choice in treating mania?

The drug is still widely used and considered a first line agent. However, its use is rapidly being decreased in favor of less toxic agents, such as valproic acid or gabapentin.

53. Describe the therapy of Tourette syndrome.

Conventional therapies include dopaminergic antagonists such as haloperidol and pimozide. Recent evidence indicates that the addition of low-dose nicotine to the regimen significantly reduces the incidence and severity of facial tics, indicating that the use of transcutaneous nicotine as adjunct therapy may improve manifestations of the disorder.

BIBLIOGRAPHY

1. Bocchetta A, Chillotti C, Severino G, et al: Carbamazepine augmentation in lithium-refractory bipolar patients: A prospective study on long-term prophlyactic effectiveness. J Clin Psychopharmac 17(2):92–96, 1997.
2. Bowden CL.: Efficacy of lithium in mania and maintenance therapy of bipolar disorder [review]. J Clin Psychiatry 61 Suppl 9:35–40, 2000.
3. Hardman J, Limbird L, Gilman A: Goodman & Gilman's The Pharmacological Basis of Therapeutics, 10th ed. McGraw-Hill Publishers, 2001.
4. Griswold KS, Pessar LF: Management of bipolar disorder [review]. Am Fam Physician 62(6):1343–1353, 1357–1358, 2000.
5. Iwata Y, Kotani Y, Hoshino R, et al: Carbamazepine augmentation of clomipramine in the treatment of refractory obsessive-compulsive disorder [letter]. J Clin Psychiatry. 61(7):528–529, 2000.
6. Katzung B: Basic and Clinical Pharmacology, 8th ed. Appleton & Lange, 2001.
7. Kudo S, Ishizaki T: Pharmacokinetics of haloperidol: An update [review]. Clin Pharmacokinet 37(6):435–456, 1999.
8. Madhusoodanan S, Brenner R, Suresh P, et al: Efficacy and tolerability of olanzapine in elderly patients with psychotic disorders: A prospective study. Ann Clin Psychiatry 12(1):11–18, 2000.
9. Madhusoodanan S, Brenner R, Alcantra A: Clinical experience with quetiapine in elderly patients with psychotic disorders. J Geriatr Psychiatry Neurol 13(1):28–32, 2000.
10. Misra LK, Erpenbach JE, Hamlyn H, et al: Quetiapine: A new atypical antipsychotic [review]. S D J Medicine 51(6):189–193, 1998.
11. Poolsup N, Li Wan Po A, de Oliveira IR: Systematic overview of lithium treatment in acute mania. J Clin Pharm Ther 25(2):139–156, 2000.
12. Schaffer A, Levitt AJ, Joffe RT: Mexiletine in treatment-resistant bipolar disorder. J Affect Disord 57(1–3):249–253, 2000.

7. DRUGS USED IN THE THERAPY OF PARKINSON'S DISEASE AND ALZHEIMER'S DISEASE

1. Describe the general principles underlying the therapy of Parkinson's disease.

This disease results in an imbalance between dopamine and acetylcholine levels in the nigrostriatal tract. Thus, effective therapy results from lowering acetylcholine levels or activity to correlate with reduced dopamine levels, or increasing dopaminergic activity to correlate with normal acetylcholine levels.

2. Why is dopamine administration not an effective therapy for Parkinson's disease?

Dopamine is ionized at physiologic pH, and does not effectively cross the blood-brain barrier. In addition, systemic administration of dopamine has effects on major organs (e.g., heart and kidney), resulting in a high degree of adverse effects.

3. Describe the pharmacodynamics of L-dopa that make it useful for the treatment of Parkinson's disease.

L-dopa is a chemical intermediate produced in the synthesis of dopamine (see Figure below). It is formed from the actions of tyrosine hydroxylase on tyrosine, and is subsequently converted into dopamine by aromatic-L-amino acid decarboxylase (LAAD, or dopa decarboxylase). This molecule is taken up into the dopaminergic nerve terminal and converted to dopamine, which is then released into the synaptic cleft. Unlike dopamine, dopa is in nonionized form at physiologic pH and thus will cross into the central nervous system (CNS).

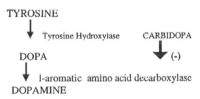

4. Describe the limitations of L-dopa therapy in patients with advanced Parkinson's disease.

The efficacy of L-dopa depends on the presence of intact nerve terminals, which are necessary to convert it to dopamine. As the disease progresses, fewer intact terminals are present. Thus, the efficacy of the drug gradually decreases with time.

5. What is the etiology of adverse effects associated with L-dopa therapy?

L-dopa is taken into both dopaminergic and noradrenergic nerve terminals, both in the CNS and periphery. Thus, peripheral levels of dopamine and norepinephrine may increase with administration of the drug, resulting in effects on the cardiovascular system, renal blood flow, and skeletal muscle function.

6. Describe the cardiovascular effects seen with L-dopa therapy.

Cardiovascular effects are primarily due to increased production of norepinephrine, and include atrial and ventricular arrhythmias, ventricular tachycardia, and atrial fibrillation. These effects are markedly reduced with concurrent administration of an inhibitor of peripheral LAAD.

7. Which drug, commonly used in the therapy of Parkinson's disease, is related to actions outside of the CNS?

Carbidopa. This drug inhibits peripheral dopa decarboxylase activity.

8. Describe the actions of carbidopa.

Carbidopa is an inhibitor of LAAD, and thus decreases the production of dopamine in a dose-dependent fashion. Because the molecule does not cross the blood-brain barrier, only peripheral LAAD is affected. Thus, the untoward effects of systemically administered L-dopa are minimized.

9. Describe the interactions of orally administered L-dopa and food.

The presence of food significantly reduces absorption of the drug, and various amino acids may also compete with the drug for transport into tissues.

10. If administered alone, how much of an orally administered dose of L-dopa will actually reach the CNS?

Only about 1 to 3 percent of the drug will actually enter the CNS. The remainder is metabolized or converted to dopamine in the periphery.

11. How does concurrently administered carbidopa affect L-dopa's efficacy?

The vast majority of administered L-dopa is converted to dopamine (or norepinephrine) in peripheral neurons. Concurrent administration of a dopa decarboxylase inhibitor, such as carbidopa, decreases the peripheral conversion of the drug to dopamine (or norepinephrine) in a dose-dependent manner. Thus, the proportion of administered drug that enters the CNS is significantly increased, resulting in increased efficacy of L-dopa. Thus, concurrent administration of carbidopa allows for lower doses of L-dopa.

12. Describe the effects of dopaminergic agonist therapy on vascular pressure.

Dopaminergic-receptor agonists, such as pergolide, pramipexole, and ropinirole cause a drop in systemic blood pressure in Parkinson's patients—decreases of up to 15mm Hg have been observed in both systolic and diastolic pressures.

13. What are limiting factors in L-dopa therapy?

Eighty percent of patients on L-dopa therapy develop dyskinesias. These are commonly manifested as choreoathetosis of the face and distal limbs. However, other manifestations, such as chorea, ballismus, myoclonus, tics, and tremors in the face and trunk may also occur. These effects are dose-related, and may also be related to the duration of therapy.

14. Describe the relationship of dose to the appearance of dyskinesias in Parkinson's patients on L-dopa therapy.

With increasing dose, the incidence of dyskinetic activity increases. In addition, with time, the effects may manifest at a constant, previously well-tolerated dose, indicating possible development of receptor suspersensitivity.

15. Is there an idiosyncratic component to the development of dyskinesias due to L-dopa therapy?

Yes. A wide patient variability has been observed.

16. Is the appearance of dyskinetic effects influenced by concurrent administration of a dopa decarboxylase inhibitor (e.g., carbidopa)?

Yes. The appearance of dyskinesias is markedly increased by the concurrent administration of carbidopa.

17. How can dyskinesias be minimized in patients on L-dopa therapy?

By removing the drug at intervals (a "drug holiday") in order to reduce the degree of receptor supersensitivity.

18. Describe the adverse psychological effects produced by L-dopa therapy.

These effects range from confusion and somnolence to depression, anxiety, and insomnia. Euphoria, delusions, and hallucinations have also been reported.

19. Describe the interaction of L-dopa and pyridoxine.

Pyridoxine acts as a cofactor in the activity of LAAD and increases the peripheral metabolism of L-dopa, resulting in a decrease in therapeutic effect.

20. Should L-dopa therapy be initiated in a patient taking a monoamine oxidase (MAO) inhibitor?

No. Therapy should not be initiated for at least 2 weeks post removal of MAO inhibitor therapy, because otherwise a hypertensive crisis may result. This effect is largely due to the increase in norepinephrine synthesis produced with L-dopa therapy, due to the uptake of L-dopa by peripheral noradrenergic nerve terminals and subsequent conversion to norepinephrine.

21. What adverse gastrointestinal effects are common with both L-dopa and bromocriptine therapy?

Nausea and vomiting due to effects on the chemoreceptor trigger zone.

22. Is bromocriptine therapy effective in patients refractory to therapy with L-dopa?

No.

23. Describe the use of bromocriptine.

Bromocriptine is considered first line treatment for Parkinson's. It is effective in conjunction with a cholinergic-lowering drug (e.g., amantadine), and is also used as monotherapy in patients undergoing a "drug holiday" from therapy with L-dopa. It may also be used as a "partial replacement" for L-dopa, allowing the dose of L-dopa to be lowered. Bromocriptine is also used to ameliorate "on-off" phenomena.

24. Does bromocriptine produce dyskinesias, such as those seen with L-dopa?

Yes, however the incidence of these events is much lower with bromocriptine.

25. What adverse psychiatric effects may be seen with bromocriptine?

Adverse psychiatric effects are similar, but increased in severity and incidence as compared with those seen with L-dopa.

26. Describe the mechanism of action and use of selegiline in the therapy of Parkinson's disease.

Selegiline is an inhibitor of monoamine oxidase B, a subtype of MAO that is selective for the degradation of dopamine. By decreasing the metabolism of dopamine in the substantia nigra, levels of dopamine increase and the DA/ACh ratio is improved.

27. Discuss the potential advantages of using selegiline in the therapy of Parkinson's disease.

The production of free radical species may contribute to the degeneration of dopaminergic neurons in the substantia nigra of Parkinsonian patients. Selegiline may directly result in decreased production of reactive oxygen species (hydrogen peroxide, superoxide anion, hydroxyl radical) in dopaminergic neurons, resulting in a decreased rate of neuronal degeneration. The ability of the drug to slow the progression of Parkinson's disease is, however, uncertain.

28. Describe the role of catechol-O-methyl transferase (COMT) in L-dopa therapy and why inhibition of COMT might be beneficial in the therapy of Parkinson's?

L-dopa can be metabolized by COMT to 3-methyl dopa. This metabolic pathway becomes active when neuronal pathways that convert dopa to dopamine are blocked by dopa decarboxylase inhibitors. The actions of COMT not only reduce circulating levels of L-dopa, which decreases the effectiveness of the drug, but the metabolite produced—3-methyl dopa—reduces the effect of L-dopa, because it competes with the drug for transport across cell membranes, particularly those of the intestinal mucosa, and structures of the blood-brain barrier. Thus, inhibition of COMT may increase the absorption of orally administered L-dopa, and also increase the proportion of drug entering the CNS.

29. Discuss the actions and use of tolcapone in the therapy of Parkinson's disease.

This drug is a COMT inhibitor that may be helpful late in the course of Parkinson's disease when combined with other therapies.

30. Discuss the mechanism of action of amantadine and its use in the therapy of Parkinson's.

This drug is an antiviral agent that also has anti-Parkinsonian effects. It has been shown to increase levels of dopamine (the mechanism is uncertain, although an increase in dopamine release has been documented), and also has anticholinergic effects. The end result is a positive effect in normalizing the ratio between cholinergic and dopaminergic effects in the substantia nigra.

31. Is amantadine suitable for monotherapy of Parkinson's disease?

No. The therapeutic effects of the drug are short-lived and the drug has severe adverse effects.

32. Discuss the therapeutic advantages of antimuscarinic therapy in the treatment of Parkinson's disease.

Antimuscarinic drugs are useful as adjunct therapy in Parkinson's, as they are useful in decreasing muscle rigidity and tremor, and attenuating the poverty of movement seen with the disease (e.g., bradykinesia). In addition, these drugs reduce undesirable effects of increased cholinergic activity, such as sweating and salivation.

33. Which major adverse effects are seen with oral antimuscarinic therapy?

Common adverse effects include xerostomia, blurred vision, parotitis, nausea/vomiting, drowsiness, dizziness, and mental confusion.

34. Do adverse effects of anticholinergic agents differ with the route of administration?

Yes. In addition to common adverse effects, parenteral administration may produce effects such as hypotension, decreased muscle coordination, and euphoria.

35. What is the primary therapeutic use of biperiden?

Biperiden is an antimuscarinic agent that may be administered orally or parenterally as adjunct therapy for Parkinson's disease. This drug attenuates extrapyramidal affects produced in other disease states and may be useful in the therapy of drug-induced extrampyramidal symptoms (e.g., with phenothiazines) as well.

36. Describe the use of procyclidine in Parkinson's treatment.

Procyclidine is an orally administered antimuscarinic agent used in adjunct therapy of Parkinson's disease.

37. Compare the adverse effects of biperiden and procyclidine.

Procyclidine has fewer adverse effects in therapeutic doses—the major adverse effect is xerostomia. Biperiden may produce CNS effects, such as euphoria, hypotension, and changes in motor coordination.

38. Describe the cardiovascular effects of trihexyphenidyl.

This antimuscarinic agent has vagolytic effects, and thus may produce tachycardia. Postural hypotension may also be seen.

39. Describe the dose-related CNS effects of trihexyphenidyl.
In small doses, the drug causes a net depression of the CNS. In larger doses, an atropine-like excitation of the CNS is manifested.

DRUGS USED IN THE THERAPY OF ALZHEIMER'S DISEASE

40. What is the clinical use of rivastigmine?
This drug is an acetylcholinesterase inhibitor used in the therapy of mild to moderate Alzheimer's dementia.

41. Why is donepezil particularly useful in the therapy of Alzheimer's disease?
Donepezil has an affinity for CNS acetylcholinesterase, over cholinesterases in the periphery. It is thus more selective, and is associated with fewer adverse effects.

42. Describe the use of donepezil in the therapy of Alzheimer's disease.
It is primarily used in the therapy of early to moderate stages of the disease.

43. Why is donepezil less useful for therapy in the late stages of Alzheimer's disease?
Its primary mechanism of action is to reduce metabolism of released acetylcholine, thus maintaining elevated levels of the transmitter. As neuronal degeneration progresses, fewer intact nerve terminals are present, less ACh is released, and the drug is less effective.

44. Does therapy with acetylcholinesterase inhibitors affect the underlying dementia associated with Alzheimer's disease?
No. The elevated levels of ACh in the cerebral cortex and limbic system may increase cognition and memory. However, the underlying mechanisms and progression of the disease remain unchanged.

BIBLIOGRAPHY

1. Barboi AC, Goetz CG: Parkinson's disease [review]. Clin Neuropharmacol 22(4):184–191, 1999.
2. Bradford HF, Zhou J, Pliego–Rivero B, et al: Neurotrophins in the pathogenesis and potential treatment of Parkinson's disease [review]. Adv Neurol 80:19–25, 1999.
3. Brooks DR: Anticholinergic drugs used in Parkinson's disease: An overlooked class of drugs from a pharmacokinetic perspective [review]. Journal of Pharmacy & Pharmaceutical Sciences 2(2):39–46, 1999.
4. Brooks DJ: Dopamine agonists: their role in the treatment of Parkinson's disease [editorial][review]. J Neurol Neurosurg Psychiatry 68(6):685–689, 2000.
5. Factor SA, Molho ES: Transient benefit of amantadine in Parkinson's disease: The facts about the myth [review]. Mov Disord 14(3):515–517, 1999.
6. Felician O, Sandson TA: the neurobiology and pharmacotherapy of alzheimer's disease. J Neuropsychiatry Clin Neurosci 11:19–31, 1999.
7. Hardman J, Limbird L, Gilman A: Goodman & Gilman's The Pharmacological Basis of Therapeutics, 10th ed. McGraw-Hill Publishers, 2001.
8. Hobson DE, Pourcher E, Martin WR: Ropinirole and pramipexole, the new agonists [review]. Can J Neurol Sci 26 Suppl 2:S27–S33, 1999.
9. Holm KJ, Spencer CM: Entacapone: A review of its use in Parkinson's disease [review]. Drugs 58(1):159–177, 1999.
10. Jankovic J: New and emerging therapies for Parkinson disease [review]. Arch Neurol 56(7):785–790, 1999.
11. Katzung, B: Basic and Clinical Pharmacology, 8th ed. Appleton & Lange, 2001.
12. Kennedy–Malone LM, Loftus SL: Parkinson's disease [review]. Lippincott's Primary Care Practice 3(2):169–173, 1999.
13. Lam YW: Clinical pharmacology of dopamine agonists [review]. Pharmacotherapy 20(1 Pt 2):17S–25S, 2000.
14. Leicht MJ, Mitchell SD: Catechol-O-methyltransferase inhibitors: New options for Parkinson's disease [review]. S D J Med 52(8):295–297, 1999.
15. LeWitt PA: New drugs for the treatment of Parkinson's disease [review]. Pharmacotherapy 20(1 Pt 2):26S–32S, 2000.

16. Mendis T, Suchowersky O, Lang A, et al: Management of Parkinson's disease: A review of current and new therapies [review]. Can J Neurol Sci 26(2):89–103, 1999.
17. Micek ST, Ernst ME: Tolcapone: A novel approach to Parkinson's disease [review]. Am J Health Sys Pharm 56(21):2195–2205, 1999.
18. Poewe W: Recent advances in the drug treatment of Parkinson's disease [editorial review]. Curr Opin Neurol 12(4):411–415, 1999.
19. Przuntek H: Non-dopaminergic therapy in Parkinson's disease [review]. J Neurol 247 Suppl 2:II19–II24, 2000.
20. Rascol O: The pharmacologic therapeutic management of levodopa-induced dyskinesias in patients with Parkinson's disease [review]. J Neurol 247 Suppl 2:II51–57, 2000.
21. Rinne UK, Gordin A, Teravainen HT: COMT inhibition with entacapone in the treatment of Parkinson's disease [review]. Adv Neurol 80:491–494, 1999.
22. Rivest J, Barclay CL, Suchowersky O: COMT inhibitors in Parkinson's disease [review]. Can J Neurol Sci 26 Suppl 2:S34–S38, 1999.
23. Sit SY: Dopamine agonists in the treatment of Parkinson's disease past, present and future [review]. Curr Pharm Des 6(12):1211–1248, 2000.
24. Stacy M: Pharmacotherapy for advanced Parkinson's disease [review]. Pharmacotherapy 20(1 Pt 2):8S–16S, 2000.

8. OPIATE PHARMACOLOGY

CLASS	STRONG AGONIST	MODERATE AGONIST	PARTIAL AGONIST	ANTAGONISTS
Phenanthrines	Morphine (Potent analgesia)	Codeine	Nalbuphene	Nalorphine
	Hydromorphone	Oxycodone	Buprenorphine	Naloxone
	Oxymorphone	Hydrocodone		Naltrexone (Long acting)
Phenylheptylamines	Methadone (No euphoric effects)	Propoxyphene (CNS effects)		
Phenylpiperidines	Meperidine (Potent euphoria)	Diphenoxylate (Limited CNS effects)		
	Fentanyl (Neuroleptanesthes)			
Benzomorphans			Pentazocine	
Morphians	Levorphanol		Butorphanol	Levallorphan

1. Discuss the general mechanism of action of opiate agonists.

These drugs attach to one or more opiate receptors, each of which can produce different effects. The binding affinity and potency of a drug on a particular receptor subtype determines the effect of the drug.

2. What are the major opiate receptors and their proposed actions?

The three opiate receptors so far characterized are the mu (m), kappa (k), and delta (d) receptors. The receptor producing the most familiar opiate effects is the m receptor. Binding to this receptor produces euphoric effects, analgesia, physical dependence, and respiratory depression. Binding of a drug to the d receptor produces many of the "negative" effects of opiates, such as dysphoria. The k receptor mediates aggressive tendencies. All three receptors appear to be involved in analgesia.

3. What are the major central nervous system (CNS) effects of opiates?

To varying degrees (depending on the individual drug) the following may be seen: Sedation, euphoria (or dysphoria, depending on the patient), analgesia, anesthesia, miosis, antitussis, nausea and vomiting, and respiratory depression.

4. What determines the degree of CNS effects seen with a particular opiate?

All opiates produce CNS effects. However, the degree to which they are seen depends on the dose of drug that enters the CNS. Thus, factors that allow the drug to cross the blood-brain barrier more efficiently will result in increased CNS effects. These include molecular structure, degree of ionization at physiologic pH, and the partition coefficient of the drug molecule. The degree of CNS effects seen may also depend on receptor selectivity.

5. What are the direct peripheral effects of opiate drugs?

Primarily effects on the gastrointestinal system. These include decreased bowel motility and decreased gastric acid secretion. It is also believed that there is a vestibular component to the emetic action of opiate drugs.

6. Discuss the physical addiction of opiates.

Physical addiction is receptor-mediated. Opiates exhibit tolerance, so a progressive increase in dose must be maintained over time in order to continue to achieve desired effects. This effect is manifested by a decrease in receptor number and sensitivity. Upon withdrawal, the receptor number and relative sensitivity to endogenous opiates is insufficient for normal bodily function. In addition, opiates affect all organ systems, particularly the heart and skeletal muscle. Abrupt withdrawal may precipitate convulsions and cardiovascular/cardiopulmonary abnormalities, particularly as a result of altered levels of norepinephrine. Gastrointestinal disturbances may also be manifested, and, because nociceptive levels are also affected, hyperalgesia may also result.

7. Discuss the psychologic addiction of opiates.

The psychologic addiction is distinct from the physical addiction, and results from a dependence on the euphoric effects produced by the drug. This results in drug cravings.

8. What are the general indications for opiate therapy?

Analgesia is the major use clinically. However, these drugs may be used during surgery to decrease reflex cough during inhalation anesthesia, as antidiarrheals, for sedation, and in some types of anesthesia.

9. Describe the types of analgesia produced by opiate drugs.

Opiates decrease the perception of pain by two general mechanisms:
1. neural input from the periphery is suppressed at the level of the cord; and
2. a dissociative effect (e.g., euphoria) is produced, which lessens the overall perception of pain.

10. At what level is opiate analgesia primarily mediated?

Opiates have a profound effect at the level of the spinal cord, decreasing sensation from the periphery.

11. Explain the medullary actions of opiates in analgesia.

In addition to the inhibition of neurotransmission by pain relays in the spinal cord, opiates act at medullary sites to disinhibit neurons that are inhibitory to transmission in pain relays. Thus, these inhibitory neurons are activated and further inhibit neuronal transmission within pain relays.

12. Describe how the respiratory depression of opiate drugs is mediated.

Respiratory depression is mediated at the level of the brain stem—primarily at medullary centers. Skeletal muscle rigidity produced by the drugs may also play a role.

13. Discuss the relationship between algesic level and opiate-induced respiratory depression.

There is in inverse relationship between manifestation of opiate-induced respiratory depression and the degree of pain stimulus present. Thus, when analgesic effects decrease the pain stimulus at high doses, respiratory depression may suddenly be manifested. In the same way, respiratory depression induced by opiate overdose may be delayed by the induction of a painful stimulus.

14. What are the effects of opiate analgesics on sleep?

At analgesic doses, these drugs disrupt both REM and nonREM sleep.

15. What are the ramifications of therapy with the phenanthrene class of opiate drugs (e.g., morphine) in the elderly?

This class of opiate agonist drugs has a strong sedative effect, particularly in the elderly. This effect may synergize with similar effects produced by other drugs (e.g., antihistamines), and, in combination with sedative hypnotic drugs, may induce a deep sleep state.

16. What physiologic effects are manifested with opiate-induced depression of medullary respiratory centers?

The decrease in respiratory rate and depth results in a decrease in blood oxygen (pO_2) and a corresponding increase in carbon dioxide (pCO_2), which may result in systemic acidosis.

17. Why should a patient with cranial trauma not be administered morphine or other strong opiate agonists?

The respiratory depression produced by these drugs results in an increase in plasma acidity, as carbon dioxide (CO_2) is converted to carbonic acid. This acidosis results in a reflex vasodilatation in the brain, resulting in increased intracranial pressure.

18. Does tolerance develop to the CNS effects of opiate agonists?

Yes, with the exception of miosis, tolerance is developed to all effects of opiate agonists. Thus, progressively higher doses are required to produce the desired level of effect.

19. What adverse effects of opiates are seen on the cardiovascular system?

Very few direct effects are seen. The most common effect is hypotension, which is seen in susceptible individuals. This effect is most pronounced with concurrent therapy involving drugs that stimulate the release of histamine. Opiate-induced changes in sympathetic activity may also precipitate cardiac irritability and an increase in cardiac output.

20. Discuss the effects of opiate agonists on the gastrointestinal system.

These drugs exert effects on both the CNS and enteric nervous system to produce a decrease in gastric motility, an increase in smooth muscle tone, and decreased secretion of gastric acid (HCl).

21. Discuss the effects of opiate agonists on the renal system.

Opiate agonists mediate a decrease in renal perfusion. In addition, they stimulate the release of antidiuretic hormone (ADH), which results in an increase in urine output.

22. Explain the effects of opiate agonists on a patient with a renal calculus.

Therapy with these drugs may worsen the patient's condition, as they mediate an increase in ureteral tone.

23. What might be the effect of opiate administration during parturition?

Opiates delay parturition and prolong labor by decreasing the tone of the uterus. This effect is mediated by both peripheral and central mechanisms.

24. Discuss the effects of opiates on the fetus during parturition.

The opiate-induced delay in parturition could result in deoxygenation of the fetus. In addition, these drugs readily cross the placenta and can accumulate in the fetus, causing depression of the fetal respiratory system.

25. Explain the effect of opiate agonists on the release of endogenous hormones.

These drugs act at the level of the hypothalamus to increase the release of vasopressin (ADH), prolactin, and growth hormone. Conversely, levels of luteinizing hormone are decreased.

26. Explain the occurrence of pseudo-allergic reactions with opiate administration.

Some opiate agonists stimulate the release of histamine, causing redness and itching of skin.

27. How are opiate drugs metabolized?

These drugs are metabolized by cytochrome P_{450}. Those drugs with exposed hydroxyl groups on the ring structure (e.g., morphine) are glucuronidated, while those with ester groups (e.g., heroin) are hydrolyzed. One or more active metabolites may be produced.

28. Why is dextromethorphan, an opiate agonist, allowed to be sold over-the-counter?

This drug does not cross the blood-brain barrier and thus has no euphoric effects. It does not promote psychologic or physical addiction.

29. Compare the relative potencies of morphine and meperidine.

Morphine and meperidine are both considered to be strong agonists. However, meperidine crosses into the CNS much more readily than does morphine, and therefore has a greater euphoric potency. Morphine is more potent at the spinal level and is a more potent analgesic.

30. Why is morphine administered by a parenteral route?

This drug has a high first-pass effect. It thus has poor oral bioavailability due to rapid glucuronidation during its first pass through the liver.

31. Distinguish the relative CNS effects of morphine, loperamide, and codeine.

Morphine is a strong agonist that crosses easily into the CNS. It is highly potent with regard to CNS effects, such as euphoria and medullary respiratory depression. Codeine is also a strong to moderate agonist, but does not cross the blood-brain barrier well. Thus, higher doses are needed to achieve CNS effects. Loperamide has little ability to cross into the CNS and is unlikely to produce CNS effects at any dose. It is thus sold over-the-counter.

32. Compare the effects of methadone and meperidine.

These drugs are both strong agonists and have similar peripheral effects. However, methadone does not produce euphoria and, therefore, does not promote psychological addiction.

33. Discuss the use of methadone in the treatment of chronic pain.

Methadone is a second-line choice in the treatment of chronic pain. It is highly bioavailable by oral and rectal routes, and has no euphoric effects (is not psychologically addictive).

34. Does methadone produce active metabolites?

No. The lack of active metabolites allows predictable effects with a given dosage.

35. When is methadone useful as a replacement drug for patients on other strong agonist opiates (e.g., morphine)?

Methadone is useful in patients who have developed tolerance to other opiate agonists or have developed intractable side effects due to opiate therapy.

36. Describe the properties of diphenoxylate.

This drug is used primarily as an antidiarrheal, in conjunction with atropine. It has limited ability to cross the blood-brain barrier, but in high doses can cause CNS effects and euphoria.

37. Describe the principal use of dextromethorphan.

This opiate agonist is used as an antitussive. It does not cross into the CNS and thus does not promote psychologic addiction.

38. What are the advantages of using dextromethorphan, rather than codeine, as an antitussive?

Both drugs are excellent antitussives. However, codeine promotes a much higher degree of constipation than does dextromethorphan. In addition, codeine has abuse potential, as it has the ability to cross into the CNS in high doses.

39. How is the dispensing of opiates regulated?

The degree of regulation of opiate drugs is directly proportional to their potency with regard to CNS effects. Those potent agonists with a high degree of CNS effects, such as morphine and meperidine, are strictly regulated (class II), whereas drugs with less ability to cross into the CNS, such as codeine, diphenoxylate and propoxyphene, are less strictly regulated (class III-V). Those drugs with little or no CNS activity, such as loperamide and dextromethorphan are not strictly regulated, and may be sold over-the-counter.

40. Describe the use of fentanyl in anesthesia.
Fentanyl is used in combination with droperidol to produce dissociative anesthesia, or neuroleptanesthesia.

41. Describe the effect of opiate analgesics on skeletal muscle.
Opiate analgesics may cause rigidity in skeletal muscle.

42. Describe the possible impairment of respiration seen with neuroleptanesthesia.
The use of fentanyl may cause severe chest compressions, due to the induction of skeletal muscle rigidity.

43. What is the proposed mechanism by which opiate analgesics decrease anxiety, restlessness, and subjective perception of fear?
These effects are related to sympathetic activity (norepinephrine). Opiate analgesics that cross into the CNS and are potent at the m receptor inhibit the activity of the locus ceruleus, reducing sympathetic activity.

44. Discuss the advantages of using morphine in the treatment of acute pulmonary edema.
The decrease in norepinephrine output mediated by opiates at the level of the locus ceruleus results not only in decreased anxiety, but also decreases arterial and venous tone (resulting in decreased preload and afterload). This in turn reduces ventricular filling, resulting in the increased force of contraction of ventricular muscle and more efficient ventricular ejection. The increase in left ventricular ejection fraction results in less pulmonary tension, a decrease in pulmonary capillary filtration, and decreased edema.

45. What are the possible effects of intravenous (IV) fentanyl on the release of histamine?
Fentanyl, a strong opiate agonist, is unlikely to stimulate histamine release after IV administration.

46. Discuss the interactions of opiate agonists with monoamine oxidase (MOA) inhibitors.
Opiates mediate an increase in body temperature, which, when combined with the effects of increased adrenergic activity due to the inhibition of MOA could produce a hyperpyrexic coma.

47. Discuss the interactions of opiate agonists with antipsychotics.
Both drugs produce sedation, and so would synergize, causing profound CNS effects. In addition, the hypotensive effects of antipsychotics would be markedly potentiated by the decrease in sympathetic activity produced by opiate agonists, causing severe cardiovascular complications. Both drugs affect skeletal muscle and medullary centers, as well, and may synergize to cause severe respiratory depression.

48. Discuss the interactions of opiate agonists with sedative-hypnotic drugs.
Both opiate agonists and sedative-hypnotic drugs produce CNS depression (resulting in sedation). Used concurrently, these drugs synergize to cause profound CNS depression.

MIXED AGONIST-ANTAGONIST DRUGS

49. Discuss the actions of the morphine-type mixed agonist-antagonist drugs (e.g., buprenorphine).
These drugs have low intrinsic m agonist activity but have a high affinity for the m receptor. Thus, they act as partial agonists at the m receptor, producing analgesic and CNS effects similar to those of morphine, but at a lower potency.

50. Explain the actions of buprenorphine.
This drug is a morphine-type mixed agonist-antagonist opioid. It exerts analgesic effects by acting as partial agonist at the m receptor, and has little affinity for k receptors.

51. Which drugs are included in the nalorphine-type mixed agonist-antagonist opiates?
This class of drugs includes butorphanol, nalbuphine, and pentazocine.

52. Discuss the agonist-antagonist receptor properties of the nalorphine-type drugs.
These drugs act as agonists at k receptors and antagonists at m receptors. However, the level of potency of these drugs is generally less than that produced by a pure agonist or antagonist. Therefore, because these drugs are competitive in binding, they may act as partial agonists or antagonists as well.

53. What are the major adverse affects of the nalorphine-type mixed agonist-antagonist opiates?
These drugs have a high incidence of undesirable psychologic effects, such as hallucinations, sleep disturbances, and anxiety.

54. Discuss the use of mixed agonist-antagonist drugs in the therapy of drug addiction.
The mixed agonist-antagonist opiates produce negligible euphoric effects. However, other receptor-mediated effects are similar to those of morphine. Therefore, the physical manifestations of opiate withdrawal are minimized, and psychologic dependence is not exacerbated.

OPIATE ANTAGONISTS

55. Compare the effects of naloxone and naltrexone.
Naloxone and naltrexone are both competitive opiate antagonists. Naloxone has a very short half-life while the duration of action of naltrexone is several days.

56. Which opiate antagonist is most likely to be used to treat symptoms of opioid overdose in a nonaddicted patient receiving analgesic therapy?
Nalmefene—a parenterally administered pure opiate antagonist.

57. What is a simple diagnostic procedure for the determination of opiate overdose?
Administration of naloxone. It has a brief duration of action and will quickly reverse miosis produced by opiate administration but not miosis produced by other means.

58. Why is naltrexone used in the therapy of opiate withdrawal?
Naltrexone is particularly useful in outpatient therapy for withdrawal, as it has a long half-life ($T\frac{1}{2} = 10$ hours) and a single dose can block the euphoric effects of opiates up to 48 hours. This helps to prevent the patient from procuring opiate drugs outside of the therapy milieu and "getting high."

59. Is naloxone administered orally?
No. It must be given parenterally for peak efficacy, as it has a high first-pass effect.

60. How is naloxone metabolized?
It is metabolized mainly by hepatic cytochrome P_{450} and glucuronide conjugation.

61. How is naltrexone administered?
Naltrexone may be administered orally or parenterally.

62. Discuss the possible use of naltrexone in the therapy of alcohol withdrawal.

Naltrexone has recently been approved for use in the therapy of chronic alcoholism, as it decreases the craving for alcohol. This is possibly due in part to alterations in sympathetic activity.

63. Describe the effects seen with administration of naloxone to a severely opiate-intoxicated patient.

The patient will recover consciousness rapidly, but, due to the high degree of intoxication and short half-life of naloxone, will quickly relapse into a comatose state within 60 to 90 minutes. A drug with longer duration of action would be indicated in this case.

64. Describe the use of nalmefene.

Nalmefene, a derivative of naltrexone, is used in therapy of opiate overdose.

65. What is the duration of action of nalmefene?

This drug has a long half-life (8–10 hours) and a long duration of action.

66. Will opiate antagonists affect a person to whom exogenous opiates have not been administered?

No. They are essentially inert. This allows the drugs to be used in diagnosis of opiate overdose without fear of systemic disruption.

67. Describe the reversal of opiate effects seen with the intravenous administration of an opiate antagonist.

Reversal of effects is rapid, occurring within 1 to 3 minutes. Normalization of pupil size, respiration, and consciousness is seen very rapidly.

68. Is tolerance exhibited to the effects of opiate antagonists?

No. Tolerance is not seen with chronic administration, and withdrawal of the drug does not precipitate adverse physiologic effects in non-opiate-dependent persons.

69. Are opiate antagonists equally potent among all opiate receptors?

No. In general, they are most potent at the m receptor, with varying effects at the other receptors.

BIBLIOGRAPHY

1. Corey PJ, Heck AM, Weathermon RA: Amphetamines to counteract opioid-induced sedation [review]. Ann Pharmacother 33(12):1362–1366, 1999.
2. Garrido MJ, Troconiz IF: Methadone: A review of its pharmacokinetic/pharmacodynamic properties [review]. J Pharmacol Toxicol Methods 42(2):61–66, 1999.
3. Gebhart GF, Su X, Joshi S, et al: Peripheral opioid modulation of visceral pain [review]. Ann N Y Acad Sci 909:41–50, 2000.
4. Hardman J, Limbird L, Gilman A: Goodman & Gilman's The Pharmacological Basis of Therapeutics, 10th ed. McGraw-Hill Publishers, 2001.
5. Katzung, B: Basic and Clinical Pharmacology, 8th ed. Appleton & Lange, 2001.
6. Kest B, Sarton E, Dahan A: Gender differences in opioid-mediated analgesia: Animal and human studies [review]. Anesthesiology 93(2):539–547, 2000.
7. Manzanares J, Corchero J, Romero J, et al: Pharmacological and biochemical interactions between opioids and cannabinoids [review]. Trends Pharmacol Sci 20(7):287–294, 1999.
8. Quock RM, Burkey TH, Varga E, et al: The delta-opioid receptor: Molecular pharmacology, signal transduction, and the determination of drug efficacy [review]. Pharmacol Rev 51(3):503–532, 1999.
9. Rawal N: Epidural and spinal agents for postoperative analgesia [review]. Surg ClinNorth Am 79(2):313–344, 1999.
10. Schiller PW, Weltrowska G, Schmidt R, et al: Subtleties of structure—agonist versus antagonist relationships of opioid peptides and peptidomimetics [review]. J Recept Signal Transduc Res 19(1–4):573–588, 1999.
11. Stefano GB, Goumon Y, Casares F, et al: Endogenous morphine [review]. Trends Neurosci 23(9):436–442, 2000.

12. Terenius L: From opiate pharmacology to opioid peptide physiology [review]. Ups J Med Sci 105(1):1–15, 2000.
13. Vaccarino AL, Olson GA, Olson RD, et al: Endogenous opiates: 1998 [review]. Peptides 20(12): 1527–1574, 1999.
14. White JM, Irvine RJ: Mechanisms of fatal opioid overdose [review]. Addiction 94(7):961–972, 1999.

III. Cardiovascular Pharmacology

Patricia K. Anthony, Ph.D., Judith Kautz, R.N., M.S., C. Andrew Powers, Ph.D., and Rebecca Thoms, R.N., N.P.

9. AUTONOMIC NERVOUS SYSTEM PHARMACOLOGY

1. Discuss the relationship between the sympathetic system (norepinephrine) and the parasympathetic system (acetylcholine).

The relationship between the two systems is complicated. The actions of one system tend to oppose those of the other (the "Yin-Yang" effect) but are by no means mutually exclusive. An extremely important concept in this area is that pharmacologic inhibition of either system simply allows the activity of the opposing system to predominate. For example, administration of a muscarinic antagonist (e.g., atropine) would result in sympathetic effects, and administration of an antagonist to either the α_1 or β_1 receptor would result in parasympathetic effects of the particular organ or tissue. The same is not true, however, of an α_2-receptor antagonist (see following).

2. What are the physiologic effects of acetylcholine on the heart?

Acetylcholine (ACh) decreases the rate of firing of the sinoatrial (SA) node (**negative chronotropic effect**) and the rate of conduction through the atrioventricular (AV) node and ventricular conduction system (**negative dromotropic effect**), resulting in bradycardia. The force of contraction of the heart muscle is also reduced (**negative inotropic effect**), resulting in decreased ejection fraction and decreased cardiac output.

3. What are the effects of acetylcholine on bodily secretion and excretory functions?

The effects of ACh on bodily secretions and excretion are generally stimulatory. They may be remembered with the mnemonic "SLUD"— increased **s**alivation, **l**acrimation, **u**rination and **d**efecation.

4. What are the physiologic and cellular effects of norepinephrine (or epinephrine) on the heart?

Norepinephrine affects calcium flux within cardiac muscle tissue and conductive tissue, resulting in a positive inotropic and dromotropic effect. It also increases the rate of firing of the SA node, resulting in an increase in heart rate (positive chronotropic effect).

5. Describe the actions of the α_1-adrenergic receptor.

The α_1 receptor causes smooth muscle contraction, through the actions of the inositol phosphate and diacylglycerol cascade.

6. Describe the actions of the α_2-adrenergic receptor.

The α_2 receptor is a regulatory receptor, which acts by inhibition of adenylate cyclase and subsequent decrease in cAMP. α_2-receptors are located primarily on the membrane of the adrenergic nerve terminus, where they act to decrease norepinephrine release from the neuronal ending. α_2-receptors are also located on the nucleus tractus solitarius (NTS) of the hypothalamus, which regulates systemic sympathetic outflow.

7. Discuss the cellular actions of the β_1 receptor.

The β_1 receptor acts through stimulation of adenylate cyclase, which results in an increase in the levels of cyclic adenosine monophosphate (cAMP). This results in phosphyorylation of ion channels and increased conductance.

8. Discuss the major actions of the β_1 receptor.

β_1 receptors on the sinoatrial node increase the frequency of firing of the SA node through a cascade resulting in the phosphorylation of sodium channels and increased sodium conductance. In the kidney, these receptors stimulate the release of renin, which initiates the renin-angiotensin cascade and results in the formation of angiotensin II, which contributes to an increase in local and systemic blood pressure. In lipocytes, these receptors stimulate the breakdown of fats and, in muscle and liver tissue, the breakdown of glycogen, resulting in an increase in blood sugar.

9. Discuss the actions of the β_2 receptor

β_2 receptor stimulation results in stimulation of adenylate cyclase and increased cAMP. This receptor mediates relaxation of smooth muscle in vessel walls and in bronchioles. It also may stimulate increased cardiac output.

10. What would be the physiologic result of administering an α_2-receptor agonist rather than an α_2 receptor antagonist?

An agonist at the sympathetic α_2 receptor decreases norepinephrine release and produces parasympathetic effects (e.g., bradycardia, increased micturition, vasodilatation, etc.) because the α_2 receptor is a regulatory receptor. An antagonist would increase norepinephrine release and produce sympathetic effects. It is useful to remember this concept when predicting the adverse effects of an α_2-receptor agonist used for hypertension (e.g., clonidine).

11. What are the differential sensitivities to epinephrine of the various adrenergic receptors?

Epinephrine is approximately equipotent on the α_1, α_2, and β_1 receptors. However, the β_2 receptors are much more sensitive to the drug. This sensitivity is offset in the vasculature by fewer β_2 receptors present, but becomes an issue with dose and rate of administration.

12. Why do the effects of epinephrine differ between patients?

The effects of epinephrine can be unpredictable, due to idiosyncratic differences in the number of β_2 receptors present, and the differential sensitivity of receptors.

13. Why are epinephrine and norepinephrine administered by the parenteral route?

Both epinephrine and norepinephrine have a high first-pass effect, and are rapidly inactivated if given orally.

14. Explain the physiologic ramifications of the rate of administration of epinephrine as compared to norepinephrine.

Because of the differential receptor sensitivity, a low dose, or slow administration, of epinephrine will stimulate the sensitive β_2 receptors more than the less sensitive α_1 receptors, producing a net vasodilatation. A high dose or rapidly administered dose will stimulate both receptor subtypes maximally and produce a rapid vasoconstriction, which, in a normotensive patient, could precipitate a hypertensive crisis.

Norepinephrine, because of its negligible effect (generally considered to be none) on the β_2 receptor does not produce this response. Therefore, the effect of norepinephrine is independent of dose or rate of administration, and is manifested as vasoconstriction.

15. What are the pharmacologic differences between epinephrine and norepinephrine?

Both epinephrine and norepinephrine have potent activity on the α_1, α_2, and β_1 receptors. Norepinephrine has slightly more activity on the α_1 receptor than epinephrine, but stimulation of the adrenergic β_2 receptor is negligible. Thus the effects of norepinephrine are more predictable.

16. What is "epinephrine reversal?"

Epinephrine stimulates all four adrenergic receptors, and the actions of the α_1 receptor (vasoconstriction) are opposed to those of the β_2 receptor (vasodilatation). Therefore, if epinephrine is given in pharmacologic doses, blood pressure rises, due to the action on the α_1 receptor. If an antagonist to the α_1 receptor (e.g., prazosin) is subsequently administered, the blood pressure will show a precipitous drop, due to the inhibition of the α_1 receptor-mediated vasoconstriction in the face of the vasodilatation produced by the β_2 receptor, which has not been affected. Thus, the action is reversed from vasoconstriction and increased pressure to vasodilatation and a precipitous decrease in pressure.

17. Compare the synthesis of epinephrine, norepinephrine, and dopamine.

The synthesis pathway is initially the same for all three agents (see Figure). The amino acid tyrosine is acted upon by tyrosine hydroxylase to form DOPA, which then is converted to dopamine, through the actions of dopa decarboxylase (1-aromatic amino-acid decarboxylase). The pathway stops at this point in dopaminergic neurons. In chromaffin cells and noradrenergic neurons, the pathway continues further, with dopamine being converted to norepinephrine by dopamine-β-hydroxylase in the secretory granule. The pathway continues further only in adrenal chromaffin cells, where norepinephrine is converted to epinephrine by phenylethanolamine-N-methyltransferase (PNMT). The length of the pathway and the particular humoral agent produced is a function of the enzymes available within the particular cell.

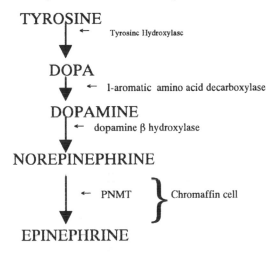

Synthesis of epinephrine.

18. How are the actions of norepinephrine terminated?

Norepinephrine (NE) is taken up into the nerve terminus of the adrenergic neuron by neuronal reuptake mechanisms ("pumps"). It is then degraded intracellularly, by monoamine oxidase (MAO) (primarily MAO$_A$, a mitochondrial enzyme) to form dihydroxymandelic acid. This is further inactivated by the tissue enzyme catechol-O-methyl transferase (COMT). Transmitter remaining in the synaptic cleft is rapidly degraded, first by COMT, located on postsynaptic membranes, to form normetanephrine. This in turn is taken into the neuron and converted to 3-methoxy, 4-hydroxy mandelic acid (VMA) through the actions of MAO (see Figure, top of next page).

19. Describe the hepatic metabolism of catecholamines.

Plasma catecholamines undergo a rapid phase I reaction with cytochrome P$_{450}$ followed by a phase II methylation reaction involving adenosyl methionine and cytosolic methyltransferases.

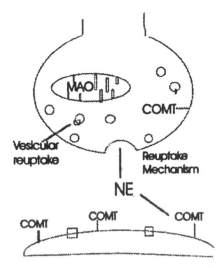

Schematic representation of norepinephrine metabolism at the level of the neuron.

20. Are epinephrine and norepinephrine subject to the same reuptake and degradation mechanisms?

Yes. Epinephrine may also be taken into the adrenergic nerve terminus and degraded by MAO_A. It is also degraded by tissue COMT. The end product of the degradation of both epinephrine and norepinephrine is VMA.

21. Discuss the ramifications of the pharmacologic inhibition of MAO_A.

Inhibition of this enzyme allows intracellular concentrations of NE to increase to the point where reuptake mechanisms are no longer effective, and precipitate a leaching out of NE and an increase in tissue and blood concentrations. In addition, the metabolites of epinephrine and norepinephrine produced by the actions of COMT still have pharmacologic activity, until acted upon by MAO, so actual degradation is minimized severely. The increased levels of epinephrine, norepinephrine, and their metabolites (metanephrine and normetanephrine, respectively) result in tachycardia, increased cardiac output, increased blood sugar, and vasoconstriction. The cardiovascular effects may ultimately precipitate a hypertensive crisis.

22. What is the nicotinic acetylcholine receptor?

The nicotinic receptor is found primarily in post effector ganglion cell membranes and also in the postsynaptic motor endplate. It is a transmembrane channel, or sodium **ionophore**, composed of five polypeptide subunits. Upon conformational change, the channel opens and allows the entrance of sodium into the cell, resulting in excitatory action potentials. The channel is opened upon the binding of acetylcholine or a nicotinic agonist to the receptor protein. This event occurs extremely rapidly—the channel opens and closes in a matter of milliseconds, resulting in an extremely rapid and short-lived depolarization.

23. Discuss the effects of muscarinic receptor stimulation.

Stimulation of muscarinic receptors in the heart results in bradycardia, due to a slowing of conduction through the AV node, a decrease in firing of the SA node, and decreased force of cardiac muscle contraction. Muscarinic stimulation increases bladder tone, and muscarinic effects on smooth muscle may produce bronchoconstriction (particularly in patients with pulmonary disease), vasodilatation, increased exocrine secretions, and increased peristalsis. In the CNS, muscarinic receptor stimulation is involved in cognizance and motor function.

24. How are the actions of acetylcholine terminated?

ACh released from cholinergic neurons may be returned to the neuron by reuptake mechanisms. However, the majority of the ACh molecules are quickly degraded in the synaptic cleft by acetylcholinesterase, which splits the molecule into acetate and choline. These may then be taken up into the cholinergic neuron by reuptake mechanisms and recycled. ACh in plasma is quickly degraded by plasma esterases.

25. What are the pharmacologic uses of acetylcholine?

ACh is rapidly degraded by plasma esterases if administered parenterally, and degraded in the stomach if given orally. Thus, the pharmacologic uses of acetylcholine are limited to topical use in glaucoma.

CARDIAC REFLEXES

26. Discuss the role of cardiac reflexes in the therapeutic use and efficacy of drugs that affect the sympathetic nervous system.

Cardiovascular function is in part regulated by cardiac reflexes (e.g., the baroreceptor reflex) that sense changes in pressure and compensate with inhibition or stimulation of the sympathetic nervous system. These reflexes act in a manner contrary to the desired effects of a large number of drugs and must be anticipated when administering a particular drug. Drugs that lower systolic pressure by rapid vasodilatation (e.g., α_1 receptor antagonists), for example, will initially produce the desired therapeutic result, but the effects of the drug will quickly be attenuated, due to stimulation of the baroreceptor reflex. With constant therapy, however, the baroreceptors will "reset" at a lower level, increasing the efficacy of the drug.

27. What is the role of cardiac reflexes in the therapeutic use and efficacy of drugs that affect the parasympathetic nervous system?

Drugs that affect the parasympathetic nervous system tend to produce a high degree of baroreceptor-mediated responses under normal usage. Thus, their responses are typically limited in duration, irrespective of drug half-life. This may not apply when the drug is used under life threatening conditions (e.g., the use of atropine in the resuscitation of cardiac failure), because the baroreceptor reflex is set at normal levels of tension.

28. Discuss the mechanism of cardiac reflexes in the therapeutic use of parasympathetic nervous system agonists.

Parasympathetic agonists produce a relatively unopposed baroreceptor response. The decrease in systolic pressure produced by the administration of a parasympathetic agonist produces a reflex tachycardia and vasoconstriction, both of which are relatively unopposed by the drug, which itself has no sympathetic receptor involvement.

29. Discuss the mechanism of cardiac reflexes in the therapeutic use of parasympathetic nervous system antagonists.

Use of a muscarinic antagonist blocks the actions of the parasympathetic nervous system in a dose-dependent manner, leaving the actions of the sympathetic nervous system relatively unopposed by cardiac reflexes. Administration of a parasympathetic (muscarinic) antagonist will result in sympathetic effects (e.g., tachycardia, increased cardiac output). Normally, this would precipitate an increase in parasympathetic activity, due to baroreceptor reflexes. The level of ACh secretion may increase, however, because receptors are blocked and physiologic actions normally seen with an increase in ACh are blocked in a dose-dependent manner, leaving the actions of the sympathetic system dominant. Tachycardia and increased cardiac output are seen, and peripheral resistance remains increased.

30. Which classes of autonomic drugs are less likely be affected by cardiac reflexes?

α_2-receptor agonist drugs, such as clonidine and α-methyl dopa, will not be affected by cardiac reflexes—indeed, they inhibit compensatory reflexes because they block sympathetic outflow from the NTS, inhibiting baroreceptor mediated reflex response.

BIBLIOGRAPHY

1. Cabral AM, da Silva IF, Gardioli CR, et al: Chronic activation of central alpha 2-adrenoceptors prevents hypertension in DOCA-salt rats. Auton Neurosci 82(3):146–153, 2000.
2. Chow FA, Seidler FJ, McCook EC, et al: Adolescent nicotine exposure alters cardiac autonomic responsiveness: Beta-adrenergic and m2-muscarinic receptors and their linkage to adenylyl cyclase. Brain Res :878(1–2):119–126, 2000.
3. Dampney RA, Tagawa T, Horiuchi J, et al: What drives the tonic activity of presympathetic neurons in the rostral ventrolateral medulla [review]? Clin Exp Pharmacol Physiol 27(12):1049–1053, 2000.
4. Elenkov IJ, Wilder RL, Chrousos GP, et al: The sympathetic nerve—an integrative interface between two supersystems: The brain and the immune system [review]. Pharmacol Rev 52(4):595–638, 2000.
5. Gobel I, Trendelenburg AU, Cox SL, et al: Electrically evoked release of ((3)H)noradrenaline from mouse cultured sympathetic neurons: Release-modulating heteroreceptors. J Neurochem 75(5): 2087–2094, 2000.
6. Hardman J, Limbird L, Gilman A: Goodman & Gilman's The Pharmacological Basis of Therapeutics, 10th ed. McGraw-Hill Publishers, 2001.
7. Kandel ER, Schwartz JH, Jessel TM: Principles of Neuroscience. Elsevier Publishers, 2000.
8. Katzung B: Basic and Clinical Pharmacology, 8th ed. Appleton & Lange, 2001.
9. Lohmeier TE, Lohmeier JR, Haque A, et al: Baroreflexes prevent neurally induced sodium retention in angiotensin hypertension. Am J Physiol Regul Integr Comp Physiol 279(4):R1437–1448, 2000.
10. Porges WL, Hennessy EJ, Quail AW, et al: Heart-lung interactions: The sigh and autonomic control in the bronchial and coronary circulations. Clin Exp Pharmacol Physiol 27(12):1022–1027, 2000.
11. Rosol TJ, Yarrington JT, Latendresse J, et al: Adrenal gland: Structure, function, and mechanisms of toxicity. Toxicol Pathol 29(1):41–48, 2000.
12. Shukla VH, Dave KR, Katyare SS: Effect of catecholamine depletion on oxidative energy metabolism in rat liver, brain and heart mitochondria; use of reserpine. Comp Biochem Physiol C Pharmacol Toxicol Endocrinol 127(1):79–90, 2000.

Websites:
Clinical Pharmacology 2000: http://cp.gsm.com
Medline plus: http://medlineplus.nlm.nih.gov/
Medscape Multispecialty Journal Room: http://pharmacotherapy.medscape.com/Home/Topics/multispecialty/directories/dir-MULT.JournalRoom.html
Medscape Pharmacotherapy News (cardiology):
http://cardiology.medscape.com/home/topics/pharmacotherapy/directories/dir-PHAR.News.html

10. DRUGS THAT AFFECT THE PARASYMPATHETIC NERVOUS SYSTEM

1. Discuss the general mechanism of action of direct muscarinic agonists.

These drugs stimulate muscarinic receptors, resulting in organ-specific effects such as miosis of the eye, stimulation of peristalsis and increased secretion of stomach acid, increased secretion of exocrine glands, and cardiovascular depressant effects (e.g., negative inotropic, chronotropic and dromotropic actions). These agents have varying degrees of selectivity toward the muscarinic receptor—there is crossreactivity between nicotinic and muscarinic receptors with most agents.

2. How is the action of a muscarinic agonist terminated?

In general, these agents are degraded by cholinesterases. This may include acetylcholinesterases, plasma cholinesterases, and tissue cholinesterases.

3. What confers the specific properties (e.g., receptor selectivity, cholinesterase resistance) of a cholinergic agonist?

Specific structure-function relationships. For example, certain structural domains are responsible for binding to the nicotinic receptor and muscarinic receptor. Also, structural modifications that block the binding site for one receptor subtype result in a selectivity of the drug for the other subtype. In the same way, modifications that result in steric hindrance to the cholinesterase binding site will confer cholinesterase resistance.

4. What are the adverse gastrointestinal effects of muscarinic agonists?

These agents increase peristaltic tone, resulting in increased incidence of diarrhea, nausea, vomiting, and excessive production and expulsion of gasses.

5. Discuss the interactions of muscarinic agonists and drugs such as clemastine, diphenhydramine, methdilazine, and promethazine.

These drugs are H_1-blockers, and have antimuscarinic activity. Thus, concurrent administration decreases the potency of a muscarinic agonist.

6. Discuss the use of acetylcholine (ACh) as an ophthalmic agent.

This drug is used to produce miosis during ophthalmic surgery. The muscarinic action of the drug results in contraction of the circular muscles of the iris (leading to miosis) and contraction of the ciliary muscle (resulting in accommodation). These effects are short-lived, lasting approximately 10 minutes (see Table below).

Therapeutic Properties of Choline Esters

DRUG	RECEPTOR SELECTIVITY	PLASMA HALF-LIFE
Acetylcholine	Non-selective	Short—rapidly hydrolyzed
Carbachol	Non selective	Long not hydrolyzed
Bethanechol	Muscarinic selective	Medium—slowly hydrolyzed
Methacholine	Muscarinic selective	Short—rapidly hydrolyzed

7. Explain the intravenous use of acetylcholine.

Acetylcholine is not used intravenously, as it is degraded almost immediately by plasma cholinesterases.

8. Which cholinergic agonists in clinical use are classified as choline esters?
Methacholine, bethanechol, and carbachol (a carbamate ester).

9. Explain the structure-function properties of methacholine
Methacholine is a choline ester with an added methyl group. This methyl group is conjugated to the portion of the structure that normally would convey specificity for the nicotinic receptor, blocking access to the site. Thus, this agent is a selective muscarinic agonist and has negligible nicotinic activity.

10. Why is carbachol long-acting?
Carbachol is a carbamate ester. The presence of the carbamate moiety on the drug structure provides steric hindrance to the cleavage site for cholinesterases, making the drug cholinesterase resistant.

11. Describe the receptor selectivity of carbachol.
Carbachol is a non-selective agent, and will act as an agonist at either muscarinic or nicotinic receptors.

12. Discuss the properties of bethanechol.
Bethanechol has a chemical structure that is intermediate between those of methacholine and carbachol. It is thus both long acting and selective for muscarinic receptors.

13. Describe the mechanism of action of bethanechol.
It is a direct acting muscarinic agonist and acts by competitive stimulation of the muscarinic cholinergic receptor.

14. Is bethanechol administered by bolus injection?
No. It is resistant to plasma cholinesterases, as compared to acetylcholine, and is not degraded. Therefore, rapid infusion may precipitate circulatory collapse. This drug is administered orally.

15. Does bethanechol have central nervous system (CNS) effects?
No. It has a quaternary amine structure and does not cross the blood-brain barrier.

16. What are the clinical uses of bethanechol?
Bethanechol may be used to treat urinary retention and stimulate GI motility. It is also used in the treatment of postpartum and postoperative nonobstructive urinary retention, and to counteract the antimuscarinic effects of phenothiazines and tricyclic antidepressants (e.g., bladder dysfunction).

17. Explain the contraindications to the use of bethanechol in cardiac patients.
Bethanechol, like any muscarinic agent, has negative inotropic, chronotropic and dromotropic effects. It may also cause systemic vasodilatation, decreased TPR, and dramatically lowered blood pressure. In a healthy person, sympathetic reflexes would compensate for these effects. However, such reflexes would worsen symptoms in a patient with cardiovascular dysfunction. Bethanechol's use is therefore contraindicated in patients with pronounced bradycardia, hypotension, coronary artery disease, or any type of cardiac disease.

18. Discuss the contraindications to the use of bethanechol in hyperthyroid patients.
Thyroid hormone sensitizes the heart to catecholamines. Because bethanechol is a muscarinic agent, it would cause a decrease in heart rate and systemic pressure, triggering an increase in catecholamine secretion. Thus, the combination of elevated catecholamines and increased catecholamine sensitivity could lead to abnormal heart function (e.g., arrhythmias).

19. Is bethanechol or carbachol contraindicated in patients with lung disease?

Yes. As muscarinic agents, these drugs mediate bronchoconstriction, and would therefore be contraindicated in these patients, particularly those with asthma or chronic obstructive pulmonary disease (COPD).

20. Does spinal cord injury affect the actions of bethanechol on urinary retention?

No. It is a receptor agonist.

21. What are the clinical indications for carbachol?

Carbachol is used as an ophthalmic agent, in the reduction of intraocular pressure. The drug induces miosis, and is therefore also used to counteract the effects of sympathetic agents in the eye.

22. What are the clinical uses of pilocarpine?

Pilocarpine is used as a miotic agent in the therapy of glaucoma, and is also used in the therapy of xerostomia caused by drugs with a high degree of antimuscarinic effects.

23. Describe the effects of orally administered pilocarpine.

Pilocarpine administered orally stimulates secretions of exocrine glands.

24. Discuss the pharmacokinetics of pilocarpine.

Pilocarpine is highly protein-bound, to both serum and tissue proteins. Degradation occurs via plasma cholinesterases and acetylcholinesterase. Elimination is primarily renal.

25. What are the clinical uses of metoclopramide and cisapride?

These drugs are muscarinic agonists, used to stimulate gastrointestinal (GI) motility and bladder function.

26. Discuss the mechanism of action of indirect cholinergic agonists.

Acetylcholinesterase binds to acetylcholine and cleaves the molecule into acetate and choline. The indirect cholinergic agonists bind to the ACh binding site on the enzyme, thus inhibiting acetylcholinesterase activity. This results in elevated levels of ACh and increased cholinergic effects.

27. What determines the duration of action of indirectly acting cholinergic agonists?

The strength of the enzyme-agent interaction is the major determinant of the duration of activity. Those agents that weakly bind to the ACh binding site (e.g., edrophonium) are easily reversible, whereas those that bind covalently, such as the carbamate esters, are removed with difficulty and thus have a longer duration of action. (See Table below.)

Selected Cholinesterase Inhibitors

DRUG	DURATION OF ACTION	NEUROLOGICAL ACTION
Edrophonium	Short acting/reversible	CNS activity
Carbamates	Intermediate acting/reversible	
Neostigmine		No CNS activity
Physostigmine		CNS activity
Piperidines (e.g., donepezil)	Long acting/reversible	CNS activity
Organophosphates	Irreversible	CNS activity

28. Why are organophosphates considered irreversible indirect cholinergic agonists?

These agents phosphorylate the active site of acetylcholinesterase. Once the phosphorylation is stable, it is not reversible within the length of time that the enzyme is active (the inactivation extends for the life of the enzyme). (See Table above.)

29. What is the approximate half-life of an irreversible indirect agonist?
Approximately 100 hours.

30. Describe the clinical uses of edrophonium.
Edrophonium is very short-acting, so is not used for treatment. Its major uses are in diagnostic procedures, such as the diagnosis of myasthenia gravis. It is also used to reverse the effects of competitive neuromuscular blockade (e.g., d-tubocurarine) after surgery.

31. Describe the adverse effects of edrophonium.
Edrophonium has the same adverse (cholinergic) effects as other cholinesterase inhibitors. However, the short duration of the drug does not allow for manifestation of these effects. Thus, observed adverse effects are negligible.

32. Explain the dangers of using atropine to ameliorate the symptoms of cholinergic intoxication from cholinesterase inhibitors.
Atropine may mask the signs of a cholinergic crisis, which is a life-threatening event.

33. Which cholinesterase inhibitors are most likely to cause hypersensitivity reactions?
Cholinesterases that contain bromide, such as pyridostigmine, neostigmine, and demecarium may cause hypersensitivity reactions.

34. Describe *"acetylcholinesterase myopathy."*
Prolonged, high doses of acetylcholinesterases (AChEs) have been shown to cause ultrastructural changes in skeletal muscle and motor endplate in experimental animals. In addition, the increase in available ACh initiates a negative feedback response, resulting in a decrease in ACh synthesis, and a decrease in post-junctional receptor sensitivity and density. Withdrawal of terminal neuronal branches from the motor endplate has been observed as well. These changes may result in an observable decrease in skeletal muscle function.

35. Describe the clinical uses of neostigmine and physostigmine.
Both of these agents are carbamate esters and have similar properties. Neostigmine is a quaternary amine and therefore carries a charge at physiological pH. This prevents the drug from entering the CNS. Thus, neostigmine is more useful in the therapy of conditions in the periphery, such as myasthenia gravis. Physostigmine, a tertiary amine, does not carry a charge, and thus has central effects. This drug is useful in conditions with a central etiology, such as atropine overdose.

36. Why would physostigmine be less useful than neostigmine in the therapy of myasthenia gravis?
The central effects of physostigmine could mediate adverse effects, such as motor impairment and cognitive changes. Physostigmine also has less potency at the neuromuscular junction than does neostigmine.

37. Is physostigmine useful in the therapy of Alzheimer's disease?
Yes. The increased levels of acetylcholine in the limbic system may result in an increase in cognizance. A sustained-release form of physostigmine salicylate (Synapton®) has completed phase III investigation for the treatment of Alzheimer's disease as of August 1996.

38. Explain the use of physostigmine in the treatment of tricyclic-induced anticholinergic toxicity.
Physostigmine, administered intravenously (IV), may be useful in the amelioration of life threatening anticholinergic effects due to tricyclics.

39. Why is physostigmine not the drug of choice for treatment of tricyclic overdose?

Physostigmine has the potential for induction of seizure activity. In addition, the increase in cholinergic activity does not significantly affect the bradycardia caused by the "quinidine-like" effects of tricyclics.

40. Compare low-dose and high-dose administration of physostigmine.

At low doses, physostigmine acts primarily at muscarinic cholinergic synapses and within the CNS. Effects on the neuromuscular junction are relatively low. At higher doses, physostigmine may actually cause a depolarizing blockade at the neuromuscular junction, due to the accumulation of high levels of acetylcholine. In the same way, the increase in ACh levels seen with high-dose physostigmine may also mediate a depolarizing blockade at autonomic ganglia, resulting in altered autonomic effects. In the same way, the drug may directly potentiate CNS depression.

41. What is the primary use of physostigmine?

This drug is commonly used in the therapy of glaucoma. It produces miosis and contraction of the ciliary muscle, which allows drainage from the canals of Schlemm, decreasing intraocular pressure.

42. How is systemic physostigmine administered?

Physostigmine must be administered parenterally for systemic therapy. It is normally administered IV or intramuscularly (IM).

43. How quickly are the effects of physostigmine seen?

Effects are seen in less than five minutes after parenteral administration.

44. Describe the metabolism and duration of action of physostigmine.

The drug is metabolized by systemic cholinesterases. Its duration of action is therefore fairly short— around 2 hours if given parenterally, and 12 to 36 hours with topical administration to the eye.

45. What problems are associated with the acridine-type cholinesterase inhibitors (e.g., tacrine)?

These drugs are associated with hepatotoxicity. They also have an extensive first-pass effect when administered orally.

46. Why is donepezil particularly useful in the therapy of Alzheimer's disease?

Donepezil has an affinity for CNS acetylcholinesterase, over cholinesterases in the periphery. It is thus more selective, and is associated with less adverse effects.

47. Is donepezil bound to plasma proteins?

Yes. It is highly protein-bound (96 percent), primarily to albumin, but also to $\alpha_1$glycoprotein.

48. Describe the metabolism and elimination of donepezil.

Donepezil is metabolized by isoenzymes 2D6 and 3A4 of hepatic cytochrome P_{450}. The drug may then be glucuronidated. Excretion is primarily renal, with some unchanged drug detectable in the urine. Excretion may also occur through the bile and feces.

49. Does donepezil have active metabolites?

Yes.

50. Describe and list organophosphate drugs in clinical use.

Organophosphates have the potential for extreme toxicity and thus are mainly used topically in the therapy of glaucoma. These include echothiophate, demecarium, and isoflurophate.

51. Describe the symptoms of cholinesterase inhibitor intoxication.

These are simply symptoms of extreme parasympathetic activity: bradycardia, hypotension, bowel and bladder dysfunction, miosis, and dyspepsia. Difficulty in breathing may also be present, due to increased secretions and bronchiolar constriction. Muscle weakness and confusion may also be present due to depolarizing blockade (which further exacerbates difficulty in breathing). With extreme doses, death may ensue from respiratory failure.

52. Describe the possible therapies available in organophosphate intoxication.

If the patient is treated within 24–36 hours after exposure, the cholinesterase reactivator pralidoxime may be effectively administered, and the effects reversed in a time-dependent manner. Otherwise, supportive care and cholinergic antagonists may be used to prolong life until new enzyme can be synthesized.

53. Describe the actions of pralidoxime.

The irreversible cholinesterase inhibitors are deemed irreversible due to the strength of the bond between the phosphoryl group (added to the enzyme by the drug) and the active site of the enzyme. This strong binding is not immediate, but occurs over time. Initially, the interaction between phosphoryl group and enzyme is relatively weak. The reactivator, pralidoxime, has a greater affinity for the phosphate than does the enzyme, and will thus disrupt the bonding process and free the enzyme. However, at 30 minutes after exposure, the bond between the enzyme and phosphate becomes progressively stronger and the drug becomes less effective, until finally, after 24 to 48 hours, the phosphorylation is stable and reactivation is no longer possible.

54. Explain the result of administration of succinylcholine to a patient taking donepezil.

Succinylcholine produces a depolarizing blockade in skeletal muscle. The increased amount of acetylcholine produced by the administration of an inhibitor of acetylcholinesterase increases this blockade. Thus, circulatory and respiratory collapse may ensue. In addition, succinylcholine is metabolized by cholinesterases that may be inhibited by acetylcholinesterase inhibitors, causing the activity and duration of action of the drug to increase.

CHOLINERGIC ANTAGONISTS

55. How are cholinergic antagonists categorized?

These drugs are categorized by the number of side chains on the chemical structure that attach to the nitrogen (common in all structures of this group). The compounds may be tertiary amines (three side chains) or quaternary amines (four side chains). This classification determines the general properties of each group.

56. Which cholinergic antagonists are classified as tertiary amines?

Atropine, benztropine, dicyclomine, scopolamine, and trihexyphenidyl are all tertiary compounds. Tertiary amines do not carry a charge at physiologic pH, and thus will cross into the CNS and placenta.

57. Which cholinergic antagonists are classified as quaternary amines?

Glycopyrrolate, ipratropium, and propantheline. These agents carry a charge at physiologic pH and are less likely to cross into the CNS and placenta.

58. Which anticholinergic agents are used in the therapy of Parkinson's Disease?

Benztropine and trihexyphenidyl are the anticholinergics most often used for parkinsonism, primarily because the effects of these drugs are less peripheral and more central. Thus, adverse effects are lower with these agents.

59. What is the primary use of quaternary amines such as dicyclomine and propantheline?

These drugs are most commonly used as GI and/or genitourinary (GU) antispasmodics. Propantheline, an older drug, is used less frequently.

60. Describe the oral bioavailability of the quaternary amine antimuscarinics.

These drugs have low bioavailability, due to the presence of a polar, charged side group. This makes these drugs useful for gastrointestinal dysfunction (e.g., as antiulcer or antispasmodic agents).

61. What are the common adverse effects of antimuscarinic drugs?

Dryness of the mucous membranes, gastrointestinal upset, decreased sweating; mydriasis, and cycloplegia. In addition, tachycardia, constipation, confusion, and urinary retention are seen.

62. Describe the symptoms of antimuscarinic toxicity.

Antimuscarinic toxicity manifests as excessive sympathetic activity. This may include excessive cardiovascular stimulation (e.g., tachycardia, angina, arrhythmias), and CNS stimulation (e.g., anxiety, insomnia, restlessness). Other CNS effects may also occur, such as headache, ataxia, disorientation, hallucinations, delirium, coma, dizziness, excitement, agitation, and confusion.

63. Describe the mechanism of action of atropine.

Atropine is a competitive antagonist at the muscarinic receptor. It thus competes with acetylcholine for receptor binding and blocks activity at the receptor.

64. Describe the isomeric composition of atropine.

Atropine consists of l-hyoscyamine, which manifests all antimuscarinic activity, and d-hyoscyamine, which manifests no antimuscarinic activity.

65. Does atropine cross the blood-brain barrier?

Yes. It thus has CNS activity.

66. Does atropine have the same degree of effect on all peripheral organs?

No. Receptor sensitivity differs among the various organs, making atropine effects dose-dependent. The most sensitive receptors are those of the salivary, bronchial, and sweat glands. Next are the receptors in the eye and heart, followed by the receptors in the GI tract.

67. Discuss the effects of therapeutic doses of atropine on the cardiovascular system.

Atropine blocks the effects of acetylcholine in a dose-dependent manner. Thus, the effects of the sympathetic system are seen. At therapeutic doses, tachycardia, increased cardiac output, and an increase in systemic blood pressure may be seen.

68. What effects of atropine are seen at low doses?

At lower doses, a paradoxical decrease in heart rate and cardiac output is seen, due in part to cardiac reflexes.

69. What systemic effects may be seen with high-dose atropine administration?

At high doses, atropine may affect nicotinic receptors in autonomic ganglia, causing sympathetic effects such as restlessness, agitation, and delirium.

70. Does atropine produce CNS depression?

No. Sedation and effects on REM sleep are not seen.

71. Describe the effects of atropine on the respiratory bronchioles.

Atropine is a potent bronchodilator because it inhibits the acetylcholine-mediated release of cyclic guanosine 3c,5c-monophosphate (cGMP) from mast cells. In addition, it reduces secretions from respiratory airways.

72. Describe the uses of atropine in asthmatics.

Atropine may be useful in the treatment of exercise-induced bronchospasm in asthmatics.

73. How is atropine administered?

Atropine may be administered orally, by inhalation, or by injection (usually intramuscular).

74. Describe the distribution of atropine.

Atropine is widely distributed, and crosses the fetal-placental barrier.

75. Describe the metabolism and elimination of atropine.

Atropine is metabolized by the liver and eliminated through the urine. Secondary routes of elimination include excretion through the bile and expired air.

76. Are the effects of atropine short-lived?

Not particularly. The elimination half-life is 12.5 hours.

77. Why is atropine useful in treating organophosphate toxicity?

Atropine blocks the muscarinic receptors at effector organs, resulting in a decrease in acetylcholine mediated decreases in cardiac output, miosis, and GI function. In addition, the drug crosses into the CNS, and is therefore effective against organophosphate-mediated CNS effects as well.

78. Discuss the use of atropine as adjunct therapy in the reversal of neuromuscular blockade.

The reversal of neuromuscular blockade usually involves the administration of an AChE inhibitor, which increases circulating acetylcholine and reduces the effects of competitive blockade. Atropine administration decreases the systemic effects of acetylcholine produced by the cholinesterase inhibitor, without affecting the blockade reversal (because atropine does not affect skeletal muscle in normal therapeutic doses).

79. Define "*atropine flush*."

An intense flushing of the face and trunk that can occur 15 to 20 minutes following IM injection. This phenomenon is most common in children.

80. Is atropine therapy indicated in a patient with angina?

No. The resulting positive inotropic effect of atropine may result in increased oxygen demand and may exacerbate angina.

81. Describe the adverse effects associated with atropine.

Xerostomia, and general decrease in exocrine secretions; constipation, due to the inhibition of the actions of acetylcholine on the gastrointestinal system; dyspepsia; tachycardia; and anginal pain, due to an increase in contractile force of cardiac muscle. In addition, common adverse effects include urticaria, flushing of the skin, photophobia, thirst, nausea and vomiting, leukocytosis, fever, and urinary retention secondary to decreased tone and amplitude of contractions of the ureters and bladder.

82. Is the appearance of Stevens-Johnson syndrome associated with atropine therapy?

Yes, but the instances are rare.

83. Is atropine therapy indicated for all forms of glaucoma?

No. Atropine therapy should be avoided in closed-angle glaucoma because the resulting cycloplegia and mydriasis may increase intraocular pressure.

84. Should atropine be used in patients with concurrent GI infections?

Atropine should be administered with caution in these cases, as the resulting decrease in peristalsis subsequent to atropine therapy may decrease elimination of the organism and prolong the infection.

85. What is the common clinical use of atropine?

Atropine, as well as glycopyrrolate, are routinely used before surgery or invasive procedures to reduce secretions, particularly those in the respiratory tract. Atropine is commonly used in conjunction with opiates, to reduce cholinergic effects produced by opiates.

86. What is the primary clinical use of cyclopentolate and tropicamide?

Cyclopentolate and tropicamide are ophthalmologic agents, and are used frequently because of their relatively short duration of action.

87. Describe the clinical uses of glycopyrrolate.

Glycopyrrolate is used as an antispasmodic agent in GI dysfunction. It is also used prior to general anesthesia to reduce GI and pulmonary secretions and lessen the chance of acid aspiration during surgery.

88. Does hyoscyamine cross the blood-brain barrier?

Yes. It also crosses the fetal-placental barrier, and into breast milk.

89. Which antimuscarinic agent is prescribed for relief of both neurogenic and non-neurogenic bladder disorders ("overactive bladder")?

Oxybutynin, a tertiary amine class of antimuscarinic agent.

90. Discuss the pharmacologic properties of oxybutynin that make it effective in the control of bladder dysfunction.

This drug possesses not only antimuscarinic activity, but is also antispasmodic as well. It also manifests local anesthetic activity.

BIBLIOGRAPHY

1. Albuquerque EX, Alkondon M, Pereira EF, et al: Properties of neuronal nicotinic acetylcholine receptors: Pharmacological characterization and modulation of synaptic function. J Pharmacol Exp Ther 280(3):1117–1136, 1997.
2. Bayguinov O, Hagen B, Sanders KM: Muscarinic stimulation increases basal Ca(2+) and inhibits spontaneous Ca(2+) transients in murine colonic myocytes. Am J Physiol Cell Physiol 280(3): C689–C700, 2001.
3. Bibevski S, Zhou Y, McIntosh JM, et al: Functional nicotinic acetylcholine receptors that mediate ganglionic transmission in cardiac parasympathetic neurons. J Neurosci 20(13):5076–5082, 2000.
4. Conroy WG, Berg DK: Neurons can maintain multiple classes of nicotinic acetylcholine receptors distinguished by different subunit compositions. J Biol Chem 270(9):4424–4431, 1995.
5. Cowl CT, Prakash UB, Kruger BR: The role of anticholinergics in bronchoscopy. A randomized clinical trial. Chest 118(1):188–192, 2000.
6. Cuevas J, Berg DK: Mammalian nicotinic receptors with alpha7 subunits that slowly desensitize and rapidly recover from alpha-bungarotoxin blockade. J Neurosci 18(24):10335–10344.
7. De Biasi M, Nigro F, Xu W: Nicotinic acetylcholine receptors in the autonomic control of bladder function. Eur J Pharmacol 393(1–3):137–140, 2000.
8. Hardman J, Limbird L, Gilman A: Goodman & Gilman's The Pharmacological Basis of Therapeutics, 10th ed. McGraw-Hill Publishers, 2001.
9. Katzung B: Basic and Clinical Pharmacology, 8th ed. Appleton & Lange, 2001.
10. Kirkby DL, Jones DN, Barnes JC, et al: Effects of anticholinesterase drugs tacrine and E2020, the 5-HT(3) antagonist ondansetron, and the H(3) antagonist thioperamide, in models of cognition and cholinergic function. Behav Pharmacol 7(6):513–525, 1996.
11. McEntee WJ, Crook TH: Cholinergic function in the aged brain: implications for treatment of memory impairments associated with aging. Behav Pharmacol 3(4):327–336, 1992.

12. Niemann JT, Stratton SJ: Endotracheal versus intravenous epinephrine and atropine in out-of-hospital "primary" and postcountershock asystole. Crit Care Med 28(6):1815–1819, 2000.
13. Shih TM, McDonough JH: Efficacy of biperiden and atropine as anticonvulsant treatment for organophosphorus nerve agent intoxication. Arch Toxicol 74(3):165–172, 2000.
14. Skaddan MB, Kilbourn MR, Snyder SE, et al: Acetylcholinesterase inhibition increases in vivo N-(2-[18F] fluoroethyl)-4-piperidyl benzilate binding to muscarinic acetylcholine receptors. J Cereb Blood Flow Metab 21(2):144–148, 2001.
15. Smith RD, Grzelak ME, Coffin VL: Methylatropine blocks the central effects of cholinergic antagonists. Behav Pharmacol 5(2):167–175, 1994.
16. Taylor SC, Peers C: Three distinct Ca(2+) influx pathways couple acetylcholine receptor activation to catecholamine secretion from PC12 cells. J Neurochem 75(4):1583–1589, 2000.
17. Zubieta JK, Koeppe RA, Frey KA, et al : Assessment of muscarinic receptor concentrations in aging and Alzheimer disease with [11C] NMPB and PET. Synapse 39(4):275–287, 2001.

Websites:
Clinical Pharmacology 2000: http://cp.gsm.com
Medline Plus: http://medlineplus.nlm.nih.gov/medlineplus/
Medscape Multispecialty Journal Room: http://pharmacotherapy.medscape.com/Home/Topics/multispecialty/directories/dir-MULT.JournalRoom.html
Medscape Pharmacotherapy News (cardiology):
http://cardiology.medscape.com/home/topics/pharmacotherapy/directories/dir-PHAR.News.html

11. DRUGS THAT AFFECT THE SYMPATHETIC NERVOUS SYSTEM

1. Describe the potential toxicities of sympathomimetic drugs used as pressor agents.

These agents produce marked increases in blood pressure that may precipitate cerebral edema, cerebral hemorrhage, and pulmonary edema. Because of the decrease in vessel diameter, total peripheral resistance is increased, which increases afterload. This increases oxygen demand to the myocardium and may precipitate angina. Prolonged therapy may cause myocardial damage.

2. What would be the result of norepinephrine administration on a normotensive patient?

Because of the action on both arterial and venous α_1 receptors, a potent increase in systemic blood pressure would be seen. Both systolic and diastolic pressures would be elevated. Because norepinephrine has negligible activity on the β_2 receptor, no vasodilatation would be seen. Thus, pulse pressure would not increase. (See Figure.)

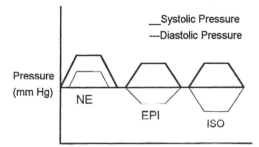

Relative changes in systolic pressure, diastolic pressure and pulse pressure between agonists.

3. What is the effect of the administration of epinephrine on a normotensive patient?

Epinephrine produces a potent increase in systolic pressure, but diastolic pressure would increase only slightly, or not at all, due to the action on the β_2 receptor.

4. Why do α_1 agonists such as norepinephrine and methoxamine produce a large increase in diastolic pressure?

Veins are capacitance vessels, which, due to venous compliance, function as blood "reservoirs." The vessel walls contain α_1 receptors that regulate smooth muscle contraction, but few β receptors are present. Because norepinephrine has potent α_1 activity, it therefore not only acts to constrict arterioles (which results in an increase in systemic pressure) but constricts veins, as well, forcing blood reserves into systemic circulation. This increases circulating blood volume, resulting in an increase in diastolic pressure.

5. Explain the ramifications of norepinephrine administration in a severely hypotensive patient.

Norepinephrine may rapidly increase systolic and diastolic pressure in a severely hypotensive patient, which is a desirable effect. However, because of the potent alpha activity of the drug, blood flow to major organs, particularly the kidney, is decreased. In a severely hypotensive patient, this may precipitate renal failure. Thus, norepinephrine would not be a first choice drug in the therapy of such a patient.

6. What is the mechanism of action of ephedrine?

Ephedrine stimulates all four sympathetic receptors, and has potent α_1 activity. It acts primarily at the receptor level. It may also be taken up into the adrenergic nerve ending, by cellular reuptake mechanisms, and subsequently taken into the adrenergic vesicle by the secretory vesicular pump, where it causes the systemic release of norepinephrine.

7. Does ephedrine normally have major central nervous system (CNS) effects?

No. The drug is charged at physiological pH, and thus does not cross the blood-brain barrier well.

8. Describe the structural relationship between ephedrine and amphetamines

The structures of ephedrine and amphetamine differ only in two aliphatic side chain groups (See Figure). Thus, ephedrine is easily converted into methamphetamine.

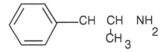

Amphetamine

Ephedrine

9. Describe the pharmacological uses of ephedrine and its advantages over epinephrine administration.

Ephedrine is useful in the therapy of hypotension, bronchospasm, Stoke-Adams syndrome, and narcolepsy. It is also included in preparations for topical application in the eye, and in over-the- counter (OTC) cold preparations for use as a decongestant. It is administered orally, unlike epinephrine, and has a longer duration. It does, however, have more CNS effects than epinephrine.

10. Describe the result of frequent dosing with ephedrine.

The drug exhibits a tolerance effect. If used repeatedly, the drug becomes less effective, as the receptors become desensitized. Thus, progressively higher doses are required for comparable efficacy.

11. How is ephedrine intoxication distinguished from intoxication with another β sympathomimetic?

Most sympathomimetics produce mydriasis that is abolished by light reflexes. The mydriasis produced by ephedrine is not abolished by the application of light. Accommodation is also not affected by ephedrine, unlike with other sympathomimetics.

12. Describe the effects of systemic acidosis in ephedrine intoxication.

Ephedrine is a weak base and is therefore ionized at acidic pH. Thus, systemic acidification accelerates excretion of the drug.

"SELECTIVE" ALPHA-1-RECEPTOR AGONISTS

13. Explain the mechanism of action of α_1 agonists as decongestant agents.

When used topically as a nasal decongestant, the drug comes in direct contact with the nasal mucosa, causing vasoconstriction within mucosal vessels that have dilated due to the vasodilatory actions of histamine. These vessels are partially blocking the nasal passages, trapping mucoid discharge. Reduction of vessel size allows drainage and promotes freer breathing.

14. What are the pharmacologic uses of the topical administration of an α_1 agonist?

These drugs are used topically to promote hemostasis. They may also be used as decongestants, or in the therapy of hemorrhoids to shrink blood vessels in the affected area and thus decrease swelling. Because the administration is topical and localized, there are few systemic effects when administered in proper dosage.

15. Describe the effect of α_1 agonists on intracellular calcium.

The activation of the inositol phosphate cascade results in the release of calcium form intracellular stores and an increase in cytoplasmic calcium.

16. Discuss the therapeutic uses of phenylephrine

Given intravenously, phenylephrine is useful in the therapy of paroxysmal atrial tachycardia (PAT), or as a pressor agent in hypotensive states. Used topically, it reduces blood vessel diameter and thus is useful as a decongestant, hemostatic agent, or to reduce swelling of inflamed tissues, or as a mydriatic. It is also used systemically in the therapy of frequent urination.

17. Is phenylephrine inactivated by catechol-O-methyl transferase (COMT)?

No. It is not a catechol derivative. The refractivity to inactivation by COMT accounts for its long duration of action, as compared to other agents.

18. Describe the differential effects of phenylephrine on systemic arteries and veins.

Phenylephrine markedly constricts arterioles, with little effect on veins.

19. Describe the effect of systemic administration of phenylephrine on blood volume and systemic pressure.

Due to its lack of effect on venous compliance, the drug has little or no effect on circulating blood volume. It does, however, have a potent effect on arterial smooth muscle. Thus, it increases systolic blood pressure to a greater degree than diastolic blood pressure.

20. Discuss the mechanism of action of phenylephrine in the therapy of PAT.

Because of its rapid vasoconstrictor activity, the drug produces a marked reflex bradycardia, due to stimulation of vagal reflexes. The increase in vagal tone increases the threshold for firing of the sinoatrial (SA) node and atrial tissue, resulting in a slower rate of firing and atrial conduction.

21. Discuss the mechanism of action of phenylephrine in differential blood flow.

Because of the vagal influence and the selective stimulation of α_1 receptors, phenylephrine causes a selective change in blood flow. Blood flow is decreased to most organs and to skeletal muscle; however, coronary blood flow is increased.

22. Explain the effects of differential administration of phenylephrine.

For maximum effect, the drug must be administered slowly because it is metabolized quickly upon reaching the hepatic portal circulation. Rapid injection will cause the dose to reach the liver faster, and the drug will be rapidly inactivated. For example, if the drug is given intravenously, a rise in systemic blood pressure will be seen which will last about 20 minutes. In contrast, if it is given subcutaneously, which allows the drug to be absorbed more slowly into the body, the increase in blood pressure will last over 50 minutes.

23. Describe the differential actions of mephentermine on systemic blood pressure.

Mephentermine acts to increase both systolic and diastolic pressure. Stimulation of α_1 receptors produces a contraction of the smooth muscle in the walls of both arteries and veins.

Contraction of veins forces reserved blood into circulation, which increases diastolic pressure, while the increased circulating blood volume, coupled with arteriolar constriction (which increases the total peripheral resistance), increases systolic pressure. The drug simultaneously causes norepinephrine to be released from sympathetic nerve terminals, which increases cardiac output and antagonizes the effects of vagal compensation.

24. Are the effects of mephentermine dose-dependent?

Yes. Moderate doses result in vasopressor effect and an increase in heart rate and cardiac output. Large doses, or doses administered too quickly, rapidly increase blood pressure and stimulate baroreceptor reflexes. In this case, the drug may actually depress cardiac function and decrease heart rate and cardiac output.

25. Discuss the potential CNS toxicity of mephentermine.

Like the effects on the cardiovascular system, effects on the CNS are also dose-dependent. With moderate doses (15–45 mg IM), there is little effect on the CNS, but, as the dose increases, or if the drug is given IV in a rapid infusion, CNS effects are prominent. These effects initially include sedation, mental depression, and incoherence, but may progress to more serious effects, such as convulsions. Both the cardiovascular and CNS effects are reversible, however, if the drug therapy is discontinued.

26. Discuss the toxicity of metaraminol.

Metaraminol produces a decrease in blood flow to major organs such as the brain and kidney, which, with prolonged therapy, could result in oxygen depravation and toxicity to these organs. This effect is independent of blood pressure or cardiac output—blood flow to these organs may not resume, even after blood pressure and/or cardiac output have been significantly raised.

27. What are the contraindications of use of metaraminol?

Metaraminol is contraindicated for use in patients who have compromised renal function, a CNS dysfunction, or head trauma. It may also be contraindicated in patients who have emphysema or congestive heart failure, as constriction of the pulmonary vessels can occur, resulting in elevated pulmonary pressure and pulmonary edema.

28. Should metaraminol be administered to a patient with head trauma?

No. The administration of metaraminol may result in a decrease in cerebral blood flow that will result in inadequate removal of waste products and carbon dioxide. This will lead to a reflex vasodilatation within the brain, and increased intracranial pressure.

29. What are the physiologic effects of methoxamine administration?

Methoxamine, a selective α_1-receptor agonist, primarily constricts arterioles, rather than veins, and produces a pronounced reflex bradycardia. When given by intravenous or intramuscular injection, it causes a rise in both systolic and diastolic pressure that persists for 60 to 90 minutes.

30. What is the primary use and mechanism of action of midodrine?

Midodrine is a selective venopressor, and thus is efficacious for the therapy of orthostatic hypotension.

31. Explain why oxymetazoline might be preferred to relieve decongestion in a hypertensive patient.

Oxymetazoline stimulates α_1 receptors to promote vasoconstriction, but also has significant affinity for the α_{2A} receptor. It thus mediates a central inhibition of norepinephrine release. Even though decongestant medications may be given intranasally, which avoids the majority of systemic adverse effects, some drug will always be absorbed through the mucosa or swallowed, and a "pure" α_1 receptor agonist could exacerbate hypertension. This potential is ameliorated with oxymetazoline, due to the effect on the α_{2A} receptor.

32. Does xylometazoline have a central effect?

No. Xylometazoline does not have the α_2 agonist effect of oxymetazoline, even though both are similar drugs.

ALPHA-1-RECEPTOR ANTAGONISTS

33. Discuss the mechanism of action of α_1-receptor antagonists.

The α_1 antagonists in clinical use primarily bind to the α_1 receptor in a competitive manner. Once bound to the receptor, the drug inhibits binding of endogenous catecholamines (e.g., epinephrine and norepinephrine) to the receptor and thus inhibits stimulation of the receptor and associated physiologic events. Because the receptor binding is reversible, however, the drug dissociates, allowing endogenous ligand binding. Thus, efficacy is increased with dose, as the greater the number of antagonist molecules, the greater the probability that an antagonist molecule, and not the endogenous ligand, will occupy the receptor site.

34. Which α antagonists are quinazoline compounds?

Doxazosin, prazosin and terazosin are members of the quinazoline class.

35. If a patient is allergic to prazosin, should terazosin be prescribed instead?

No. There is cross-sensitivity between the drugs of this class.

36. What CNS effects might be seen with the use of α_1 antagonists?

Effects which may be due to lack of oxygen, such as fatigue, headache, and sedation, as well as muscle dysfunctions such as paresthesias, kinetic dysfunction, and ataxia. Excitatory effects such as anxiety, depression, and insomnia may also be seen.

37. What adverse cardiovascular effects may be seen with α_1 antagonists?

Baroreceptor reflex effects, such as tachycardia, palpitation, and arrhythmia; effects due to decreased tension, such as edema, and postural hypotension; and effects due to decreased oxygen delivery, such as peripheral ischemia, dizziness, syncope, vertigo, and lightheadedness.

38. Are anticholinergic effects associated with α_1 antagonists?

Yes. Cross-reactivity with the muscarinic receptor may result in classic anticholinergic effects such as constipation, dry mouth, and dyspepsia.

39. Describe the pharmacokinetics of doxazosin.

Doxazosin is highly protein-bound (greater than 98 percent), and is metabolized by the liver. These metabolites may either be pharmacologically active or inactive. Metabolites may be excreted through the bile or the urine.

40. Describe the pharmacologic uses of doxazosin.

Doxazosin is used in the therapy of primary hypertension, and is also effective in treatment of benign prostatic hypertrophy (BPH).

41. Are there serious complications associated with the use of α_1 antagonist therapy for hypertension?

Yes. Patients taking α_1 antagonists, particularly doxazosin, as antihypertensive therapy have been shown to have a 25 percent increase in cardiovascular events, and a two-fold increase in heart failure rate. An increase in the propensity for stroke has also been observed in these patients, as compared to patients using diuretics as primary therapy.

42. Describe the clinical uses of phentolamine.

Phentolamine may be used in the therapy of BPH, to reduce the size of the tumor by decreasing blood flow. It is also useful as a local infiltrate in the prevention of systemic absorption of extravasated IV norepinephrine and in the therapy of pheochromocytoma.

43. Why does phentolamine produce a large amount of cardiac stimulation?

Phentolamine potently blocks both α_1 and α_2 receptors. Thus, a decrease in pressure mediated by α_1 blockade activates the baroreceptor reflex, which increases sympathetic tone. The physiologic compensation mechanism is normally initiated by the α_2 receptor, which is now blocked by the drug.

44. Is phentolamine a pure antagonist?

No. It has agonist activity at both H_1 and H_2 receptors, and also at muscarinic receptors.

45. Describe the receptor pharmacology of phenoxybenzamine.

Phenoxybenzamine is a noncompetitive antagonist. It binds primarily to the α_1 receptor, for up to 48 hours or more. It is, however, relatively nonselective and binds to a variety of receptors, including histamine (H_1), acetylcholine, and serotonin receptors.

46. Describe the pharmacologic use of phenoxybenzamine and phentolamine in the management of pheochromocytoma.

Phenoxybenzamine is administered preoperatively, to control hypertensive episodes due to manipulation of the tumor, while phentolamine is used to reverse hypertensive episodes during surgical manipulation of the tumor. Phentolamine may also be used in the diagnosis of pheochromocytoma, because a precipitous drop in systemic pressure will be seen upon administration.

47. Describe the major adverse effect associated with the use of selective α_1-receptor antagonists for chronic hypertension.

Because of the selectivity for the α_1 receptor, the major adverse effect of these drugs is postural hypotension. This is due to inhibition of the α_1 receptor-mediated contraction of venous smooth muscle, which is normally under sympathetic control. This effect is usually most severe with the initial dose.

ALPHA-2-RECEPTOR AGONISTS AND ANTAGONISTS

48. Discuss the mechanism of action of clonidine.

Clonidine has a high affinity for the regulatory α_2 receptor. Thus, as an α_2-receptor agonist, it mediates a decrease in sympathetic outflow both from the noradrenergic nerve terminus, and through the central α_2 receptor located on the nucleus tractus solitarius of the hypothalamus.

49. Discuss the mechanism of action of clonidine in the therapy of primary hypertension.

The stimulation of the regulatory (α_2) receptor by clonidine results in a decrease in sympathetic outflow and a decrease in blood pressure. Because the drug blocks the regulatory receptor, the resulting decrease in pressure is not subject to compensation by the action of baroreceptor reflexes. (See Appendix B for review of physiology.)

50. Describe the use of α_2 agonists in the therapy of narcotic addiction.

α_2 agonists, such as clonidine, are frequently used in the therapy of narcotic withdrawal (as well as nicotine addiction) because a central α_2 receptor is involved in mediating a decrease in the psychologicl sensation of drug "craving."

51. What is the clinical effect of α_2 agonists on thrombosis?

α_2 Agonist drugs cause platelet aggregation and may promote vascular infarcts in susceptible patients. This effect may be due to a decrease in the levels of platelet cyclic adenosine monophosphate (cAMP).

52. What are the effects of α_2 agonists on transmembrane ionic flux?

These drugs mediate an increase in potassium flux, due to an increase in the number of opening potassium channels. A decrease in calcium flux is also seen, due to the closing of membrane calcium channels.

53. Explain the effects of abrupt withdrawal of clonidine therapy.

The decrease in circulating catecholamines due to prolonged clonidine administration mediates a supersensitivity of receptors. When clonidine therapy is abruptly withdrawn, catecholamine levels rebound, reflex activity overcompensates, and this, combined with the supersensitivity of receptors, produces an exaggerated response to stimulation and a dramatic increase in blood pressure. A hypertensive crisis may ensue within 12 to 24 hours after drug withdrawal.

54. Discuss the use of α_1 receptor antagonist therapy in conjunction with clonidine withdrawal.

The administration of an α_1 receptor antagonist decreases stimulation of the inositol phosphate cascade in vascular smooth muscle and attenuates the dramatic rise in blood pressure.

55. Explain the importance of proper dosage interval in clonidine therapy.

Clonidine must be dosed at intervals that allow for a "wearing off" of the drug. This tends to decrease the effect of receptor supersensitivity and reflex overcompensation.

56. What effects will be seen with frequent dosing of clonidine?

If the dosage interval is too short, rebound sympathetic effects may be seen—tachycardia, sweating, anxiety, insomnia, and heart palpitations.

57. Discuss the withdrawal of therapy with beta-blockers combined with clonidine.

β receptor antagonists increase the rebound effect, particularly the nonselective agents that block the β_2 receptor, and must be withdrawn before clonidine therapy is discontinued.

58. Explain the pharmacology of α-methyldopa.

α-Methyldopa is taken up into the adrenergic nerve terminus and enters the norepinephrine synthesis pathway. It is converted, by dopa decarboxylase, into α-methylnorepinephrine, a potent α_2 agonist. α-Methyldopa is generally considered to be a pro-drug.

59. Explain the receptor selectivity of α-methyldopa.

α-Methyl dopa, when converted to α-methylnorepinephrine, has a preference for binding of α_2 receptors in the midbrain.

60. Would α-methyldopa therapy be an appropriate choice for a patient on carbidopa therapy?

Yes. While α-methyldopa may be converted to α-methylnorepinephrine in both central and peripheral adrenergic neurons, the major antihypertensive effect of the drug is in the midbrain. Because carbidopa does not cross the blood-brain barrier, the drug would not affect levels of central α-methylnorepinephrine.

61. Should α-methyldopa be administered concurrently with antidepressants?

No. Monoamine oxidase (MAO) inhibitors and tricyclics decrease the effect of the drug.

62. Describe the interactions of α-methyldopa with antipsychotics and antiparkinsonian drugs.

The toxicities of antipsychotics and lithium are increased when combined with α-methyldopa therapy. The drug also blunts the therapeutic effects of levodopa in the therapy of parkinsonism, due to competition for neuronal dopa decarboxylase.

63. Is orthostatic hypotension a common side effect of α_2 agonists?

No. These drugs mediate a decrease in sympathetic activity, rather than blocking a specific receptor site. Sympathetic reflexes also are inhibited.

64. Describe the actions of guanfacine.

Guanfacine is an α_2 agonist drug that is similar to clonidine in mechanism of action, toxicity and side effects. It is administered orally. The duration of action is longer than that of clonidine (16–20 hours) and so is normally administered once per day.

65. Describe the mechanism of action of guanabenz.

Guanabenz, like clonidine, is an α_2 adrenergic receptor agonist. In addition, it has a slight ganglioplegic action in the periphery.

66. Why is loading dose administered with the onset of guanabenz therapy?

The drug is highly protein-bound. Therefore, an increased dose must be administered to achieve therapeutic levels in the plasma.

67. What is yohimbine?

Yohimbine is an α_2 antagonist derived from the bark of the yohimbé tree. Although the drug has little current therapeutic use, α_2 antagonists are being evaluated for use in the therapy of diabetes and depression.

BETA-RECEPTOR AGONISTS AND ANTAGONISTS

68. What are the indications for therapy with salmeterol xinafoate?

Salmeterol is indicated for use in long-term maintenance treatment of chronic asthma. It is also used in the therapy of reversible obstructive airway disease (including nocturnal asthma), and in prevention of exercise-induced bronchospasm.

69. Is salmeterol indicated for use in pediatric patients?

No. The drug is used in prevention of bronchospasms in patients over 12 years of age.

70. Describe the pharmacokinetic parameters of salmeterol.

Salmeterol is significantly bound to plasma proteins. The drug is cleared by hepatic metabolism.

71. Describe the actions of isoproterenol.

Isoproterenol activates both β_1- and β_2-adrenergic receptors, resulting in an increase in heart rate and force of contraction, which lead to an increase in cardiac output. Increased renin secretion is also seen due to effects on the β_1 receptor, which contributes to an increase in systemic pressure. The resulting increase in systemic pressure is offset by a decrease in total peripheral resistance mediated by the β_2 receptor. Relaxation of bronchial smooth muscle is also seen.

72. Describe the effects of beta agonists, such as epinephrine and ephedrine, on blood glucose.

These drugs stimulate glycogenolysis and gluconeogenesis, due to stimulation of hepatic and lipocytic β_1 receptors.

73. Would administration of a beta agonist be an appropriate choice for a diabetic patient?

Selective agonists for the β_2 receptor would be appropriate, but those that stimulate the β_1 receptor should be used with caution, due to the effects on blood sugar.

74. Would administration of a beta agonist be the best choice for a hypertensive patient in congestive heart failure?

No. Although these drugs may be used, the actions of such drugs on the β_1 receptor would increase the production of angiotensin II, which may exacerbate hypertension.

75. Is isoproterenol an appropriate choice for inhalation therapy?

No. Although it may be used, it is readily absorbed from the lung, limiting dosage due to peripheral side effects.

76. Why is isoproterenol not a good choice for administration by slow infusion?

The drug rapidly oxidizes in the presence of water or oxygen and could be inactivated over the period of a slow infusion.

77. What would be the advantage of isoproterenol therapy over other beta agonists in a diabetic patient?

Isoproterenol, like any beta agonist, stimulates glycogenolysis and gluconeogenesis. However, it is unique in that it also stimulates insulin secretion to some degree, which opposes the increase in blood sugar. The drug consequently has less of a hyperglycemic effect than other β_1 agonists.

78. What is the dose-limiting toxic effect of isoproterenol?

The most serious toxic effect of the drug is its ability to cause or exacerbate cardiac arrhythmias. Indeed, overdosage of isoproterenol inhalation therapy (0.4 mg or above per dose) can be fatal.

79. Is the *"epinephrine reversal"* phenomenon seen with norepinephrine or other cardiostimulatory drugs, such as isoproterenol?

No. For this phenomenon to occur, the drug must be active at both the α_1 receptor and β_2 receptor. Norepinephrine (NE) has no β_2 activity, and isoproterenol is a pan-beta (β_1, β_2 receptor) agonist, without α_1 activity. Thus, the effects of these drugs are not reversed by the administration of an α_1 antagonist, and no dramatic lowering of blood pressure is seen (the effects of NE are blocked, to some degree, but not reversed).

80. Discuss the mechanism of action of β_1-receptor antagonists on the heart.

These drugs decrease heart rate and contractility, resulting in decreased cardiac output.

81. Discuss the effects of β-blockers on the cardiac action potential.

β-Blockers inhibit the catecholamine-induced increase in the slope of phase 4 depolarization. The slope is thus decreased, which effectively lengthens the time to threshold and the subsequent action potential. This results in a decrease in heart rate.

82. Describe the differential effects of β-blockers on heart rate.

These drugs block the catecholamine-induced increase in heart rate. Therefore, little effect is seen on resting heart rate. The major decrease is seen in tachycardia induced by exercise or emotional stimuli.

83. What effect do β_1-receptor antagonists have on the production of angiotensin II?

Antagonism of the β_1 receptor results in decreased renin release, which leads to a decrease in the production of angiotensin II.

84. Discuss the indirect effect of β_1-receptor antagonists on fluid volume.

The decrease in angiotensin II release mediated by these drugs leads to a decrease in aldosterone levels. This results in a decrease in salt and water retention, leading to a decrease in plasma volume.

85. Explain the dangers of beta-blocker therapy in the diabetic patient.

The adrenergic responses to hypoglycemia (the "warning signals") are mediated by the sympathetic nervous system (e.g., tachycardia, restlessness). Beta blockade masks these symptoms, so that a decrease in blood sugar may go unnoticed by the patient. Long-term therapy with beta-blockers may also lead to insulin resistance.

86. What effects do beta-blockers have on serum lipids?

In general, beta-receptor antagonists have a detrimental effect on the serum lipid profile. Triglyceride levels are sharply increased, as are low-density lipoproteins (LDL) levels, while high-density lipoproteins (HDL) levels may be decreased. This effect is lessened, or even reversed, with drugs that have intrinsic sympathomimetic activity (e.g., pindolol, acebutolol).

87. Describe the negative effects of beta-blockers.

In general, the adverse effects are related to decreased cardiac output and decreased tissue perfusion. Patients may exhibit symptoms of congestive heart failure (CHF), or worsening of existing CHF, exacerbation of vascular disease (e.g., intermittent claudication), fatigue, bradycardia, cold in the extremities, and fatigue. Alterations in conduction may produce atrioventricular (AV) nodal dissociation or exacerbation of AV nodal blockade. Drugs that block β_2 receptors may also produce bronchospastic effects, and should be avoided in patients with lung dysfunction or asthma.

88. Describe the effects of propranolol on AV nodal potassium currents.

Propranolol causes an outward flux of potassium (a "quinidine-like" action), which tends to partially hyperpolarize cardiac tissues. This results in slowed conduction through the AV node.

89. Contrast the effects of low-dose and high-dose propranolol on cardiac excitability.

In low therapeutic doses, the drug produces a decrease in conduction rate through β_1 receptor blockade and an increase in outward potassium flux. In high doses, the drug depresses sodium permeability, causing a local, anesthetic-like effect.

90. Discuss the half-life of propranolol.

Propranolol has a very short half-life (2–6 hours) and is thus administered four times a day.

91. Describe the effects of rapidly infused propranolol.

Propranolol given by rapid infusion causes peripheral vasodilatation, resulting in hypotension.

92. What are the adverse effects of propranolol?

Cardiodepressant effects, such as bradycardia and decreased force of myocardial contraction. AV blockade and asystole may also be seen. The AV block may be reversed by IV atropine. However, asystolic effects are not reversible by catecholamines.

93. Discuss the effects of abrupt discontinuation of propranolol therapy.

Abrupt discontinuation of the drug may precipitate angina or vasospastic infarct. These effects appear to be due to cardiac receptor up-regulation, caused by chronic therapy with β-blockers.

94. What unusual characteristic does acebutolol posses?

This drug, while it is a beta receptor antagonist, has intrinsic sympathomimetic activity.

95. Discuss the pharmacologic uses of timolol.

Timolol is a nonselective β-receptor antagonist that is used topically in the therapy of glaucoma. The antagonism of β receptors on the radial muscle of the iris results in miosis, which facilitates drainage of humor into the canals of Schlemm. Timolol is also used in the therapy of angina and vasospastic infarct.

96. Differentiate between the cardioselective (β_1) antagonist drugs.

Metoprolol and atenolol are relatively long-acting cardioselective agents, whereas esmolol is a short-acting agent, with a half-life of about nine minutes.

97. What accounts for the short half-life of esmolol?

The chemical structure of esmolol contains an ester linkage that is rapidly degraded by plasma and erythrocytic esterases.

98. Discuss the pharmacodynamics of esmolol.

Upon continuous infusion of esmolol, steady-state is rapidly achieved. Upon termination of the drug infusion, however, effects are rapidly discontinued, due to the rapid inactivation of the drug by blood esterases. Thus, the drug is safer to use in critically ill patients.

99. Discuss the actions and uses of pindolol.
Pindolol is a partial β-receptor agonist. It has weak agonist activity, particularly at the β_2 receptor, but acts as an antagonist in the presence of norepinephrine or epinephrine (see Figure below). It may thus be used in the therapy of inappropriate norepinephrine secretion. Due to its ability to weakly stimulate the β_2 receptor while blocking the β_1 receptor, it is also useful in the therapy of hypertension.

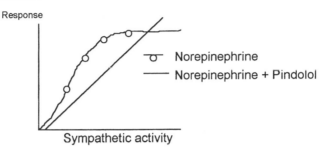

Graphic representation of the effects of a partial agonist on physiologic response.

100. Discuss the advantage of the use of sympatholytic drugs that have partial beta activity.
These partial agonist drugs (e.g., pindolol, acebutolol. carteolol, celiprolol, and penbutolol), like the beta antagonists, are useful in the therapy of hypertension and angina. They do, however, tend to cause less bradycardia and lipid abnormalities than do beta antagonist drugs.

101. Describe the pharmacologic actions of prenalterol.
Prenalterol is a partial agonist that is selective for the β_1 receptor.

102. Which drug has antagonist effects at both alpha and beta receptors?
Labetalol is an antagonist at both α_1 and β_1 receptors. It has partial agonist activity at the β_2 receptor.

103. What are the clinical uses of labetalol?
Oral labetalol is used in the therapy of a wide variety of forms of hypertension. It is also used IV for the treatment of hypertensive crises, in coronary bypass surgery, angioplasty, therapy of pheochromocytoma, and in general prevention of perioperative and preoperative hypertension. It is also used to prevent sympathetic effects with the withdrawal of clonidine therapy.

104. Describe the pharmacokinetics of labetalol.
Labetalol undergoes an extensive first-pass effect and is rapidly metabolized by the liver and excreted as glucuronidated metabolites. The first-pass effect and degree of drug metabolism is decreased by hepatic disease or by concurrent administration of a drug which decreases the activity or amount of cytochrome P_{450}, such as cimetidine.

105. Which beta-blockers exhibit quinidine-like activity?
Propranolol, timolol, betaxolol (to some degree), labetalol and pindolol all promote alterations in membrane ionic conduction and a local anesthetic action.

106. Discuss the interactions of over-the-counter cold medications with β-blockers.
OTC cold medications, or other medications that contain drugs with α_1 agonist activity (e.g., ephedrine, phenylpropanolamine), should be avoided with β antagonist therapy, as they may precipitate acute hypertension. This is due to the vasoconstrictor actions of the α_1 agonist that are unopposed in the presence of a drug with β_2 antagonist activity.

DOPAMINERGIC DRUGS

107. Discuss the differential receptor stimulation with low-dose and high-dose dopamine.

At low doses, the drug primarily stimulates the D_1 receptor. At high therapeutic doses, dopamine stimulates adrenergic receptors, primarily the cardiac β_1 receptor and vascular α_1 receptor.

108. Discuss the physiologic effects of low-dose dopamine administration.

In low therapeutic doses, or with the initial dose, dopamine produces relatively little change in total peripheral resistance. It produces vasodilatation in selective vascular beds, primarily the renal, coronary, and mesenteric. Glomerular filtration rate (GFR) is increased, and sodium excretion increases.

109. Discuss the physiologic effects of high-dose dopamine administration.

At higher doses or faster rates of infusion, dopamine produces an increase in total peripheral resistance (TPR) and cardiac output, resulting in an increase in systemic pressure. The vasoconstriction produced may also selectively decrease perfusion to the kidney, heart, and mesentery. Dopamine also releases norepinephrine from neuronal endings, which increases the pressor effect.

110. What are the major indications of dopamine therapy?

Dopamine therapy is useful in patients with decreased cardiac output, or patients in hypovolemic shock. In low doses, it increases perfusion to major organs, decreasing the probability of organ failure.

111. What are pharmacologic contraindications to dopamine therapy?

Concurrent therapy with MAO inhibitors may precipitate a hypertensive crisis. The dose of dopamine should be reduced to approximately 10 percent of the therapeutic dose in this case. Concurrent therapy with tricyclics may also produce an untoward response, depending on the patient.

112. Explain why dopamine is not administered orally.

It is rapidly degraded by both MAO and COMT.

113. Discuss dopamine administration and its duration of effect.

Dopamine is normally administered by IV drip. The general effect of the drug is very brief, so the effects may be controlled by the dose and rate of administration.

114. Describe the effect of dopamine administration on systolic, diastolic, and pulse pressures.

Due to the lack of effect on TPR and venous capacitance, diastolic pressure is not significantly increased. Due to the increase in cardiac output, systolic pressure and pulse pressure are increased.

115. What are the pharmacologic effects of dobutamine?

Dobutamine is a selective β_1 agonist. It therefore increases cardiac output, renal perfusion, and total peripheral resistance. Perfusion pressure is also increased, due to effects on the renin-angiotensin system.

116. Why is dobutamine dispensed in a racemic mixture?

The two isomers of dobutamine have opposing effects at the α_1 receptor. The "+" isomer of dobutamine has antagonist activity at the α_1 receptor, while the "−" isomer has agonist activity. The two isomers are thus dispensed as a racemic mixture, to avoid the pharmacologic variable of alpha-receptor activity.

SYMPATHOPLEGIC DRUGS

117. Describe the mechanism of action and use of reserpine

Reserpine depletes circulating catecholamines, particularly norepinephrine. The drug is taken into the adrenergic neuron and subsequently binds to the adrenergic vesicle, inhibiting the vesicular pump. Because NE is normally taken back into the neuron after release, sequestered in vesicles, and reused, the inhibition of the vesicular pump leaves the salvaged NE unsequestered, and vulnerable to the actions of mitochondrial monoamine oxidase. It is then quickly metabolized, leaving norepinephrine stores depleted. The depletion of circulating catecholamines makes the drug useful in the control of hypertension.

118. Is there an advantage to using high daily doses of reserpine?

No. An increase in daily dose produces more side effects than therapeutic effects. Because the restoration of depleted catecholamine stores is very slow, only a small dose is needed for therapeutic effect.

119. Why is reserpine often combined with a thiazide diuretic (e.g., chlorthiazide)?

The diuretic and sympathoplegic drugs work synergistically to lower blood pressure, by lowering both cardiac output and fluid volume. The depletion of circulating catecholamines by reserpine mediates a decrease in cardiac output and TPR, decreasing systolic pressure. If fluid volume remains high, however, systolic pressure may not be reduced to adequate levels, and diastolic pressure may still be elevated, resulting in peripheral edema. The addition of the diuretic results in a lower blood volume, further lowering of arterial pressure, and a decrease in edema. Thiazides are particularly useful due to their effect on glomerular filtration rate.

120. Is reserpine active at a central level?

Yes. It is primarily active in the periphery, but does have central effects.

121. What are the major side effects of reserpine?

Reserpine may mediate depression, due to its effects on both catecholaminergic and serotonergic reuptake and storage. Parasympathomimetic effects such as increased secretion of gastric acid, intestinal hypermotility, miosis, and male sexual dysfunction may also be seen.

122. Are the effects of reserpine immediate?

No. Effects may not be seen for 2 to 3 weeks after onset of therapy, and may persist for as long as 3 weeks after discontinuation of therapy.

123. Explain the mechanism of action of guanethidine.

Guanethidine is taken up into the adrenergic nerve terminal and competes with norepinephrine for sites on the vesicular pump. Thus, it decreases the sequestration of norepinephrine, and is itself concentrated within the secretory vesicle. Within the vesicle, it mediates vesicular destruction.

124. What is the differential postural effect of guanethidine in the therapy of hypertension?

Because the drug affects the capacitance of veins, as well as vasodilatation, therapy is more effective in an upright state, rather than a supine position. In susceptible patients (e.g., diabetics with autonomic neuropathy) the drug causes severe orthostatic hypotension.

125. What is the mechanism of action of metyrosine?

Metyrosine is α-methyl tyrosine, which competes with tyrosine for sites on tyrosine hydroxylase—the enzyme responsible for the rate-limiting step in catecholamine biosynthesis. Thus, it decreases catecholamine biosynthesis, resulting in a decrease in circulating levels of catecholamines. Metyrosine is a tyrosine hydroxylase inhibitor.

126. What is the primary clinical use for metyrosine?

Metyrosine is used in the therapy of pheochromocytoma.

127. Are urinary catecholamines or metabolites seen with metyrosine therapy?

No. The drug suppresses urinary excretion of catecholamines and their metabolites.

BIBLIOGRAPHY

1. Abe H, Nagatomo T, Kohshi K, et al: Heart rate and plasma cyclic AMP responses to isoproterenol infusion and effect of beta-adrenergic blockade in patients with postural orthostatic tachycardia syndrome. J Cardiovasc Pharmacol 36 Suppl 2:S79–S82, 2000.
2. Burke WJ, Li SW, Zahm DS, et al: Catecholamine monoamine oxidase a metabolite in adrenergic neurons is cytotoxic in vivo. Brain Res 891(1–2):218–227, 2001.
3. Collister JP, Osborn JW: The chronic infusion of hexamethonium and phenylephrine to effectively clamp sympathetic vasomotor tone: A novel approach. J Pharmacol Toxicol Methods 42(3):135–147, 1999.
4. Ferlay A, Charret C, Galitzky J, et al: Effects of the perfusion of beta-, beta2-, or beta3-adrenergic agonists or epinephrine on in situ adipose tissue lipolysis measured by microdialysis in underfed ewes. J Anim Sci 79(2):453–462, 2001.
5. Granados G, Garay-Sevilla ME, Malacara JM, et al: Plasma epinephrine and norepinephrine response to stimuli in autonomic neuropathy of type 2 diabetes mellitus. Acta Diabetol 37(2):55–60, 2000.
6. Hardman J, Limbird L, Gilman A: Goodman & Gilman's The Pharmacological Basis of Therapeutics, 10th ed. McGraw-Hill Publishers, 2001.
7. Henaff M, Hatem SN, Mercadier JJ: Low catecholamine concentrations protect adult rat ventricular myocytes against apoptosis through cAMP-dependent extracellular signal-regulated kinase activation. Mol Pharmacol 58(6):1546–1553, 2000.
8. Hjalmarson A: Cardioprotection with beta-adrenoceptor blockers: Does lipophilicity matter? Basic Res Cardiol 95 Suppl 1:I41–I45, 2000.
9. Jayachandran M, Hayashi T, Sumi D, et al: Up-regulation of endothelial nitric oxide synthase through beta(2)-adrenergic receptor: The role of a beta-blocker with NO-releasing action. Biochem Biophys Res Commun 280(3):589–594, 2001.
10. Katzung B: Basic and Clinical Pharmacology, 8th ed. Appleton & Lange, 2001.
11. Kendall MJ: Clinical trial data on the cardioprotective effects of beta-blockade. Basic Res Cardiol 95 Suppl 1:I25–I30, 2000.
12. Kitajima T, Okuda Y, Mishio M, et al: Acute cigarette smoking reduces vasodilative effect induced by sympathetic block in dogs. Reg Anesth Pain Med 26(1):41–45, 2001.
13. Limon-Boulez I, Bouet-Alard R, Gettys TW, et al: Partial agonist clonidine mediates alpha(2)-AR subtypes specific regulation of camp accumulation in adenylyl cyclase II transfected DDT1-MF2 Cells. Mol Pharmacol 59(2):331–338, 2001.
14. Mehta JL, Li D: Epinephrine upregulates superoxide dismutase in human coronary artery endothelial cells. Free Radic Biol Med 30(2):148–153, 2001.
15. Mesquita ET, Deus FC, Guedes CR, et al: Effects of propranolol on the QT dispersion in congestive heart failure. Arq Bras Cardiol 73(3):295–298, 1999.
16. Ohtsuka T, Hamada M, Hiasa G, et al: Effect of beta-blockers on circulating levels of inflammatory and anti-inflammatory cytokines in patients with dilated cardiomyopathy. J Am Coll Cardiol 37(2):412–417, 2001.
17. von Kanel R, Dimsdale JE: Effects of sympathetic activation by adrenergic infusions on hemostasis in vivo [review]. Eur J Haematol 65(6):357–369, 2000.
18. Wilhelmi BJ, Blackwell SJ, Miller JH, et al: Do not use epinephrine in digital blocks: Myth or truth? Plast Reconstr Surg 107(2):393–397, 2001.

Websites:

Clinical Pharmacology 2000: http://cp.gsm.com
Medline plus: http://medlineplus.nlm.nih.gov
Medscape Multispecialty Journal Room: http://pharmacotherapy.medscape.com/Home/Topics/multispecialty/directories/dir-MULT.JournalRoom.html
Medscape Pharmacotherapy News (cardiology):
http://cardiology.medscape.com/home/topics/pharmacotherapy/directories/dir-PHAR.News.html

12. CALCIUM CHANNEL BLOCKERS

1. Describe the role of calcium in atrioventricular (AV) nodal depolarization.

Conduction through the calcium-dependent portions of the AV node is dependent on extracellular calcium flux. The initial AV nodal depolarization results in changes in membrane potential that result in the opening of voltage-gated (type "L") calcium channels. This allows the rapid influx of calcium into the cell, resulting in changes in membrane potential. Because the membrane potential for calcium is more positive than the resting potential, the membrane becomes more excitable as calcium enters the cell.

2. Why might intracellular calcium increase the potential for arrhythmias?

Because cardiac cells do not sequester appreciable amounts of intracellular calcium, the cytosolic calcium remaining after depolarization triggers the sodium-calcium transporter, which pumps out calcium in exchange for sodium in a 1:2 ratio. This increases the resting membrane potential closer to depolarization threshold, making it hyperexcitable. This results in early afterpotentials, and an increased probability of ventricular arrhythmias, particularly if intracellular calcium is high (i.e., a large influx of calcium has occurred during depolarization.

3. Discuss the therapeutic use of calcium channel blockers.

These agents are useful in the therapy of hypertension and angina (see Table). Cardioselective drugs (e.g., verapamil) may be useful in the therapy of arrhythmias. Lesser uses include therapy of drug resistance in oncologic therapy (e.g., verapamil) and prevention of ischemic damage in stroke victims (e.g., lipophilic drugs such as nimodipine).

DRUG	CLASS	PRIMARY USE	DURATION	PROTEIN BINDING
Nifedipine	Dihydropyridine	Angina, hypertension	4 h	90%
Nimodipine	Dihydropyridine	CNS	2 h	
Nicardipine	Dihydropyridine	Angina, hypert, Raynaud's	8 h	95%
Nisoldipine	Dihydropyridine	Angina, hypertension	7–12 h	99%
Nitrendipine	Dihydropyridine		5–12 h	
Felodipine	Dihydropyridine	Hypertension	11–16 h	99%
Amlodipine	Dihydropyridine	Angina, hypertension	35 h	93%
Isradipine	Dihydropyridine	Hypertension	12 h	99%
Verapamil	Diphenylalkylamine	Angina, hypertension, SVT	8–10 h	90%
Diltiazem	Benzothiazepine	Angina, hypertension, PST	4–6 h	70–80%
Bepridil	Not classified—class I & III antiarrhythmic properties	Stable angina	24–64 h	99%

4. Discuss the mechanism of action of calcium channel blockers.

These drugs block voltage-gated (type "L") calcium channels in a dose-dependent manner.

5. Describe how blockade of calcium channels is accomplished.

The drugs bind to depolarized (open) channels, from the inner (cytosolic) side of the cell membrane.

6. Do all classes of calcium channel blocker bind to the same receptor on the channel?

No. Binding sites for drugs of the dihydropyridine class are separate from those of other calcium channel blockers.

7. Do calcium channel blockers affect serum calcium concentration?
No. These agents affect transmembrane calcium flux.

8. Discuss the adverse effects of calcium channel blockers.
Adverse effects include flushing, constipation, edema, dizziness, and nausea.

9. Describe the action of calcium channel blockers on vascular smooth muscle.
These drugs decrease calcium influx, thus causing muscle relaxation and vasodilatation. The degree of vasodilatation produced depends on the selectivity of the individual drug.

10. Can calcium channel blockers affect neuronal function?
Yes. Type "L" voltage-gated channels are present in neuronal membranes, and certain drugs (e.g., verapamil) may affect neuronal function.

11. Do calcium channel blockers precipitate bronchospasm?
No. They are, therefore, safe to use in patients with asthma.

12. Do calcium channel blockers affect skeletal muscle?
No. Voltage-gated calcium channels are found only in smooth and cardiac muscle. Excitation-contraction coupling in skeletal muscle depends on the release of intracellular calcium from the sarcoplasmic reticulum.

13. What effect might changes in physiologic pH (e.g., ischemia, injury) have on the action of calcium channel blockers?
Because the drugs must bind at the inner surface of the membrane, they must first-pass through the membrane. Changes in pH would affect the degree of ionization of the drug and thus change the proportion of drug able to cross the membrane. Thus, potency of the drug would vary with tissue pH.

14. Does therapy with calcium channel blockers increase life expectancy in patients with cardiovascular dysfunction?
No. These drugs are effective in amelioration of symptoms, but do not affect the underlying disease.

DIHYDROPYRIDINES

15. Which drugs are included in the dihydropyridine class of calcium channel blockers?
This class includes vasoactive drugs, such as nifedipine, nicardipine, felodipine, nimodipine, and amlodipine.

16. What is the differential action of dihydropyridine-type calcium channel blockers?
This class of drug has prominent vascular effects, rather than cardiac effects. Effects on the vasculature are mainly arterial and there is little effect on veins.

17. Are drugs of the dihydropyridine class useful in the therapy of arrhythmias?
No, due to the selectivity of these drugs for calcium channels in the vasculature. They have limited cardiodepressant or dromotropic effects.

18. Which drug of the dihydropyridine class is considered the most potent?
Isradipine.

MISCELLANEOUS CALCIUM CHANNEL BLOCKERS

19. Which calcium channel blocker bears a similarity to the benzodiazepines?
Diltiazem, a calcium channel blocker of the benzothiaprine class.

20. Describe the mechanism of action of bepridil.

Bepridil, an atypical calcium channel antagonist, has antiarrhythmic activity, in addition to actions on the calcium channel. In addition to blockade of calcium channels, blockade of both sodium and potassium channels is manifested, which results in unique actions on cardiac tissue.

21. Which calcium channel blockers are most effective in the control of supraventricular arrhythmias?

Verapamil and diltiazem, as they have the highest efficacy in blockade of nodal calcium channels.

22. Identify and characterize the calcium channel blocker most effective in the therapy of Wolff-Parkinson-White syndrome.

Verapamil is most effective, as it slows conduction in the AV node and interrupts reentry pathways.

23. Which calcium channel blocker is used in the therapy of subarachnoid hemorrhage?

Nimodipine, as it is lipophilic and crosses the blood-brain barrier into the CNS. This drug is useful in the therapy of ischemic neuronal injury.

CARDIAC EFFECTS

24. Contrast the degree of depression of sinoatrial (SA) node firing among calcium channel blockers.

Members of the dihydropyridine class of calcium channel blocker drugs (e.g., nifedipine, nisoldipine) have intrinsically less effect on the cardiac conduction system than other classes. In particular, verapamil has a high degree of SA nodal and AV nodal blockade, and diltiazem has a somewhat lower effect. Bepridil blocks both sodium and potassium channels, and also causes both SA nodal and AV nodal blockade.

25. Describe the effects of verapamil on the cardiac action potential.

Verapamil has a high degree of effect on nodal conduction, and therefore affects the action potential. Blockade of calcium channels results in an increase in the time required to reach the membrane potential for calcium, resulting in a dose-dependent lengthening of phase 2.

26. Describe the effects of nifedipine on the cardiac action potential.

Nifedipine, like other dihydropyridines, does not have an appreciable effect on cardiac tissue or conduction. Therefore, there is limited effect on the cardiac action potential.

27. Can the effects of calcium channel blockers on cardiac conduction be decreased by the administration of a β_1-receptor agonist?

Yes. Beta agonists increase calcium influx into nodal tissue.

28. Contrast the sympatholytic effect of nifedipine, verapamil and diltiazem.

Diltiazem has a marked sympatholytic effect, possibly due to the inhibition of calcium influx into the noradrenergic neuron, which is required for neurotransmitter release. Verapamil has less of an effect, and nifedipine appears to have little or no sympatholytic action.

29. Why are some calcium channel blockers associated with a high degree of reflex tachycardia?

Drugs that have a high degree of sympatholytic activity are generally not associated with reflex sympathetic effects. Drugs with a low degree of sympatholytic activity (e.g., nifedipine) produce significant reflex activity.

30. Is bepridil useful as an antiarrhythmic?

Yes. It is has class I and class III antiarrhythmic activity. It is, however, proarrhythmic and must be used with caution.

31. Discuss the actions of bepridil on calcium-calmodulin binding.

Bepridil blocks the binding of calcium to calmodulin, thus decreasing the intracellular actions of calcium.

32. What types of calcium channels are inhibited by the actions of bepridil?

Physiologic effects of both receptor-mediated and voltage-gated calcium channels are inhibited, due to the actions of the drug on calcium-calmodulin binding.

33. Describe the effect of bepridil on the cardiac action potential.

Bepridil prolongs phase 2 of the cardiac action potential, due to the inhibition of calcium flux. The potential may also decrease in amplitude (phase 0) with the inhibition of fast sodium channels. A decrease in the slope of phase 3, due to the potassium channel blockade and decreased slope of phase 4, may also be evident. The net effect is a prolongation of the action potential and an increase in ERP.

34. What adverse effects might result from bepridil administration that are related to its effect on the cardiac action potential?

The prolongation of the cardiac action potential caused by bepridil (particularly the prolongation due to changes in the slope of phase 3 and 4) increases the incidence of torsades de points.

35. Is bepridil highly protein-bound?

Yes, up to 99 percent bound, primarily to α_1-glycoprotein.

36. Does nisoldipine decrease AV nodal conduction?

No. Nisoldipine has no clinical effect on AV conduction.

37. Discuss the half-life of nimodipine as it relates to the dosage interval of the drug.

This drug shows a nonlinear rate of clearance. Thus, even though true half-life of nimodipine is approximately 8 to 9 hours, it must be administered frequently (every 4 hours) to maintain therapeutic levels, as there is an initial rapid decline in plasma concentrations below therapeutic level.

38. Does verapamil have active metabolites?

Yes. It is metabolized by the liver to norverapamil, a potent metabolite.

39. Discuss the activity of norverapamil.

Norverapamil has negligible actions on cardiac conduction, but has potent vasodilatory activity.

40. Explain the advantage of administering verapamil as a racemic mixture.

Verapamil is normally supplied as a 1:1 mixture of D and L isomers. The advantage of this may be that, because first pass metabolism of verapamil is stereoselective, with preferential metabolism of the L-isomer, the L-isomer is metabolized first, generating the active (vasodilatory) metabolite. Thus, the remaining drug isomer retains cardiodepressant activity, while the primary metabolite, norverapamil, contributes significant vasodilatory activity, balancing the cardiodepressant effect. This results in reduced cardiac work and myocardial oxygen consumption. In addition, it contributes to an increase in cardiac perfusion and oxygen delivery.

41. Describe the common adverse effects of verapamil.

Constipation, headache, pruritus, mild nausea, nervousness, and peripheral edema are most common. More serious effects, such as hypotension, bradycardia, and asystole may also result, particularly if the drug is administered in combined therapy with a β-blocker.

42. Compare the actions of felodipine to those of nifedipine.

Both of these drugs belong to the dihydropyridine class of calcium channel blockers. However, felodipine has greater selectivity for vascular smooth muscle relative to myocardial muscle than does nifedipine.

43. Is felodipine useful in the therapy of angina?

Felodipine would be useful in antianginal therapy due to its coronary vasodilatory actions, but its potent vasodilatory activity elicits a reflex tachycardia that increases myocardial oxygen consumption.

44. Describe the oral bioavailability of felodipine.

Oral bioavailability of this drug is extremely low (< 20 percent) due to an extensive first-pass metabolism.

45. Does isradipine cause reflex tachycardia?

No reflex tachycardia is seen with chronic therapy.

46. Compare the duration of action of nifedipine and isradipine.

Isradipine has a significantly longer duration of action than nifedipine.

47. Is nifedipine distributed bound to proteins?

Yes, the drug is highly protein-bound (up to 98%).

48. Discuss the metabolism and elimination of nifedipine.

Nifedipine is almost 100 percent metabolized in the liver, and excreted through the urine as inactive conjugates.

49. What are the clinical uses of diltiazem?

Diltiazem is used in the therapy of Prinzmetal's angina, variant angina, stable angina pectoris, hypertension, and paroxysmal supraventricular tachycardia (PSVT). In addition, the drug is effective in the management of atrial fibrillation and flutter (through cardiodepressant effects and partial AV nodal blockade), and is useful in prophylaxis following angioplasty.

50. Describe the bioavailability of diltiazem.

Diltiazem has a first-pass effect, which reduces bioavailablity. Bioavailability may be improved, however, with the use of the sustained release form of the drug.

51. Does diltiazem have active metabolites?

Yes. The drug is extensively metabolized, producing both inactive metabolites and the active metabolite desacetyldiltiazem, which has coronary vasodilatory activity.

52. Which calcium channel blockers have a long half-life, suitable for once-a-day (q. d.) dosing?

Amlodipine, felodipine, and bepridil.

53. Contrast the half-life of amlodipine with that of nifedipine.

The half-life of nifedipine is 2 to 5 hours, making repeated dosing necessary. The duration of amlodipine is much longer ($T\frac{1}{2}$ = 35 hours), and is administered once daily.

BIBLIOGRAPHY

1. Barrere-Lemaire S, Piot C, Leclercq F, et al: Facilitation of L-type calcium currents by diastolic depolarization in cardiac cells: Impairment in heart failure. Cardiovasc Res: 47(2):336–349, 2000.
2. Bech J, Madsen JK, Kelbaek H: Amlodipine reduces myocardial ischaemia during exercise without compromising left ventricular function in patients with silent ischaemia: A randomised, double-blind, placebo-controlled study. Eur J Heart Fail 1(4):395–400, 1999.

3. Hardman J, Limbird L, Gilman A: Goodman & Gilman's The Pharmacological Basis of Therapeutics, 10th ed. McGraw-Hill Publishers, 2001.
4. Kakinoki S, Nomura A, Takechi S, et al: Effects of short- and longacting calcium channel blockers on the relationship between blood pressure and physical activity. Am J Hypertens 14(1):66–69, 2001.
5. Katzung B: Basic and Clinical Pharmacology, 8th ed. Appleton & Lange, 2001.
6. Minamino T, Kitakaze M, Papst PJ, et al: Inhibition of nitric oxide synthesis induces coronary vascular remodeling and cardiac hypertrophy associated with the activation of p70 S6 kinase in rats. Cardiovasc Drugs Ther 14(5):533–542, 2000.
7. Nakamura T, Obata J, Onitsuka M, et al: Benidipine, a long-acting calcium-channel blocker, prevents the progression to end-stage renal failure in a rat mesangioproliferative glomerulonephritis. Nephron 86(3):315–326, 2000.
8. Sabbatini M, Vitaioli L, Baldoni E, et al: Nephroprotective effect of treatment with calcium channel blockers in spontaneously hypertensive rats. J Pharmacol Exp Ther 294(3):948–954, 2000.
9. Sabbatini M, Leonardi A, Testa R, et al: Effect of calcium antagonists on glomerular arterioles in spontaneously hypertensive rats. Hypertension 35(3):775–779, 2000.
10. Sogabe T, Mori T, Ohura M, et al: Venodilatory effect of pranidipine, a calcium channel blocker, monitored with perfluorocarbon in vivo (19)F-NMR spectroscopy. Magn Reson Imaging 18(8): 1011–1016, 2000.
11. Zhabyeyev P, Missan S, Jones SE, et al: Low-affinity block of cardiac K(+) currents by nifedipine. Eur J Pharmacol 401(2):137–143, 2000.

13. DIRECT VASODILATORS

1. Discuss the major drugs used as vasodilators, and the levels at which they act.

- Drugs that act primarily at the venous level. These include most nitrates.
- Drugs that act primarily at the arterial level (e.g., hydralazine and calcium channel antagonists). These are potent vasodilators.
- Drugs that have actions at both arterial and venous levels. This group includes sodium nitroprusside α_1-receptor antagonists, and angiotensin-converting enzyme (ACE) inhibitors.

2. Which vasodilators are considered direct vasodilators?

Those drugs that affect vascular smooth muscle directly (non-receptor-mediated) are included in this category. It is believed that these drugs all act by a mechanism similar to that of nitrates.

3. Should vasodilators be used in patients with recent myocardial infarct?

No. The reduction in blood pressure could result in reduction of coronary perfusion and extension of the infarct.

NITRATES

4. Describe the mechanism of action of nitrates.

These drugs are converted to nitric oxide within smooth muscle. The nitric oxide produced interacts with the reducing environment of the cytoplasm (e.g., thiols) forming nitroso-thiols. These agents then activate guanylate cyclase, which catalyzes conversion of guanylate triphosphate (GTP) to cyclic guanylate monophosphate (cGMP), which inhibits calcium binding, inhibits the activity of myosin light chain kinase, and thus prevents smooth muscle contraction (thus promoting relaxation).

5. What are the clinical uses of nitrates?

Nitrate compounds (e.g., nitroglycerin, isosorbide mononitrate) may be used in the reducing esophageal spasm, managing heart failure, and decreasing postoperative hypertension.

6. What is the significance of nitrates in acute situations?

These drugs tend to act very quickly to promote vessel relaxation and are thus useful in acute situations. They are used in the therapy of acute attacks of angina (e.g., nitroglycerine), and may be useful during a hypertensive crisis (e.g., sodium nitroprusside).

7. Are nitrates vasodilators?

Not in the strict sense. These drugs primarily dilate veins, more than arteries. Some drugs in the class, such as sodium nitroprusside, also have significant vasodilatory activity.

8. Explain the actions of nitrates on the heart.

Nitrates primarily decrease venous tone that results in increased coronary perfusion. In addition, venodilation results in decreased filling of the heart, and decreased preload. Afterload may also be decreased, proportionate with the degree of arterial dilation of the particular drug. The net result is a decrease in myocardial stretch leading to increased cardiac output (due to Starling's law), decreased myocardial oxygen consumption, and an increase in coronary perfusion.

9. Explain the relationship between nitrates and adrenergic neurotransmitters.

The vasodilatory action of nitrates is antagonistic to the effects of norepinephrine at the α_1 receptor.

10. What is the duration of action of glycerol trinitrate (nitroglycerin)?
It is particularly short—only 30 minutes.

11. Does tolerance develop to the actions of nitroglycerin?
Yes, if large doses are given, or if dosage is constant. Thus, nitroglycerine is best suited for intermittent (acute) therapy.

12. Discuss the bioavailability of nitroglycerin.
This drug is poorly bioavailable (< 10 percent). It is therefore administered sublingually or transdermally.

13. Describe the distribution of nitroglycerin.
Nitroglycerin is widely distributed and has a high volume of distribution.

14. Is nitroglycerin protein bound?
Yes. It is approximately 60 percent plasma protein bound.

15. What is the half-life of nitroglycerin?
The half-life of the parent drug is 1–3 minutes.

16. Does nitroglycerin have active metabolites?
Yes. The metabolites of nitroglycerin are 1,3- and 1,2-glyceryl dinitrate.

17. Compare the activity of nitroglycerin to its metabolites.
The active metabolites produced are much less potent than the parent compound. However, the half-lives are much longer—extending to as much as 40 minutes.

18. How are the metabolites of nitroglycerin eliminated?
The metabolites are excreted renally.

19. Describe the clinical uses of sodium (Na) nitroprusside.
This drug is useful in the treatment of peripheral vasospasm secondary to ergot alkaloid overdose, and as an adjunct in the treatment of valvular regurgitation.

20. How is sodium nitroprusside administered? Explain.
Na nitroprusside must be administered intravenously, due to its short half-life. It is administered in short infusions to limit toxic effects.

21. Can a specific blood pressure be achieved with sodium nitroprusside?
Yes. Any pressure within a physiologic range can be achieved, by titrating the amount of drug administered (i.e., the flow rate of the infusion).

22. Explain the use of sodium nitroprusside in the therapy of pheochromocytoma.
Sodium nitroprusside is used to control paroxysmal hypertension (due to catecholamine release from manipulation of the tumor) during surgery secondary to pheochromocytoma.

23. Why does diuresis occur with sodium nitroprusside therapy?
Peripheral vasodilatation includes dilation of the renal artery and increased renal blood flow, promoting an increase in glomerular filtration rate (GFR) and increased urine output.

24. Discuss the effects of Na nitroprusside on intracranial pressure.
This drug can cause vasodilatation in the brain, resulting in an increase in intracranial pressure. It is, therefore, contraindicated in patients with cranial injury or encephalopathy.

25. Are the effects of Na nitroprusside affected by sympathetic output?

Yes. α_1-receptor stimulation causes direct vasoconstriction, which antagonizes the effects of the drug.

26. Is sodium nitroprusside given on an outpatient basis?

No. The drug must be given under supervision, as the hypotensive effects can be severe.

27. Are the effects of Na nitroprusside affected by sympathetic antagonists?

No, as the mechanism of action of the drug is completely independent of sympathetic involvement.

28. Describe the breakdown of nitroprusside and its potential toxicity.

The structure of nitroprusside contains cyanide (HCN). After administration, the drug rapidly interacts with sulfhydryl groups in cell membranes, and, in erythrocytes, reacts with thiols and hemoglobin to form methemoglobin. This results in the release of cyanide, which is extremely toxic. The toxicity of the released cyanide is prevented by the buffering of the cyanide radicals by the methemoglobin, resulting in the formation of cyanomethemoglobin. Cyanide radicals remaining are converted hepatically to thiocyanate, which is then excreted renally.

29. Discuss the limiting factors (with regard to adverse effects) to administration of sodium nitroprusside.

The primary limiting factor is adequate hemoglobin, although renal and hepatic competence are also of prime importance.

30. What is the physiologic tolerance level to sodium nitroprusside? Explain.

A normal patient can tolerate up to 450–500 µg of drug per kilogram of body weight. This figure depends on the buffering capacity and amount of methemoglobin available to buffer the cyanide produced by the drug.

31. Why would the use of nitroprusside be contraindicated in patients with severe renal disease?

The drug produces cyanide, and cyanide congeners, which are excreted renally. Renal impairment would result in an increase in the plasma levels of these compounds and toxicity.

32. What is the primary clinical use of isosorbide mononitrate?

Isosorbide mononitrate is taken orally for the therapy of angina. As a venodilator, it would also be beneficial in the therapy of hypertension and heart failure, but would not be a first line drug for that purpose.

33. Does isosorbide mononitrate have effects on all types of smooth muscle?

Yes. Isosorbide nitrates relax all types of smooth muscle including bronchial, biliary, gastrointestinal (GI), ureteral, and uterine.

34. Does isosorbide mononitrate have a first-pass effect?

No. It is 100 percent bioavailable.

35. Describe the relationship between isosorbide mononitrate and isosorbide dinitrate.

Isosorbide mononitrate is the active metabolite of isosorbide dinitrate. It is long-acting, as compared to isosorbide dinitrate.

36. Is isosorbide mononitrate widely distributed?

No. It has a low volume of distribution.

37. Are isosorbide nitrates plasma protein-bound?

These drugs exist less than 4 percent bound to plasma proteins.

38. Describe the onset of isosorbide mononitrate.
The onset of antianginal effects occurs in 1–4 hours.

39. Discuss the inactivation of isosorbide mononitrate.
This drug is greater than 99 percent metabolized. It undergoes glucuronidation in the liver, and is excreted as glucuronide conjugates in the urine.

40. What are the adverse effects of isosorbide mononitrate?
Headache, dizziness, weakness, nausea/vomiting, and syncope. Rarely, the drug induces methemoglobinemia.

41. Describe the hypersensitivity reactions associated with isosorbide mononitrate.
These include cutaneous vasodilatation (flushing), and diaphoresis. Cardiovascular effects may include sinus tachycardia, syncope, palpitations, and ultimately cardiovascular collapse.

42. What is the basis of the headache observed with isosorbide mononitrate?
The rapid vasodilatation of cerebral vasculature caused by the drug causes an increase in intracranial pressure.

43. Do isosorbide nitrates cause orthostatic hypotension?
Yes, but this occurs in less than 1 percent of patients.

44. Discuss the duration of action of isosorbide nitrates.
The duration of action is relatively short, as the half-life is only 5 hours.

45. Discuss the toxicity of isosorbide nitrates.
Toxic effects are mainly due to adverse cardiovascular effects (e.g., hypotension, and sinus tachycardia leading to ventricular dysrhythmias).

46. What measures should a patient be taught regarding the drug nitroglycerin?
- The drug should be kept out of direct light, in a tinted bottle.
- The drug should be disposed of after 6 months.
- A radial pulse should be taken before administration of the drug. Caution is advised if the pulse is below 60.

ARTERIAL VASODILATORS

47. Describe the clinical use of minoxidil.
Minoxidil is used orally in the therapy of severe hypertension that has been shown to be refractory to therapy with other drugs.

48. Does minoxidil exhibit central nervous system (CNS) effects?
No. It is mainly a peripheral vasodilator.

49. Describe the interactions of minoxidil with the sympathetic nervous system.
The drug exhibits no blockade of adrenergic nerve terminals, nor does it affect adrenergic receptors. The actions of norepinephrine do, however, antagonize the effects of the drug at the level of the α_1 receptor.

50. Discuss the compensatory reactions to minoxidil therapy.
Reflex sympathetic activity may abolish much of the effects of the drug—reflex increases in heart rate, cardiac output, and renin release are seen with administration of the drug. This is primarily due to the potent vasodilatory actions of the drug, which cause a sudden and robust change in blood pressure.

51. Does minoxidil lead to positive changes in left ventricular hypertrophy?

No. This is primarily due to the increase in fluid volume with the drug (i.e., stimulation of the renin-angiotensin-aldosterone system).

52. Compare the absorption of oral and topical minoxidil.

The drug is well absorbed orally (> 90 percent). However, topical absorption is minimal (< 2 percent).

53. Contrast the half-life and therapeutic duration of minoxidil.

The half-life of the drug is short, about 4 hours. However, the effects of the drug persist for up to 5 days. This is ostensibly due to biochemical changes made by the drug within the vascular smooth muscle cell that have yet to be determined.

54. Describe the pharmacokinetics of minoxidil.

Minoxidil is not significantly bound to plasma proteins and is thus freely filtered into the urine. Upon passage through the liver, a significant proportion of the drug undergoes hepatic glucuronidation, and is eliminated via the kidney.

55. How is hydralazine administered?

It may be administered orally or parenterally.

56. Describe the vascular selectivity of hydralazine.

Hydralazine is selective for arterioles, and thus is a very potent vasodilator.

57. Is the vasodilatation produced by hydralazine selective for certain vascular beds?

Yes. Coronary, cerebral, splanchnic and renal blood flow are increased.

58. Does administration of hydralazine increase GFR?

No. In fact, the drug promotes fluid retention.

59. Explain the disadvantages of oral administration of hydralazine.

Hydralazine is subject to a strong first-pass effect, which reduces bioavailability. In addition, because the drug is inactivated by acetylation, bioavailability is variable among patients who may be either "slow acetylators" or "fast acetylators."

60. Discuss dosage adjustments of hydralazine in patients with compromised renal function.

The $T\frac{1}{2}$ of the drug is 4–7 hours. However, because the kidney eliminates the drug and its conjugates, a patient with compromised renal function will require reduced dosage.

61. Describe the mechanism of action of epoprostenol and its clinical use.

Epoprostenol is a prostacyclin analog that antagonizes the vasoconstrictor effect of thromboxanes. It is useful in the therapy of pulmonary hypertension.

BIBLIOGRAPHY

1. Burcham PC, Kerr PG, Fontaine F: The antihypertensive hydralazine is an efficient scavenger of acrolein. Redox Rep 5(1):47–49, 2000.
2. Chowdhary S, Vaile JC, Fletcher J, et al.: Nitric oxide and cardiac autonomic control in humans. Hypertension 36(2):264–269, 2000.
3. Fenton BM: Influence of hydralazine administration on oxygenation in spontaneous and transplanted tumor models. Int J Radiat Oncol Biol Phys 49(3):799–808, 2001.
4. Hardman J, Limbird L, and Gilman A: Goodman & Gilman's The Pharmacological Basis of Therapeutics, 10th ed. McGraw-Hill Publishers, 2001.
5. Katzung, B: Basic and Clinical Pharmacology, 8th ed. Appleton & Lange, 2001.

6. Shapira OM, Alkon JD, Macron DS, et al: Nitroglycerin is preferable to diltiazem for prevention of coronary bypass conduit spasm. Ann Thorac Surg 70(3):883-888; [discussion] 888–889, 2000.
7. Tanabe A, Naruse M, Adachi C, et al: Hydralazine decreases blood pressure and endothelin-1 mRNA expression in tissues but not cardiac weight in SHR-SP/Izm rats. J Cardiovasc Pharmacol 36(5 Suppl 1):S176–S178, 2000.

Websites:

Clinical Pharmacology 2000: http://cp.gsm.com

Medline plus: http://medlineplus.nlm.nih.gov/medlineplus/

Medscape Multispecialty Journal Room: http://pharmacotherapy.medscape.com/Home/Topics/multispecialty/directories/dir-MULT.JournalRoom.html

Medscape Pharmacotherapy News (cardiology):

http://cardiology.medscape.com/home/topics/pharmacotherapy/directories/dir-PHAR.News.html

14. THE THERAPY OF HYPERTENSION

1. Explain the rationale behind effective therapy of systemic hypertension.

Hypertension is due to an increase in vascular pressure (e.g., increased force exerted against vessel walls). Therefore, reductions in plasma volume, reduced cardiac output, and increases in vascular diameter are all effective means of reducing tension.

2. Discuss the cardiovascular ramifications of uncontrolled hypertension.

The increased pressure against vascular walls, combined with normal blood flow, produces a shearing effect on the vascular endothelium. This results in damage to endothelial cells, production of paracrine mediators, and decreased production of vasodilatory substances such as those involved in the nitrous oxide/guanylate cyclase cascade. This may result in increased incidence of vasospasm (e.g., stroke, myocardial infarct [MI]). The endothelial damage produced by the increased shear may also provide a repository for lipid substances, facilitating the formation of sclerotic plaques, which decrease vessel diameter and reduce blood flow to critical organs. In addition, increased pressure, flow rate, and total peripheral resistance (TPR) (afterload) increase ventricular stretch and may result in ventricular hypertrophy and congestive heart failure. End organ failure (e.g., liver and kidney) may also occur.

3. What is the first step in the therapy of hypertension?

Initial therapy normally begins with a reduction of plasma volume, using a diuretic.

ADRENERGIC-RECEPTOR ANTAGONISTS

4. Describe the use of a beta$_1$-receptor antagonist in the therapy of essential hypertension.

β_1-receptor (or pan-beta-receptor) antagonists, when added to the antihypertensive regimen, lower cardiac output by decreasing heart rate and force of contraction of the cardiac muscle, resulting in decreased ejection fraction. In addition, β_1-receptor antagonism decreases the release of renin from the juxtaglomerular apparatus in a dose-dependent manner, resulting in lower circulating levels of angiotensin II, a potent endogenous vasoconstrictor. The decrease in angiotensin II then results in decreased aldosterone release. This results in decreased salt and water retention, leading to a decrease in blood volume. Thus β_1-receptor antagonism has multifaceted use in the therapy of essential hypertension.

5. Discuss the advantages of using a selective β_1-receptor antagonist (e.g., atenolol, metoprolol) in the therapy of hypertension.

The β_2-receptor is involved in peripheral arterial vasodilatation, as well as bronchiolar dilatation. Thus, with the use of a nonselective antagonist, blockade of the β_2-receptor may not only decrease the amount of vasodilatation produced, and thus decrease the efficacy of the drug, but may also precipitate bronchoconstriction in susceptible individuals. Use of a selective β_1-receptor antagonist, which by definition has negligible effects on the β_2-receptor, would preclude these events.

6. Why would antihypertensive therapy with pindolol be effective?

Pindolol is a partial agonist at the β_2-adrenergic receptor, and has antagonistic actions at the β_1-receptor. Thus, cardiac output is reduced with the drug, due to β_1-receptor antagonism, and vasodilatation is increased, due to the effects of β_2-receptor stimulation.

7. Describe the mechanism of α_1-receptor antagonists in the therapy of hypertension.

These drugs decrease the activation of α_1 receptors in the peripheral vasculature, resulting in net vasodilatation and decreased TPR. In addition, venous capacitance is increased, effectively reducing available blood volume. The abrupt lowering of systemic pressure, however, may stimulate reflex release of catecholamines, resulting in reflex tachycardia and increased cardiac output that may attenuate the therapeutic effects.

8. Do drugs such as prazosin and terazosin result in reflex tachycardia?

Because these drugs selectively block the α_1-adrenergic receptor and cause negligible blockade of the α_2-receptor, reflex tachycardia is minimal, as compared to nonselective agents.

9. Describe the major adverse effect seen with the use of α_1-receptor antagonists.

The major adverse effect is postural (orthostatic) hypotension, due to the increase in venous capacitance. As α_1-receptor antagonists block receptors on both arteries and veins, both vasodilatation and a decrease in venoconstriction are seen. This results in an increase in venous capacitance. As gravity draws blood into the veins upon standing, the compensatory venoconstrictor mechanisms are blocked by the drug, resulting in pooling of blood in the extremities.

CALCIUM CHANNEL BLOCKERS

10. Describe the use of calcium channel blockers in the therapy of hypertension.

If the combination of a beta-blocker and a diuretic does not produce sufficient lowering of pressure, a calcium channel blocker (e.g., verapamil, nifedipine) may be used. This class of drugs blocks type "L" calcium channels in the myocardium and peripheral vasculature in a dose-dependent manner, resulting in decreased cardiac output and peripheral resistance (see chapter 12 for a full discussion of calcium channel blockers). The individual drugs within the class vary as to effect on cardiac muscle and/or vasculature. Therefore, the drug used dictates the relative decrease in cardiac output and/or TPR.

11. What would be an advantage of antihypertensive therapy with nifedipine as opposed to verapamil?

Nifedipine acts primarily at the level of the vasculature, and has little effect on the myocardium. Thus, the efficiency of the heart would be increased, and the work of the heart decreased. With verapamil therapy, both cardiac conduction and contractile force would be affected, resulting in a decrease in myocardial efficiency.

DIRECT VASODILATORS

12. Describe the use of a peripheral vasodilator (e.g., hydralazine) in the therapy of hypertension.

These drugs are direct vasodilators (see Chapter 13, Direct Vasodilators, for a complete discussion of direct vasodilators). They are primarily used as second line drugs in a stepwise antihypertensive regimen. Their use results in deceased arterial tone, which results in a decrease in peripheral resistance and decreased systemic pressure.

13. Explain the tolerance seen to long-term hydralazine therapy.

The decrease in blood pressure produced by the drug stimulates adrenergic activity and a concurrent increase in renin and angiotensin II. This promotes an increase in aldosterone and corresponding increase in sodium and water retention, which is not compensated for by an increase in GFR. These effects, together with the increase in stroke volume and cardiac output produced by the drug, tend to attenuate the hypotensive effects of the drug, with time.

14. Are tolerance effects to hydralazine therapy seen immediately?

No. Production of aldosterone and the increase in fluid retention and cardiac output takes time.

15. What is the major mechanism of action of sodium nitroprusside in the therapy of hypertension?

This drug acts to increase nitrous oxide levels in the vascular endothelium, which results in net vasodilatation, decreased total peripheral resistance, and a drop in systemic blood pressure.

16. Are nitrates such as nitroglycerin and isosorbide mononitrate used as antihypertensives?

No. These drugs are primarily venodilators. Doses sufficient to lower blood pressure would likely result in toxicity.

17. Describe the use of diazoxide as an antihypertensive drug.

Diazoxide is used in short-term therapy of acute attacks of malignant hypertension.

18. Describe the mechanism of action of diazoxide.

Diazoxide, is used orally as an antihypoglycemic agent. Used parenterally, it acts as an arterial vasodilator and acts to selectively relax arterial smooth muscle. Because venous capacitance is not affected, systolic pressure is reduced more than diastolic pressure, and pulse pressure is reduced.

19. Discuss the effects of diazoxide on the myocardium.

With arterial dilation produced by the drug, afterload is decreased, and ejection fraction and cardiac output are increased. The work of the heart is decreased, due to decreased afterload, and cardiac stress is decreased as efficiency increases.

DRUGS THAT AFFECT ANGIOTENSIN II

20. Describe the physiologic role of angiotensin converting enzyme.

Angiotensin-converting enzyme (ACE) is responsible for the enzymatic conversion of angiotensin I (a weak vasoconstrictor) to angiotensin II (a potent vasoconstrictor). Angiotensin II also stimulates the release of aldosterone, resulting in retention of sodium and water, and an increase in fluid volume. In addition, ACE is also responsible for the degradation of bradykinin (see Figure).

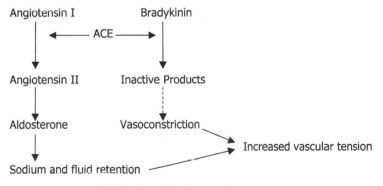

Effects of angiotensin converting enzyme.

21. Describe the use of ACE inhibitors in antihypertensive therapy.

ACE inhibitors (e.g., captopril, enalapril, lisinopril, etc.) compete with angiotensin I for binding of ACE, thus reducing the formation of angiotensin II. This results in decreased vasoconstriction. Secretion of aldosterone is also reduced, resulting in decreased fluid volume, and vasodilatation is promoted through an inhibition of the metabolism of bradykinin, a potent vasodilator. This produces a net vasodilatation, accompanied by a decrease in plasma volume, resulting in a fall in blood pressure.

22. Are ACE inhibitors a good choice as antihypertensive agents in black patients?
No. These drugs have been shown to be less efficacious in the black population than the non-black population.

23. Describe the therapeutic effects seen with telmisartan therapy.
Telmisartan and other pure angiotensin-II-receptor antagonists appear to lower both systolic and diastolic pressures with approximately equal efficacy.

24. State the effects of irbesartan therapy during periods of rest and exercise.
Irbesartan appears to reduce systolic and diastolic pressures during both rest and exercise. The primary function of the drug is to decrease peripheral resistance, with a resulting decrease in afterload. Thus, heart function is minimally affected, and the drug is equally efficacious through various types of activity.

25. Is losartan effective in the reduction of left ventricular hypertrophy (LVH) secondary to hypertension?
Yes. A substantial reduction in LVH has been observed with losartan therapy, due to the decrease in afterload produced by the drug.

26. Discuss combination therapy with trandolapril in the treatment of hypertension.
Trandolapril is used in combination with calcium channel blockers (e.g., verapamil) as a second line antihypertensive therapy. The effects of the two drugs in combination are greater than that produced by either drug alone, indicating that the effects are synergistic in the lowering of blood pressure.

27. Discuss the efficacy of trandolapril.
Trandolapril is an ACE inhibitor. It is considered a pro-drug, as hepatic metabolism produces trandolaprilat, which has approximately eight times the potency of the parent drug.

ANGIOTENSIN-II-RECEPTOR ANTAGONISTS

28. Explain the mechanism of action of angiotensin-II-receptor antagonists.
These drugs competitively bind to the angiotensin II receptor, reducing the activity of angiotensin II in a dose-dependent manner.

29. Do angiotensin-II-receptor antagonists affect heart rate?
No. Heart rate is unchanged.

30. Is saralasin a pure angiotensin II antagonist?
No. This drug has dose-dependent agonist activity as well.

31. Describe the differential administration of saralasin.
This drug must be absorbed slowly, in relatively low doses. If administration is rapid, agonist activity is produced at the angiotensin II receptor, resulting in an increase in vascular pressure.

CENTRALLY ACTING ANTIHYPERTENSIVE AGENTS

32. Discuss the mechanism of action of α_2-receptor agonists (e.g., clonidine) in the therapy of hypertension.
These drugs act as agonists the regulatory α_2-adrenergic receptor, both at the neuronal ending and at the level of the nucleus tractus solitarius (NTS). Thus, release of norepinephrine is decreased.

33. Would reflex baroreceptor responses be precipitated by the pressure decrease produced by the administration of clonidine?

No. The decrease in vascular pressure would not elicit a significant physiologic response, because the regulatory α_2 receptor on the NTS is activated by the drug and prevents the compensatory release of norepinephrine in a dose-dependent manner.

34. Discuss the activation and mechanism of action of α-methyldopa.

α-Methyldopa is taken into the adrenergic nerve terminus by the catecholamine reuptake system. It is then taken into the adrenergic vesicle and enters the catecholamine synthesis pathway. It is acted upon by dopa decarboxylase, and converted to α-methylnorepinephrine, a potent α_2-receptor agonist (see Figure). The net mechanism of the drug is therefore a centrally-mediated reduction in the release of norepinephrine.

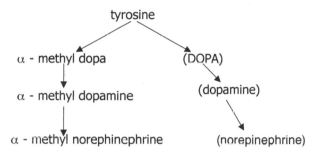

35. What is a major advantage of the use of α-methyldopa in the therapy of hypertension?

This drug is particularly useful by decreasing renal vascular resistance. Blood flow to the kidney is thus not compromised, and less end-organ damage is produced.

36. Describe the mechanism of action of reserpine.

This drug depletes neuronal stores of norepinephrine. The drug enters the adrenergic nerve terminus through the synaptic reuptake mechanism, and is transported into the adrenergic vesicle. Once in the vesicle, it displaces norepinephrine from the vesicle to the cytoplasm, where it is degraded by monoamine oxidase (MAO).

37. Does guanethidine have central nervous system (CNS) effects?

No. The effects are limited to the periphery.

DRUGS THAT ACT BY GANGLIONIC BLOCKADE

38. Discuss the mechanism of action of trimethaphan.

Trimethaphan is an antagonist at nicotinic ganglionic synapses. The drug thus blocks transmission of information through autonomic pathways in a dose-dependent manner.

39. Describe the adverse effects of trimethaphan.

This drug is both sympathoplegic and parasympathoplegic, due to blockade of nicotinic ganglia in both parasympathetic and sympathetic pathways. Thus, effects on both systems are seen. Effects due to sympathetic blockade include sedation, hypotension, and cardiovascular abnormalities, whereas those due to parasympathetic blockade include dyspepsia and constipation.

40. What is the therapeutic use of trimethaphan?

Due to the large number of adverse effects, this drug is used mainly in crisis situations (e.g., reversal of hypertensive crisis).

41. Describe the administration of trimethaphan.

This drug is administered intravenously, in a rapid bolus. Maximum efficacy is achieved only when the patient lies on an incline, with the head raised.

42. Discuss combination therapy in the treatment of essential hypertension.

The first line therapy is usually a diuretic. The addition of a beta-receptor antagonist to the regimen is preferred, although calcium channel blockers, ACE inhibitors, and angiotensin-II-receptor antagonists may also be used, depending on the properties of the actual drug chosen. The important things to consider are the age and state of health of the patient, as well as the mechanism of action of the drugs. Those drugs with similar mechanisms of action (e.g., beta blockers and calcium channel blockers) would not be a good choice for combination therapy, while drugs with disparate mechanisms (e.g., ACE inhibitors and diuretics) would synergize therapeutically, and allow lower doses of drug to be used. This would allow for greater efficacy and fewer adverse effects. In addition, doses would have to be adjusted for combination therapy, particularly in the geriatric or pediatric patient, and further adjusted in the event that the physiologic effects of one drug would affect the clearance of the other (e.g., thiazides and ACE inhibitors).

Questions 13 to 46: using the blood pressure trace (see Figure below), answer each question. Consider cardiac reflexes in your answer. Each letter represents the administration of a drug, allowing sufficient time for recovery. The drugs used are propranolol, hydralazine, clonidine, and prazosin.

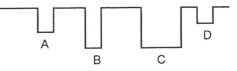

Blood pressure trace (mm Hg).

43. Which of the letters represents the administration of clonidine? Explain.

The correct choice is "C." All of the other drugs listed as potential choices elicit cardiac reflexes, which would decrease the effect of the drug. The effects of clonidine would be more sustained, because baroreceptor-mediated compensatory reflexes are blocked at the NTS level, due to the α_2 agonist activity of clonidine.

44. What is drug "A"?

"A" is propranolol. Propranolol decreases cardiac output but has little effect on peripheral resistance. Thus, initial hypotensive effects are somewhat lower than those of an α_1-antagonist, and a significant proportion of the effects are attenuated by cardiac reflexes. Reflex sympathetic activity causes vasoconstriction, which raises systemic pressure. However, due to the blockade of beta receptors by the drug, such activity does not cause increased cardiac output. Thus, initial hypotensive effects are somewhat attenuated, to a greater extent than with the other drugs presented, but not as attenuated as with a vasodilator.

45. Identify drug "B."

This drug produces significant reduction in pressure with little attenuation by cardiac reflexes. Of the drugs presented, an α_1 antagonist would be the most likely candidate, as vascular diameter is increased, causing a significant decrease in pressure. Compensatory reflex sympathetic activity is blocked at the alpha-receptor level, leaving an increase in cardiac output as the major compensatory factor.

46. Explain why the trace produced by drug "D" would be consistent with the arterial vasodilator, hydralazine.

The significant factor here is that a direct vasodilator provides little or no compensation for cardiac reflexes. The initial result is a significant lowering of pressure with arterial vasodilatation.

However, this is quickly compensated for by increased sympathetic activity. Because the drug blocks none of the sympathetic receptors, the effects of cardiac reflexes are pronounced and the effects attenuated. The other drugs presented all affect sympathetic receptors.

Questions 47 to 50: Using the diagram of a systolic pressure trace (see Figure below), answer each question.

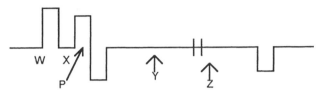

47. Of drugs "W" and "X," which is norepinephrine and which is epinephrine? Explain.

Epinephrine has agonist activity at the β_2 receptor, while norepinephrine does not. Therefore, norepinephrine administration results in a higher tension, provided both drugs are administered slowly, and at the same rate.

48. Explain what is occurring as drug "P" is administered (drug "P" is prazosin).

This phenomenon is known as "epinephrine reversal." Epinephrine, which was administered just prior to administration of prazocin, acts as an agonist at both β_2 (vasodilatory) and α_1 (vasoconstrictor) receptors. Administration of prazosin blocks the vasoconstrictor action of the α_1 receptors, leaving only the vasodilator actions of the β_2 receptor, resulting in a rapid and profound lowering of blood pressure.

49. Identify drug "Y." Why are effects of this drug substantially delayed?

Drugs used for hypertension that have markedly delayed effects are those that have effects at the nerve terminus level. This drug could be guanethidine or reserpine, but, because effects are not seen before the trace is truncated, it is likely to be α-methyldopa, because the drug requires time for the enzymatic conversion to α-methylnorepinephrine before antihypertensive effects are seen.

50. Explain why drug "Z" might be a vasodilator, such as hydralazine, but not a nitrate, such as amyl nitrate.

A vasodilator would have a slightly delayed effect, due to the processes involved in smooth muscle relaxation. If this drug were a nitrate, such as amyl nitrate, effects would be immediate, because the nitrate is converted almost instantly by the vascular endothelium into nitric oxide (NO), which increases levels of cyclic guanylate monophosphate (cGMP) and mediates vasodilatation within seconds.

51. Compare the immediacy of effect of an ACE inhibitor and an angiotensin II antagonist.

The full effects of an ACE inhibitor are slightly delayed, as compared to those of an angiotensin II antagonist. The inhibition of ACE is immediate, and the increase in circulating bradykinin follows quickly. However, the decrease in angiotensin II does not manifest as decreased blood pressure immediately. Circulating stores of angiotensin II have to be depleted before the full effect of ACE inhibition occurs. The conversion of angiotensin I to angiotensin II is decreased by these drugs in a dose-dependent manner, but there is no antagonism of existing angiotensin II. In addition, several ACE inhibitors are actually "pro-drugs" and require metabolic conversion for activation (e.g., captopril, enalapril).

BIBLIOGRAPHY

1. Bakir SE, Oparil S: Antihypertensive drug therapy in the third millennium: Are there benefits beyond blood pressure? Curr Hypertens Rep 2(3):291–294, 2000.

2. Freytag F, Schelling A, Meinicke T, et al: Comparison of 26-week efficacy and tolerability of telmisartan and atenolol, in combination with hydrochlorothiazide as required, in the treatment of mild to moderate hypertension: A randomized, multicenter study. Clin Ther 23(1):108–123, 2001.
3. Gomi T, Ikeda T, Shibuya Y, et al: Effects of antihypertensive treatment on platelet function in essential hypertension. Hypertens Res 23(6):567–572, 2000.
4. Gomi T, Ikeda T, Shibuya Y, et al: Effects of antihypertensive treatment on platelet function in essential hypertension. Hypertens Res 23(6):567–572, 2000.
5. Greenberg BH: Cardiodynamic effects and mechanisms of action of beta-blockers. Am J Manag Care (6 Suppl):S303–S307, 2000.
6. Hardman J, Limbird L, Gilman A: Goodman & Gilman's The Pharmacological Basis of Therapeutics, 10th ed. McGraw-Hill Publishers, 2001.
7. Jamerson KA: Rationale for angiotensin II receptor blockers in patients with low-renin hypertension [review]. Am J Kidney Dis 36(3 Suppl 1):S24–S30, 2000.
8. Katzung, B: Basic and Clinical Pharmacology, 8th ed. Appleton & Lange, 2001.
9. Kross RA, Ferri E, Leung D, et al: A comparative study between a calcium channel blocker (Nicardipine) and a combined alpha-beta-blocker (Labetalol) for the control of emergence hypertension during craniotomy for tumor surgery. Anesth Analg 91(4):904–909, 2000.
10. Magee LA, Duley L: Oral beta-blockers for mild to moderate hypertension during pregnancy [Cochrane review]. Cochrane Database Syst Rev 4:CD002863, 2000.
11. Mettimano M, Pichetti F, Fazzari L, et al: Combination therapy with beta-adrenergic blockade and amlodipine as second line treatment in essential hypertension. Int J Clin Pract 54(7):424–428, 2000.
12. Schmieder RE, Messerli FH: Hypertension and the heart. J Hum Hypertens 14(10-11):597–604, 2000.

15. THE THERAPY OF ANGINA

1. Explain the general goals of the therapy of angina.

Angina is a result of hypooxygenation of the myocardium. It is a function of the ratio of oxygen demand to oxygen delivery. Thus, the goals of therapy are to increase oxygen delivery to the myocardium, or, alternatively, to decrease oxygen demand commensurate with oxygen delivery.

2. Discuss the general classifications of angina.

The general classifications of angina stem from their etiologies and induction. Unstable angina (resting angina) and stable (exercise-induced) angina are both thought to be due to the formation of arterial sclerotic plaques. Unstable angina occurs at rest, i.e., anginal pain and myocardial deoxygenation occur during a relaxed state. This form of angina is most serious, as it indicates a probable infarct. Stable angina is more predictable, as is exercise-induced angina—events are precipitated by an increase in cardiac work. Variant (Prinzmetal's) angina is less common, and is due to coronary vasospasm.

3. What is the therapy for resting ("unstable") angina?

The therapy for resting angina may be an agent that increases coronary perfusion, such as a nitro compound. Alternatively, a drug that depresses cardiac function (e.g., a calcium channel blocker or beta-blocker) may be used to decrease the work of the heart.

4. Discuss therapy for Prinzmetal's angina.

This type of angina is due to coronary vasospasm, and thus would respond well to a calcium channel blocker (e.g., nifedipine or amlodipine).

5. Describe the benefits of verapamil therapy in exercise-induced ("stable") angina.

Verapamil increases exercise tolerance in patients with stable angina and reduces the frequency of anginal attacks, particularly when used in combination with nitroglycerine.

6. Describe the interaction between verapamil and nitroglycerine in the therapy of angina.

Verapamil decreases the consumption of nitroglycerine, allowing lower doses to be used. This decreases the frequency of adverse effects (e.g., headache, dizziness).

7. Describe the use of nitrates in the treatment of angina.

Nitrates are useful in treating angina because they both decrease the work of the heart and increase myocardial perfusion. In addition, they help prevent the formation of thrombi, which potentially could cause infarction.

8. How do nitrates decrease myocardial oxygen consumption?

These drugs decrease ventricular filling and increase stroke volume, effectively decreasing the work of the heart.

9. Explain the antithrombotic action of nitrates.

Nitrates are inhibitors of platelet function, by virtue of increased synthesis of cyclic guanylate monophosphate (cGMP), which is antagonistic toward cyclic adenosine monophosphate (cAMP), a necessary component of the platelet activation cascade.

10. Describe the adverse effects commonly seen with nitrate therapy.

Adverse effects include postural hypotension, syncope, nausea and vomiting, and muscle weakness. Severe hypotension and syncope are seen with less than 1 percent of patients.

11. Are hypersensitivity reactions seen with nitrates?

Yes. These include flushing of the skin, excessive sweating, sinus tachycardia, syncope, and palpitations. Severe reactions may lead to cardiovascular collapse.

12. Explain the occurrence of methemoglobinemia with nitrate therapy.

Methemoglobinemia is a rare occurrence with nitrate therapy and is characterized by cyanosis, and nausea/vomiting, progressing to shock and coma. This rare adverse effect is usually associated with high doses/overdoses of nitrate products, but can also be seen at normal therapeutic doses.

13. Does nitroglycerin increase coronary blood flow?

No. This drug increases coronary perfusion.

14. Which form of glyceryl trinitrate (nitroglycerin) would be used during an acute attack of angina?

The sublingual form, as it has a rapid onset (< 1 minute).

15. Would sublingual nitroglycerin be appropriate for maintenance therapy?

No, as the duration of action is too short. This form is used for acute attacks only.

16. Which forms of nitroglycerin are useful in maintenance therapy?

The extended release tablet form and transdermal patch or percutaneous ointment are useful in maintenance therapy, because they have a longer (or sustained release) action.

17. Does tolerance develop to antianginal therapy with isosorbide mononitrate?

Yes. Tolerance and attenuation of the vasodilatory effects of the drug may be seen. This event appears to be related to elevated plasma levels of drug.

18. Explain how tolerance to isosorbide nitrates might be minimized.

Tolerance effects are minimized in susceptible individuals by changes in dosing. Smaller doses are given at increased intervals (e.g., twice a day [BID]), and drug-free intervals are added as required.

19. Compare isosorbide dinitrate with the mononitrate form in antianginal therapy.

Both drugs have exactly the same mechanism of action. However, the onset of isosorbide mononitrate may be faster, because it takes longer for the dinitrate form to be enzymatically converted to the mononitrate form. Isosorbide dinitrate may have increased potency as a vasodilator, due to its additional nitrate group.

20. Why are potent vasodilators such as hydralazine not effective in anginal therapy?

Drugs that potently dilate arterioles can cause a phenomenon known as "coronary steal," whereby the increase in flow caused by the arteriolar dilation draws blood from unobstructed vessels and increases flow to areas already well perfused. This "steals" blood preferentially from vessels which may be obstructed (have lesser flow), and decreases perfusion in those areas which may already be ischemic.

CALCIUM CHANNEL ANTAGONISTS

21. Discuss the advantages of calcium channel antagonists in the therapy of angina.

These drugs induce vasodilatation and increase myocardial perfusion, in addition to decreasing preload and afterload (which decreases the work of the heart and thus decreases myocardial oxygen consumption). Calcium channel antagonists may also depress myocardial conduction and heart rate, resulting in an increase in diastolic perfusion time. The negative inotropic effect produced by the drugs results in decreased oxygen consumption, and lessens coronary vascular compression.

22. What are the detriments of using calcium channel blockers in angina?

The cardiodepression produced by these agents may limit the activity of the patient. In addition, most drugs of this class produce hypotension.

23. Are all calcium channel antagonists used in the therapy of angina?

No. Some drugs (e.g., isradipine, felodipine, nimodipine) have low bioavailability and are not approved for the treatment of angina. The choice of drug used depends largely on the individual requirements of the patient.

24. Describe the benefits of nifedipine therapy in angina.

Nifedipine is a vasoactive drug and thus decreases coronary spasm, allowing a greater degree of myocardial perfusion. In addition, the drug decreases afterload, which decreases the work of the heart, and preload, which decreases myocardial stretch, as well as passive coronary vascular compression. Thus, myocardial oxygen consumption is decreased and perfusion is increased.

25. Would verapamil be appropriate therapy for a patient with 1° heart block?

No. Verapamil decreases conduction velocity in the calcium dependent portion of the atrioventricular (AV) node.

26. Describe an appropriate antianginal therapy for a patient with hypotension.

A drug that has reduced vasoactive action is most appropriate in such a patient. Verapamil, diltiazem, bepridil, or a β_1 antagonist would be useful.

27. Discuss the mechanism of action and therapeutic use of amlodipine in the therapy of angina pectoris.

Amlodipine is a potent peripheral vasodilator, which decreases cardiac afterload and thus decreases cardiac work and myocardial oxygen consumption. Coronary arteries are also dilated, increasing oxygen delivery to the myocardium. Amlodipine is useful in both chronic stable angina and Prinzmetal's angina.

28. Does amlodipine decrease cardiac preload?

No. It is primarily a vasodilator, and does not affect venous capacitance.

29. Discuss the effects of amlodipine on the myocardium.

Amlodipine has little effect on myocardial tissues. It does not significantly reduce conduction, nor does it have significant negative inotropic activity.

30. Why does amlodipine not induce significant reflex tachycardia?

The drug has a gradual onset, and thus does not cause significant baroreceptor stimulation.

31. Should amlodipine be taken orally with grapefruit juice?

No. Chemical substances present in grapefruit juice inhibit cytochrome P_{450} isoenzymes involved in amlodipine metabolism. These substances decrease the first-pass metabolism of the drug and increase serum concentrations.

32. For which types of angina is bepridil effective?

Bepridil is used as a second line drug in the therapy of chronic stable angina.

33. Describe the use of bepridil in the therapy of angina.

Bepridil is used as antianginal therapy in patients with angina that has shown to be refractory to therapy with other drugs. It is not used as first line therapy, primarily due to the proarrhythmic properties of the drug.

34. Why is nicardipine useful in the therapy of angina?

Nicardipine selectively dilates cerebral and coronary vessels. Thus, myocardial blood flow and oxygen delivery are increased, but performance is not.

35. Explain why nicardipine is useful in the treatment of a patient with congestive heart failure (CHF) and angina.

Nicardipine does not decrease myocardial contractility and so would be especially useful for antianginal therapy in a patient with CHF.

36. What are the advantages of using nisoldipine for the therapy of angina?

Nisoldipine is long-acting, vasoactive, and approximately equipotent to amlodipine in the amelioration of angina.

37. Does nisoldipine have negative inotropic effects at clinical doses?

No. Effects are mainly in the vasculature.

BETA-RECEPTOR ANTAGONISTS

38. Describe the beneficial effects of beta-receptor antagonists in the therapy of angina.

These drugs block sympathetic stimulation of the myocardium, resulting in decreased heart rate and force of contraction. The decreased rate results in an increase in diastolic perfusion time and, therefore, increased oxygenation of the myocardium, while the negative inotropic effect results in a decrease in oxygen demand.

39. Compare the efficacy of propranolol and atenolol in the therapy of angina.

Atenolol is a selective β_1 receptor antagonist, and mediates a decrease in heart rate and force of contraction. This results in increased oxygen delivery and decreased myocardial oxygen consumption. β_2 receptors are relatively unaffected, so sympathetic activity results in vasodilatation and decreased afterload. Propranolol blocks vasodilatory effects with sympathetic stimulation. This may result in an increase in afterload (as compared to the effects of atenolol) and increased myocardial oxygen consumption.

40. Discuss the merits of atenolol and metoprolol as antianginal therapy.

Both of these drugs are selective antagonists at the β_1 receptor, and therefore relatively cardioselective. This results in less adverse effects in patients with diabetes and asthma.

41. Describe the beneficial effects of pindolol in antianginal therapy.

Pindolol causes a net vasodilatation, and thus decreases afterload, resulting in decreased myocardial oxygen consumption.

COMBINATION THERAPY

42. Discuss the advantages and disadvantages of combination therapy with a beta-blocker and nitrate in angina.

This combination is useful, as the two effects of the drugs synergize, allowing lower doses of each drug to be used. The cardiodepressant actions of the beta-blocker decrease the rate and force of contraction. Concurrently administered, the nitrates decrease cardiac afterload, which increases the ejection fraction of the heart and reduces end diastolic volume, in addition to decreasing myocardial oxygen consumption. Additionally, the compensatory sympathetic reflexes produced by the nitrates are inhibited by the presence of the beta receptor blockers.

43. Discuss combination therapy with atenolol and nifedipine.

These drugs synergize effects well—atenolol decreases myocardial oxygen consumption through negative inotropic and chronotropic effects, while nifedipine mediates coronary arteriolar dilatation and increased oxygen delivery. In addition, nifedipine decreases myocardial oxygen consumption by decreasing afterload. The presence of the beta-blocker also blocks reflex sympathetic effects caused by the nifedipine-mediated vasodilatation.

44. Would combination therapy with any beta-blocker and a calcium channel blocker be efficacious?

Not necessarily. The most efficacious combinations are those in which the mechanisms of action of the drugs compliment each other. For example, diltiazem, with strong cardiodepressant actions, would not be suitable in combination with propranolol, which also has negative inotropic and chronotropic activity.

45. Is antianginal combination therapy with more than one drug appropriate?

Yes, depending on the drugs involved. For example, an appropriate calcium channel blocker, beta-blocker and nitrate may be combined.

BIBLIOGRAPHY

1. Abrams JG: Medical therapy of unstable angina and non-Q-wave myocardial infarction. Am J Cardiol 86(8B):24J–33J; [discussion] 33J-34J, 2000.
2. Abrams J: Medical therapy of unstable angina and non-q-wave myocardial infarction. Am J Cardiol 86(8 Suppl 2):24–33, 2000.
3. Azevedo ER, Schofield AM, Kelly S, et al: Nitroglycerin withdrawal increases endothelium-dependent vasomotor response to acetylcholine. J Am Coll Cardiol 37(2):505–509, 2001.
4. Boon D, Piek JJ, van Montfrans GA: Silent ischaemia and hypertension. J Hypertens 18(10):1355–1364, 2000.
5. Braunwald E, Califf RM, Cannon CP, et al: Redefining medical treatment in the management of unstable angina. Am J Med 108(1):41–53, 2000.
6. Di Pastena A, Fioranelli M, Celleno D, et al: SCS in intractable angina. Minerva Anestesiol 66(11):825–827, 2000.
7. Ferguson JJ: Combining low-molecular-weight heparin and glycoprotein IIb/iiia antagonists for the treatment of acute coronary syndromes: The NICE 3 story. J Invasive Cardiol 12 Suppl E:E10–E13, 2000.
8. Hardman J, Limbird L, Gilman A: Goodman & Gilman's The Pharmacological Basis of Therapeutics, 10th ed. McGraw-Hill Publishers, 2001.
9. Holmes DR: Acute coronary syndromes: Extending medical intervention for five days before proceeding to revascularization. Am J Cardiol 86(12B):36M–41M, 2000.
10. Ishikawa K, Yamamoto T, Kanamasa K, et al: Intermittent nitrate therapy for prior myocardial infarction does not induce rebound angina nor reduce cardiac events. Secondary prevention group. Intern Med 39(12):1020–1026, 2000.
11. Jackson G: Stable angina: Maximal medical therapy is not the same as optimal medical therapy. Int J Clin Pract 54(6):351, 2000.
12. Jansen R, Niemeyer MG, Cleophas TJ, et al: Independent determinants of the efficacy of nitrate therapy. Int J Clin Pharmacol Ther 38(12):563–567, 2000.
13. Katzung, B: Basic and Clinical Pharmacology, 8th ed. Appleton & Lange, 2001.
14. Kendall MJ, Nuttall SL: Anti-oxidant therapy for the treatment of coronary artery disease. Expert Opin Investig Drugs 8(11):1763–1784, 1999.
15. Markham A, Plosker GL, Goa KL: Nicorandil. An updated review of its use in ischemic heart disease with emphasis on its cardioprotective effects. Drugs 60(4):955–974, 2000.
16. Marso SP, Bhatt DL, Roe MT, et al: Enhanced efficacy of eptifibatide administration in patients with acute coronary syndrome requiring in-hospital coronary artery bypass grafting. Circulation 102(24):2952–2958, 2000.
17. Murad MB, Henry TD. Unstable angina. Current treatment options in cardiovascular medicine. 2(1):37–54, 2000.
18. O'Connor R, Persse D, Zachariah B, et al: Acute coronary syndrome: Pharmacotherapy. Prehosp Emerg Care 5(1):58–64, 2001.
19. Pehrsson SK, Ringqvist I, Ekdahl S, et al: Monotherapy with amlodipine or atenolol versus their combination in stable angina pectoris. Clin Cardiol 23(10):763–770, 2000.
20. Pepine CJ: An ischemia-guided approach for risk stratification in patients with acute coronary syndromes. Am J Cardiol 86(12B):27M–35M, 2000.

21. Shapira OM, Alkon JD, Macron DS, et al: Nitroglycerin is preferable to diltiazem for prevention of coronary bypass conduit spasm. Ann Thorac Surg 70(3):883–888; [discussion 888–889], 2000.
22. Schwartz JS: Ischemic heart disease. Current treatment options in cardiovascular medicine. 2(1):27–36, 2000.
23. Szwed H, Sadowski Z, Kowalik LL, et al: What intervals in oral therapy of isosorbide dinitrate in various doses are sufficient to prevent nitrate tolerance? Med Sci Monit 6(4):763–768, 2000.
24. White HD: Targeting therapy in unstable angina. J Invasive Cardiol 10 Suppl D:12D–21D, 1998.
Websites:
Clinical Pharmacology 2000: http://cp.gsm.com
Medline plus: http://medlineplus.nlm.nih.gov/medlineplus/
Medscape Multispecialty Journal Room: http://pharmacotherapy.medscape.com/Home/Topics/multispecialty/directories/dir-MULT.JournalRoom.html
Medscape Pharmacotherapy News (cardiology):
http://cardiology.medscape.com/home/topics/pharmacotherapy/directories/dir-PHAR.News.html

16. THERAPY OF CARDIAC ARRHYTHMIAS

1. Describe the desired mechanism of action of an antiarrhythmic used in the therapy of atrial arrhythmias.

A drug used in the therapy of atrial arrhythmias should decrease atrial conduction and should also cause partial blockade of the atrioventricular (AV) node. This confines the arrhythmia to the atria and prevents the induction of ventricular arrhythmias. These drugs normally decrease conduction in the sodium-dependent portion of the AV node.

2. Do drugs used in the therapy of ventricular arrhythmias decrease conduction in the AV node?

No. Decreased conduction in the AV node is not desired in this case, as the influence of the sinoatrial (SA) node is necessary to keep ectopic foci in check.

3. Discuss the effect of catecholamines on the etiology of arrhythmias.

Catecholamines increase conduction rate in excitable tissue and bring the membrane potential closer to threshold. Thus, an excess of catecholamines, or sensitivity of the heart to catecholamines (e.g., by thyroid hormone) will increase the frequency of arrhythmias.

CLASS I ANTIARRHYTHMICS

4. Describe the general mechanism of action of class I antiarrhythmics.

These drugs block sodium channels. They essentially act as local anesthetics, reducing the conduction rate and amplitude of electrical impulses.

5. Describe blood dyscrasias seen with class I antiarrhythmic drugs.

Hematologic conditions caused by class I agents include hemolytic anemia (especially in patients with glucose-6-phosphate dehydrogenase [G6PD] deficiency), aplastic anemia, leukopenia, agranulocytosis, and thrombocytopenic purpura.

6. Which agents are classified as class Ia antiarrhythmics?

The prototypes for this class are quinidine, disopyramide, and procainamide. This class also includes amiodarone and the tricyclic antidepressant imipramine, which has antiarrhythmic properties.

7. Which drugs of the class Ia subset of antiarrhythmics have been shown to cause a lupus-like syndrome?

Quinidine and procainamide have both been shown to cause a syndrome resembling lupus. Symptoms may include polyarthritis, fever, and pleuritic chest pain.

8. Describe the effect of class Ia agents on action potential duration.

These drugs lengthen the duration of the action potential.

9. What is the major therapeutic use of quinidine?

Quinidine is used in the therapy of atrial arrhythmias, particularly atrial flutter and atrial fibrillation. It is also useful in other types of arrhythmias (e.g., v-tac), and is also useful in the treatment of malaria, when given intravenously.

10. Discuss in detail the effect of quinidine on the cardiac action potential.

Quinidine blocks sodium channels and also blocks potassium channels. Thus, phase 0 of the cardiac action potential is blunted, due to the sodium blockade, and the plateau phase (2) is lengthened, due to the decrease in the rate of efflux of potassium, and decreased rate of repolarization. Phase 3 is lengthened, as well, and decreased in slope, giving rise to oscillatory after-depolarizations in the resting phase (see Figure).

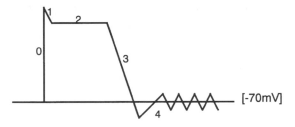

The cardiac action potential—effects of the administration of quinidine.

11. What is the significance of the oscillatory afterdepolarizations produced by quinidine?

These oscillations set the stage for the development of torsades de pointes, a potentially lethal cardiac arrhythmia.

12. What is the hallmark of quinidine toxicity?

A group of symptoms, collectively known as cinchonism. These symptoms include headache, dizziness, and tinnitus.

13. Discuss the direct actions of quinidine on the heart.

Through blockade of sodium channels, particularly in the AV node, the drug slows conduction and depresses cardiac excitability. In addition, blockade of potassium channels delays repolarization.

14. Discuss the indirect actions of quinidine on the myocardium.

Quinidine has antimuscarinic actions, and inhibits vagal tone. Thus, the increase in sympathetic activity may precipitate an increase in conduction rate and ventricular tachycardia.

15. What are the cardiac reflex actions induced by quinidine?

This drug mediates α-adrenoceptor blockade, particularly when administered rapidly. This results in vasodilatation and reflex tachycardia.

16. Describe the phenomenon of "*quinidine syncope*."

The onset of quinidine syncope is associated with a long QT interval, and includes light-headedness, fainting, and an oscillatory cardiac rhythm known as torsades de pointes.

17. Discuss the interaction of quinidine and drugs such as warfarin, digoxin, and carbamazepine.

Quinidine is highly plasma protein-bound (> 85 percent) and thus competes with other drugs that are highly protein-bound for storage sites on plasma proteins. Thus, concurrent administration of quinidine with highly plasma protein-bound drugs such as benzodiazepines, carbamazepine, warfarin and digoxin increases the plasma concentration of these drugs, leading to toxicity.

18. Does quinidine block all sodium channels?

No. The drug primarily blocks resting sodium channels. Once the membrane has been depolarized, the drug is less effective.

19. Describe the mechanism of action of procainamide.

This drug blocks both depolarized sodium channels and resting channels.

20. Compare the antimuscarinic effects of quinidine, disopyramide, and procainamide.

The antimuscarinic effects of quinidine are much more pronounced than those of procainamide. Thus, the cardiodepressant effects of procainamide are not offset by an increase in sympathetic tone. The antimuscarinic effects of disopyramide are greater than those of quinidine, thus increasing the potential for generation of ventricular tachyarrhythmias.

21. Relate disopyramide dose to toxicity.
The relationship is nonlinear. The drug is highly protein-bound, and, with increasing dose, the binding sites become saturated. Thus, with increasing saturation of binding sites, a relatively small increase in dose results in a disproportionately large increase in plasma free-drug concentration, and toxic effects are generated. Thus, total plasma concentration is not an accurate measure of potential toxicity.

22. Describe the actions of disopyramide on cardiac contractility.
Disopyramide has a strong negative inotropic action, and can produce ventricular failure in patients with preexisting left ventricular dysfunction.

23. Can disopyramide produce myocardial failure in patients with no myocardial dysfunction?
Yes. These instances are rare, but do occur.

24. What is the clinical use of disopyramide?
Disopyramide is useful in the amelioration of a variety of supraventricular arrhythmias. However, in the United States, it is only approved for use in the treatment of ventricular arrhythmias.

25. Compare disopyramide to other class Ia agents.
Of all of the class Ia agents, disopyramide has the longest half-life, is the most negatively inotropic, and causes the most anticholinergic side effects.

26. What are the prototypical drugs included in class Ib antiarrhythmics?
This class includes lidocaine, phenytoin, tocainide and mexiletine.

27. Describe the effect of class Ib agents on action potential duration.
These drugs do not affect action potential duration.

28. Are class Ib agents effective in the treatment of ventricular fibrillation?
No. These agents are the least effective of the class I agents in the therapy of lethal arrhythmias.

29. Does lidocaine cause AV nodal blockade?
No. AV nodal conduction is not impaired, making the drug useful for the therapy of ventricular arrhythmias.

30. What is the major therapeutic use of lidocaine, as a class Ib antiarrhythmic?
Lidocaine is used in the therapy of non-life-threatening ventricular arrhythmias, such as nonsustained ventricular tachycardia and frequent premature ventricular beats. It is also used as an adjunct to defibrillation and cardiopulmonary resuscitation (CPR) in patients with ventricular tachycardia and/or fibrillation.

31. Why is lidocaine administered parenterally?
This drug has a very high first-pass effect and is degraded rapidly if given orally.

32. Describe the pharmacodynamics of lidocaine.
Lidocaine is highly plasma protein-bound (40 to 70 percent) to α_1-glycoproteins.

33. Would lidocaine be suitable for administration to a patient with liver dysfunction?
No, as the drug is 90 percent metabolized by the liver.

34. Describe the half-life of lidocaine.
The half-life is very short—approximately 20 minutes in a normal patient.

35. Describe the symptoms of lidocaine toxicity.

Initially, with high dose, the patient may experience drowsiness, vertigo, twitching, and disorientation. At higher plasma concentrations (> 9 μg/ml) psychosis, convulsions, and respiratory depression are seen.

36. What are the orally active derivatives of lidocaine that are presently marketed?

Tocainide and mexiletine are orally active derivatives of lidocaine recently introduced.

37. Discuss the mechanism of action of tocainide.

This drug binds to both sodium and potassium channels, inhibiting recovery after repolarization of the membrane.

38. Describe the therapeutic uses of tocainide.

Tocainide is used in the treatment of ventricular arrhythmias including unifocal and multifocal ventricular premature contractions, coupled ventricular premature contractions, and paroxysmal ventricular tachycardia.

39. Describe the potentially lethal hematologic effects seen with tocainide therapy.

These effects are rare. They include neutropenia, leukopenia, agranulocytosis, bone marrow depression, hemolysis, hypoplastic anemia, aplastic anemia, eosinophilia, or thrombocytopenia.

40. Discuss the onset of adverse hematological effects seen with tocainide therapy.

Adverse hematological effects usually occur within 2 to 12 weeks after therapy is initiated. They are, however, reversible, as blood cell counts will return to normal with discontinuation of the drug.

41. What adverse pulmonary effects may be seen with tocainide therapy?

These events are rare, but include pulmonary fibrosis, fibrosing alveolitis, interstitial pneumonitis, pulmonary embolism, pneumonia, and pulmonary edema, and respiratory arrest.

42. What is the clinical use of mexiletine?

This drug is used to treat life-threatening ventricular arrhythmias.

43. Describe the mechanism of action of mexiletine.

This drug inhibits fast sodium channels in the myocardial cell membrane. Thus, automaticity is decreased in His-Purkinje fibers. Conduction velocity is, however, not affected.

44. Refer to the figure on the next page and describe the effect of mexiletine on the cardiac action potential and the effective refractory period (ERP).

ERP includes both the action potential duration and the time for membrane repolarization and stimulus to threshold. Mexiletine, by blocking fast sodium channels, blunts the amplitude of the cardiac action potential (phase 0 is decreased). The decrease in sodium influx and decrease in phase 0 amplitude results in a lower membrane potential as the action potential enters phase 2 and 3. This results in the membrane potential, at the end of phase 0, being closer to the membrane potential for potassium and calcium, so the influx of these ions is of shorter duration, resulting in a decrease in the length of phase 1 and 2 and a steeper slope of phase 3 repolarization. Phase 4, however, is lengthened, and the rate of rise decreased, with the decrease in the rate of sodium influx. Thus, the cardiac membrane remains relatively refractory, even after repolarization, and the ratio of the ERP to the action potential duration increases.

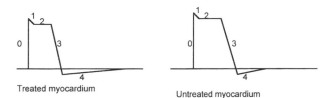

Treated myocardium

Untreated myocardium

45. List the prototypical drugs classified as class Ic antiarrhythmics.

Flecainide and encainide are prototypical class Ic agents. Also included in this class are moricizine and propafenone.

46. Discuss the effect of class Ic agents on cardiac action potential duration.

These drugs have little effect on the duration of the action potential. However, sodium current depression is much more pronounced with this subclass than with class Ia or Ib, which may result in a depression of amplitude.

47. Describe the major toxicity of class Ic agents.

These drugs have proarrhythmic effects.

48. What changes in the electrocardiogram (ECG) would be seen with administration of class Ic agents?

These agents cause a widening of the QRS complex, due to slowed conduction in the His-Purkinje system. P-R and Q-T intervals are also prolonged.

49. Does flecainide affect the influx of calcium into myocardial cells?

Yes, but this effect is only seen at high doses.

50. Is flecainide useful in the treatment of reentrant cardiac arrhythmias?

Yes. The drug is effective in the therapy of both reentrant and nonreentrant forms of cardiac arrhythmia.

51. What is the pharmacologic duration of action of flecainide?

The drug is therapeutically active for 24 to 48 hours. In patients with renal impairment, this is increased.

52. State the relationship between propranolol and propafenone.

Propafenone is a derivative of propranolol.

53. Discuss the mechanism of action of propafenone.

Propafenone, like flecainide, inhibits fast sodium channels. It also has intrinsic beta-receptor blocking activity.

54. Does propafenone exhibit β-blocking activity clinically? Explain.

The β-receptor antagonist action of propafenone is very weak as compared to true antagonists (e.g., propranolol). The plasma concentrations of the drug when used therapeutically are, however, almost 50 times that of propranolol. Thus β-receptor antagonist activity is clinically manifested.

55. Describe the actions of propafenone on the AV node.

Propafenone decreases both automaticity and conduction velocity in the AV node.

56. Discuss the inter-patient variability of orally administered propafenone.

This drug has an extensive first pass effect, and is more extensively metabolized by some patients than others. Thus, in some patients, the half-life of the drug may be as little as 2 hours, while in others it may be as much as 32 hours.

CLASS II ANTIARRHYTHMIC DRUGS

57. What is the general mechanism of action of class II antiarrhythmics?

These drugs decrease calcium flux in the AV node, and decrease the excitability of cardiac tissue. This class includes β_1-receptor antagonists (e.g., esmolol) and pan-beta receptor antagonists (e.g., propranolol).

58. Describe the use of esmolol as an antiarrhythmic drug.

Esmolol is a beta antagonist with a short half-life. Thus, it is most useful in the therapy of acute arrhythmias, and as an adjunct to surgical procedures.

59. What are the advantages of antiarrhythmic therapy with nadolol?

Nadolol has no partial agonist activity, no local anesthetic action, and is long-acting.

60. Is propranolol useful in the therapy of ventricular arrhythmias?

No. The drug decreases conduction in AV nodal tissue, which could result in exacerbation of ventricular arrhythmias. The drug is primarily used for supraventricular arrhythmias.

61. Describe the properties desirable in a β-receptor antagonist used in the therapy of arrhythmias.

Ideally, these drugs should be potent, selective for the β_1 receptor, have low to moderate lipid solubility, and be devoid of agonist activity.

CLASS III ANTIARRHYTHMIC DRUGS

62. Describe the mechanism of action of antiarrhythmics classified as class III.

The drugs prolong the cardiac action potential through increases in intracellular potassium. These drugs may achieve this result either by enhancing inward flux of potassium through changes in sodium or calcium flux, or by blocking the outward flux of potassium.

63. Describe the effect of class III antiarrhythmics on the cardiac action potential.

Phase 2 of the cardiac action potential is prolonged, due to the blockade of potassium flux decreasing the excitability of tissue and thus inhibiting the spontaneous formation of ectopic foci.

64. Are class III antiarrhythmics interchangeable?

No. Each drug has its own mechanism of action in modifying conduction.

65. Discuss the actions of bretylium on noradrenergic terminals.

Bretylium releases norepinephrine from the sympathetic ganglia and postganglionic adrenergic nerve terminals, and blocks norepinephrine reuptake.

66. How is bretylium eliminated?

Eighty percent of the drug is eliminated unchanged in the urine. Thus, dosage adjustments may be necessary in patients with renal dysfunction. Clearance of the drug is directly proportional to creatinine clearance, and thus may be predicted.

67. What is the primary clinical use of dofetilide?

Dofetilide, a recently approved class III antiarrhythmic, is primarily used in the therapy of atrial fibrillation.

68. What is the classification of ibutilide?

Ibutilide is a classified as a pure class III antiarrhythmic, with novel mechanism of action.

69. What is the mechanism of action of ibutilide?

Ibutilide increases the transport of sodium into the cardiac myocyte during the plateau phase of the cardiac action potential. The net effect of the drug is a prolongation of the action potential, and a decrease in membrane excitability, as repolarization is decreased.

70. Does ibutilide have an effect on potassium permeability?

To the extent that sodium flux is increased, potassium flux may also be decreased. However, the drug has a substantially decreased effect on the blockade of outward potassium current, as compared to that of sodium.

71. Describe the major clinical use of ibutilide.

Ibutilide is used in the therapy of atrial fibrillation and atrial flutter.

72. Does ibutilide produce hypotension?

No.

73. Does Ibutilide affect ventricular rhythm?

Ibutilide has been shown to induce ventricular tachyarrhythmias in 2 percent of patients.

74. Describe the efficacy of ibutilide in the ablation of atrial fibrillation and flutter.

Ibutilide terminates atrial fibrillation in approximately 35 percent of cases and terminates atrial flutter in a larger percentage of patients within 1 hour of administration.

75. Is there a high risk of torsades de pointes associated with ibutilide?

No. This drug has a very low risk of inducing torsades.

76. Explain the clinical use of amiodarone.

Amiodarone is useful as an antianginal agent and as an antiarrhythmic. In the United States, it is used only in the therapy of life-threatening ventricular arrhythmias.

77. Compare the mechanism of action of amiodarone with those of quinidine and disopyramide.

Quinidine primarily blocks sodium channels in the depolarized state; disopyramide has an affinity for sodium channels in both depolarized and inactive states; and amiodarone primarily blocks inactive sodium channels.

78. Compare the relative safety of quinidine and amiodarone with respect to their mechanisms of action.

Quinidine blocks open sodium channels, which decreases the rate of repolarization in a dose-dependent manner. Thus, the cardiac tissue may still depolarize normally, and the propensity for cardiac failure is lessened. Amiodarone, conversely, blocks resting channels, preventing depolarization in a dose-dependent manner. This could prevent excitation, particularly if the drug is in excess, leading to cardiac failure. Thus, this drug has a more pronounced cardiodepressant effect, as compared to quinidine, and a smaller margin of safety.

79. Explain the actions of amiodarone on peripheral vascular dilatation.

Amiodarone inhibits the activity of both vascular calcium channels, and α-adrenoceptors. Thus, a net vasodilatation is produced. This effect occurs mainly with intravenous administration.

80. Discuss the toxic effects of amiodarone on the lung.

Amiodarone can cause pulmonary fibrosis, particularly at higher dosages (> 400mg/day).

81. Describe the distribution of amiodarone.

This drug is sequestered by virtually every tissue. It may be found in major organs, and is particularly concentrated in the cornea, where it forms microcrystals appearing as brown deposits in the eye.

82. What adverse effects are seen with amiodarone?

A multitude of adverse effects are common, including cardiac effects, neurologic dysfunction (paresthesias, tremor, ataxia, cephalalgia), gastrointestinal (GI) dysfunction, lung dysfunction and hepatocellular necrosis.

83. Describe the half-life of amiodarone.

Amiodarone has an extremely long half-life—up to 103 days. It may be as long as several weeks before the effects of the drug decrease after the drug is withdrawn, due to the long half-life and tissue sequestration.

84. Does orally administered amiodarone require a loading dose?

Yes. The drug is heavily sequestered in tissue. Thus, large doses for up to 30 days are required to load the drug to therapeutic plasma concentrations. Maintenance doses are conversely quite low and may be administered once per day.

85. Is amiodarone administered intravenously?

Yes, in cases of recurring ventricular tachycardia or as emergency therapy for ventricular fibrillation.

86. Describe the actions of dronedarone.

Dronedarone is a derivative of amiodarone and has similar properties. However, it has less organ toxicity.

87. Does sotalol have proarrhythmic characteristics?

Yes.

88. How can the proarrhythmic manifestations of sotalol be minimized?

The appearance of drug-induced arrhythmias may be minimized by monitoring the QT interval lengthening, and by adjusting the dose relative to calculated creatinine.

CLASS IV ANTIARRHYTHMIC DRUGS

89. Describe the mechanism of action of class IV antiarrhythmics.

These drugs are cardiac calcium channel blockers. By decreasing calcium conduction in the calcium-dependent portions of the AV node, His' bundle and in the myocardium itself, ectopic foci can be suppressed.

90. Describe the effect of class IV antiarrhythmics on the cardiac action potential.

These drugs block the influx of calcium. Thus, phase 2 of the cardiac action potential is prolonged, because an increased amount of time is required to reach the calcium potential.

91. Would class IV antiarrhythmics be useful in ventricular arrhythmias arising from ectopic foci in the Purkinje fibers?

No. Purkinje fibers are sodium dependent, and, thus, this class of drugs would be less effective.

92. Would a calcium channel blocker such as nifedipine be useful as an antiarrhythmic agent?

No. Nifedipine has its major activity in the vasculature and has little action on the myocardium or cardiac conduction pathways.

93. Which calcium channel blocker is most effective in the therapy of paroxysmal atrial tachycardia?

Verapamil, because it slows conduction in the AV node, and prolongs the refractory period.

94. Describe the actions of verapamil in the therapy of atrial flutter and atrial fibrillation.

Due to partial blockade of the AV node, verapamil slows ventricular response in atrial flutter and fibrillation.

MISCELLANEOUS ANTIARRHYTHMIC AGENTS

95. Explain the use of magnesium as an antiarrhythmic.

Magnesium has been shown to affect the conduction of both sodium and potassium in the heart, which may be due, at least in part, to the dependence of cardiac adenosinetriphosphatase (ATPase) on magnesium. It also competes with calcium and thus decreases calcium conductance across the cardiac membranes, resulting in a prolongation of phase II of the cardiac action potential. Given intravenously, it has been shown to decrease digitalis-induced arrhythmias and torsades de pointes in susceptible patients, as well as arrhythmias produced by myocardial ischemia (e.g., due to infarction).

96. Describe the therapeutic use of adenosine.

Adenosine is most useful in the therapy of supraventricular tachycardias such as Wolff-Parkinson-White syndrome. It is not effective against "normal" atrial arrhythmias such as atrial flutter and atrial fibrillation.

97. Explain the mechanism of action of adenosine in the therapy of paroxysmal atrial tachycardia (PAT).

Adenosine is a potent vasodilator that is produced endogenously. It mediates an outward flow of potassium from adenosine-sensitive potassium channels, stabilizing cardiac membranes. This results in a decrease in the duration of the atrial action potential, as well as negative chronotropic and inotropic actions. In addition, by stabilizing excitable tissue in the AV node, the drug effectively inhibits the conversion of paroxysmal atrial tachycardia to ventricular tachycardia, which could lead to fibrillation.

98. Is adenosine therapy effective in ventricular tachycardia?

No. Once established, ventricular tachycardia is not responsive to adenosine.

99. Why would adenosine not precipitate reflex tachycardia?

Adenosine is a vasodilator, but does not precipitate reflex tachycardia due to antiadrenergic actions and a very brief duration of action.

100. What is the duration of action of intravenous adenosine?

The documented half-life is approximately 10 seconds.

101. Does adenosine precipitate hypotension?

No. Acute hypotensive episodes, such as those seen with calcium channel antagonists, are not seen, due to the brief duration of action of the drug.

102. How is adenosine eliminated?

Adenosine is taken up into erythrocytes and vascular endothelial cells and degraded by nucleases.

103. Discuss the use of digitalis glycosides in the therapy of atrial arrhythmias.

Digitalis glycosides decrease conduction in the AV node, due to a combination of effects, including increased parasympathetic outflow and changes in conductance of sodium, potassium and calcium (all of which are involved in AV nodal conduction).

Questions 104–105: The following traces of cardiac action potentials (see Figure) represent control and drug treated patients. Answer the following with regard to these traces.

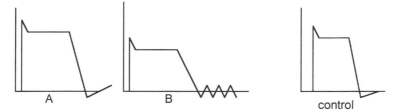

104. Patient "A" was treated with quinidine, lidocaine or verapamil. Identify the drug, and explain.

In this case, the amplitude of phase 0 is not blunted, indicating that the drug does not block fast sodium channels. Phase 2 is lengthened somewhat, consistent with a calcium channel blocker—the dose-dependent blockade of calcium channels allows less calcium to pass across the membrane per time, thus increasing the length of time taken to reach the equilibrium potential for calcium. Phase 3 is not affected, indicating that the drug has no effect on potassium flux. The drug is thus identified as verapamil.

105. Patient "B" was treated with a class I antiarrhythmic. Identify the drug, and explain.

The oscillatory afterpotentials seen post-repolarization give the first clue that the drug is quinidine. Quinidine blocks sodium channels, which is consistent with the blunting of the amplitude or phase 0, and also potassium channels, which is consistent with the lengthening of phase 2 and the decrease in the slope of phase 3. The drug is thus identified as quinidine, a class Ia antiarrhythmic.

BIBLIOGRAPHY

1. Atarashi H, Kuruma A, Yashima M, et al: Pharmacokinetics of landiolol hydrochloride, a new ultra-short-acting beta-blocker, in patients with cardiac arrhythmias. Clin Pharmacol Ther 68(2):143–150, 2000.
2. Auricchio A, Klein H: Arrhythmias in heart failure. Current Treatment Options in Cardiovascular Medicine 2(4):329–339, 2000.
3. Chaudhry GM, Haffajee CI: Antiarrhythmic agents and proarrhythmia. Crit Care Med 28(10 Suppl):N158–N164, 2000.
4. Hardman J, Limbird L, Gilman A: Goodman & Gilman's The Pharmacological Basis of Therapeutics, 10th ed. McGraw-Hill Publishers, 2001.
5. Katzung, B: Basic and Clinical Pharmacology, 8th ed. Appleton & Lange, 2001.
6. Levy S: Pharmacologic management of atrial fibrillation: Current therapeutic strategies. Am Heart J 141(2 Pt 2):15–21, 2001.
7. Lewis RV: Atrial fibrillation. The therapeutic options. Drugs 40(6):841–853, 1990.
8. Luber S, Brady WJ, Joyce T, et al: Paroxysmal supraventricular tachycardia: Outcome after ED care. Am J Emerg Med 19(1):40–42, 2001.
9. Nattel S, Hadjis T, Talajic M: The treatment of atrial fibrillation. An evaluation of drug therapy, electrical modalities and therapeutic considerations. Drugs 48(3):345–371, 1994.
10. Prystowsky EN: Management of atrial fibrillation: Therapeutic options and clinical decisions. Am J Cardiol 85(10 Suppl 1):3–11, 2000.
11. Reiffel JA: Drug choices in the treatment of atrial fibrillation. Am J Cardiol 85(10A):12D–19D, 2000.
12. Singh BN, Mody FV, Lopez B, et al: Antiarrhythmic agents for atrial fibrillation: Focus on prolonging atrial repolarization. Am J Cardiol 84(9A):161R–173R, 1999
13. Wang HE, O'connor RE, Megargel RE, et al: The use of diltiazem for treating rapid atrial fibrillation in the out-of-hospital setting. Ann Emerg Med 37(1):38–45, 2001.

17. DRUGS USED IN THE THERAPY OF CONGESTIVE HEART FAILURE (CHF)

1. Discuss the physiologic changes that are desirable in the therapy of CHF.

In heart failure, contractility is decreased, filling is increased, and ejection fraction is decreased. Thus, desirable changes include lowering afterload (to increase ejection fraction), lowering preload (to decrease filling), lowering of fluid volume, and increasing cardiac contractility.

2. Describe the effects of decreased ventricular filling in the failed heart.

A decrease in ventricular filling decreases myocardial wall tension, and decreases the stretch of myocardial fibers. This allows more efficient interaction between actin and myosin, and increased rebound force, resulting in increased ejection fraction.

3. Discuss conventional combination drug therapy for CHF.

Conventional therapy combines digoxin, diuretics, and angiotensin-converting enzyme (ACE) inhibitors. Digitalis glycosides increase cardiac contractility, diuretics decrease fluid volume and, therefore, ventricular fill volume, and ACE inhibitors (or vasodilators) decrease afterload without interfering with myocardial function. ACE inhibitors also decrease fluid volume.

DIURETICS

4. What role do diuretics play in the therapy of CHF?

Diuretics lower fluid volume, which decreases both preload and afterload. This decreases myocardial stretch and increases ejection fraction.

5. Describe the effects of torsemide or bumetanide in CHF therapy.

These drugs are loop diuretics and are extremely efficient in the lowering of fluid volume and decreasing myocardial stretch. They are also useful in reducing edema associated with CHF. The adverse effect of these drugs is the lowering of serum potassium, which may interfere with cardiac conduction in an already compromised heart.

6. Explain the use of amiloride in CHF therapy.

Amiloride has mild hypotensive effects, which are beneficial in treatment of CHF. It is also potassium sparing, and may be useful as adjunct therapy with loop diuretics.

DRUGS THAT DECREASE AFTERLOAD AND INCREASE CARDIAC EJECTION FRACTION

7. Are beta-blockers useful in the therapy of congestive heart failure and cardiomyopathy?

Yes. Beta-blockers, such as metoprolol, increase left ventricular ejection fraction, and reduce symptoms of CHF. In addition, they have been shown to increase survival rate in adults with cardiomyopathy.

8. Discuss the use of dobutamine in cardiac failure.

Dobutamine increases myocardial contractility with little effect on afterload or heart rate. It has no effect on sympathetic activity, and increases renal perfusion.

9. How is dobutamine administered?

This drug must be administered by continuous infusion, as it has an extremely short half-life. The adverse effects (e.g., tachycardia) may be controlled by the rate of infusion.

10. What is the advantage of using a selective β_1 agonist in the therapy of heart failure?

Because of its receptor selectivity (the lack of stimulation of the vasodilatory β_2 receptor), an agonist that is selective for the β_1 receptor tends to cause less reflex tachycardia than a pan-beta agonist.

11. Why would beta-blockers such as carvedilol and bucindolol be particularly useful in the therapy of CHF?

These drugs have intrinsic vasodilatory properties and reduce afterload.

12. Describe the use of hydralazine and related drugs in the therapy of CHF.

Hydralazine relaxes arteriolar smooth muscle, resulting in a decrease in afterload. This allows a greater proportion of ventricular volume to be ejected per beat, and decreases the stretch of cardiac fibers, resulting in more efficient contraction of ventricular myocytes.

13. Discuss the advantages of using ACE inhibitors in CHF.

ACE inhibitors decrease arterial tone by decreasing the production of angiotensin II and increasing bradykinin. In addition, a decrease in sodium retention by aldosterone is seen, which limits fluid retention and decreases blood volume. This in turn decreases ventricular filling and myocardial stretch.

DRUGS THAT DECREASE VENTRICULAR FILLING

14. How are nitrates useful in the management of heart failure?

These drugs cause dilation of veins. Venodilation results in a decrease in preload, and decreased ventricular filling, which decreases the load to the myocardium and increases myocardial efficiency (i.e., by Starling's law). The decrease in preload contributes to a decreased fiber stretch, and optimal actin-myosin interaction, which results in increased contractile force and increased myocardial efficiency.

15. Describe the benefits of sodium nitroprusside in the therapy of CHF.

Sodium nitroprusside improves left ventricular heart performance, with increases in cardiac index, cardiac output, and stroke volume. Heart rate also slows, and arrhythmias can be reduced or abolished.

16. Discuss the benefits of combination therapy with hydralazine and isosorbide dinitrate (IDN) in heart failure.

This combination decreases afterload (hydralazine), decreases preload (IDN) and increases myocardial oxygen delivery. It has not only been shown to improve performance in CHF patients, but it also has been shown to reduce mortality.

DRUGS THAT INCREASE CONTRACTILITY

17. Discuss the mechanism of action of digitalis glycosides in the therapy of CHF.

Digitalis glycosides block the activity of sodium-potassium adenosinetriphosphatase (ATPase). This inhibits the recovery of the cardiac myocyte from depolarization in a dose-dependent manner. This, in turn, results in a buildup of sodium within the cell and potassium outside of the cell, with successive depolarizations. The increase in intracellular sodium inhibits the membrane sodium-calcium transporter, allowing accumulation of calcium within the cell. The transporter may eventually reverse, and intracellular sodium is exchanged for extracellular calcium (see Figure). The resulting increase in intracellular calcium mediates an increase in the force of contraction of the cardiac muscle.

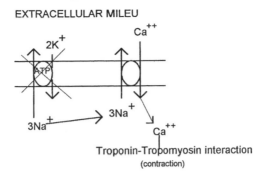

EXTRACELLULAR MILEU

Troponin-Tropomyosin interaction
(contraction)

INTRACELLULAR MILEU

Cellular actions of the cardiac glycosides—the inhibition of sodium-potassium ATPase and stimulation of the sodium-calcium transporter (bidirectional).

18. Describe the consequence of increased intracellular calcium on cardiac conduction.

Calcium overload is manifested as an early afterdepolarization of the cardiac action potential, which may result in premature depolarization of Purkinje fibers and the appearance of ventricular arrhythmias. With substantially increased calcium load, this may lead to ventricular tachyarrhythmias and death.

19. Discuss the elimination of digoxin as related to the $T\frac{1}{2}$.

Digoxin is excreted unchanged in the urine, which accounts for its relatively short half-life.

20. Discuss the elimination of digitoxin as related to the $T\frac{1}{2}$.

Digitoxin is metabolized in the liver to active metabolites. These are eliminated in the bile, and subject to enterohepatic recycling. This accounts for its relatively long half-life.

21. What is the effect of digitalis glycosides on the cardiac action potential?

Glycosides increase intracellular sodium and also extracellular potassium by inhibitory actions on sodium potassium ATPase. Thus, with chronic therapy, because intracellular sodium is increased, phase 0 may be blunted slightly. The increase in extracellular potassium results in a decrease in the rate of repolarization and thus a decrease in the slope of phase 3 of the action potential, and a "skewed" appearance. This results in a longer time for the membrane to repolarize and, accordingly, an increase in the effective refractory period. Because the objective of the drug is to increase the influx of calcium, the faster influx of calcium results in a shortened phase 2, because a shorter time is required for the membrane to reach the equilibrium potential for calcium. Finally, phase 4 is elevated and increased in slope, due to the alterations in sodium and potassium concentration. This, with chronic therapy, and particularly as toxicity is approached, results in delayed oscillatory afterpotentials (see Figure).

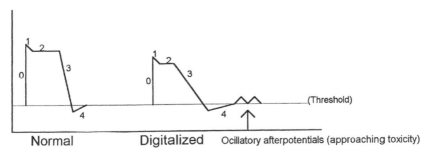

Effect of cardiac glycosides on the cardiac action potential (chronic therapy).

22. Describe the effects of digitalis toxicity.

The first sign of toxicity is bradycardia, due to the effects of the drug on the cardiac action potential. This may be accompanied by fatigue, drowsiness, mental confusion, and blurred vision. Further toxicity results in tachycardia.

23. Describe the effects of cardiac glycosides on urinary output.

In general, these drugs increase urinary output that is mainly due to improved renal circulation.

24. What is the effect of digitalis glycosides on AV nodal conduction?

These drugs decrease the rate of conduction in the AV node, due to the changes in the cardiac action potential as discussed above (increased effective refractory period [ERP]).

25. Discuss the therapeutic use of cardiac glycosides in the therapy of atrial arrhythmias.

These drugs decrease conduction in the AV node, and, thus, in therapeutic doses, mediate a partial blockade of the node. This decreases the frequency and number of ectopic foci reaching the ventricle.

26. What is the therapeutic window of digitalis glycosides?

Digitalis glycosides have a very narrow therapeutic window. Thus, accurate dosage intervals and patient compliance are critical.

27. What autonomic effects are seen at low therapeutic doses of cardiac glycosides?

These drugs sensitize nodal tissue to parasympathetic activity, resulting in a decreased rate of firing of the sinoatrial (SA) node, and a decrease in conduction.

28. Describe the effects seen with doses of cardiac glycosides in the high therapeutic range.

At doses in the high therapeutic range, these drugs stimulate sympathetic activity. Thus, an increase in excitability is seen, which may lead to arrhythmias.

29. Describe the generation of oscillatory afterpotentials by cardiac glycosides.

Cardiac glycosides increase the influx of calcium, and decrease the outflow of potassium. Because there is little sequestration of calcium in cardiac cells, intracellular calcium may increase to toxic levels, particularly with high doses of the drug, and may exchange for sodium, via the sodium-calcium exchanger. This results in an overload of intracellular sodium and calcium, which, because of the decreased outflow of potassium, is not counterbalanced. Thus, calcium overload is manifested as an early afterdepolarization of the cardiac action potential, which may result in premature depolarization of Purkinje fibers and the appearance of ventricular arrhythmias, which may result in ventricular tachyarrhythmias and death.

30. Why do toxic levels of cardiac glycosides result in bradycardia?

Digitalis glycosides cause an influx of extracellular calcium and an accumulation of extracellular potassium. The increased levels of extracellular potassium decrease the rate of repolarization of the cardiac cell. Thus, as levels of the drug approach the toxic range, accumulated extracellular potassium causes a lengthening of phase 3 of the cardiac action potential and an increase in the length of time between depolarizations. Thus, bradycardia is seen.

BIPYRIDINES

31. Describe the mechanism of action of bipyridine-type drugs (amrinone and milrinone).

These drugs mediate an inward current of calcium, possibly due to the inhibition of phosphodiesterase. In addition, they cause a release of intracellular calcium from stores in the cardiac sarcoplasmic reticulum. This increases troponin-tropomyosin interactions, and, consequently, force of contraction.

32. Discuss the use of bipyridines in the therapy of CHF.

At present, these drugs are available for short-term parenteral use only.

BIBLIOGRAPHY

1. Balaguru D, Auslender M: Vasodilators in the treatment of pediatric heart failure. Prog Pediatr Cardiol 12(1):81–90, 2000.
2. Bohm M, Maack C: Treatment of heart failure with beta-blockers. Mechanisms and results. Basic Res Cardiol 95 Suppl 1:I15–I24, 2000.
3. Hardman J, Limbird L, Gilman A: Goodman & Gilman's The Pharmacological Basis of Therapeutics, 10th ed. McGraw-Hill Publishers, 2001.
4. Gottlieb SS: Are all beta-blockers the same for chronic heart failure? Curr Cardiol Rep 3(2):124–129, 2001.
5. Katzung B: Basic and Clinical Pharmacology, 8th ed. Appleton & Lange, 2001.
6. Mabuchi N, Tsutamoto T, Kinoshita M: Therapeutic use of dopamine and beta-blockers modulates plasma interleukin-6 levels in patients with congestive heart failure. J Cardiovasc Pharmacol 36 Suppl 2:S87–S91, 2000.
7. McAreavey D, Exner DV, Curtin EL, et al: Beta-blockers in heart failure: Recently completed and ongoing clinical trials. Expert Opin Investig Drugs 9(2):415–428, 2000.
8. Metra M, Nodari S, Boldi E, et al: Selective or nonselective beta-adrenergic blockade in patients with congestive heart failure. Curr Cardiol Rep 2(3):252–257, 2000.
9. Moskowitz R, Kukin M: Current issues regarding beta-adrenergic blockade in patients with congestive heart failure: Patient selection, nonselective versus selective blockade, management of adverse effects, and indications for withdrawal of therapy. Curr Cardiol Rep 1(1):47–54, 1999.
10. Munger MA, Cheang KI: Beta-blocker therapy: A standard of care for heart failure. Pharmacotherapy 20(11 Pt 2):359S–367S, 2000.
11. Neustein S, Sampson I, Dimich I, et al: Milrinone is superior to epinephrine as treatment of myocardial depression due to ropivacaine in pigs. Can J Anaesth 47(11):1114–1118, 2000.
12. Nyolczas N, Dekany M, Fiok J, et al: Prediction of the effect of bisoprolol in dilated cardiomyopathy. Cardiovasc Drugs Ther 14(5):543–550, 2000.
13. Smith AJ, Wehner JS, Manley HJ, et al: Current role of beta-adrenergic blockers in the treatment of chronic congestive heart failure. Am J Health Syst Pharm 58(2):140–145, 2001.
14. Skrabal MZ, Stading JA, Behmer-Miller KA, et al: Advances in the treatment of congestive heart failure: New approaches for an old disease. Pharmacotherapy 20(7):787–804, 2000.
15. Winkel E, Costanzo MR: Chronic heart failure. Current Treatment Options in Cardiovascular Medicine 1(3):231–242, 1999.

18. DRUGS THAT AFFECT THE CLOTTING CASCADE

1. Refer to the figure and discuss the formation of a clot (thrombus).

The clotting cascade actually begins with the presence of an injury (or perceived injury) to the vessel wall. Platelets become activated and release endogenous mediators (e.g., adenosine 5c-diphosphate [ADP]) that cause the platelets to become "sticky" and form aggregates. In addition, the release of thromboxane A_2 causes vasoconstriction. Platelet-derived clotting factors are activated, which initiate the clotting cascade (see Figure).

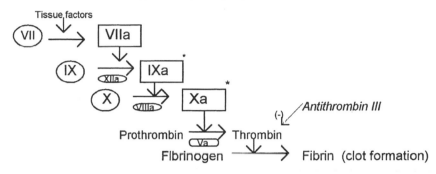

The clotting cascade. Circles denote vitamin K dependent clotting factors, ovals are clotting factors affected by endothelial cell factors (e.g., thrombomodulin). Starred factors are inhibited by the actions of heparin and antithrombin III.

2. Describe the clotting cascade.

The clotting cascade is a sequential conversion of inactive plasma factors to active factors, resulting in the ultimate conversion of soluble fibrinogen to insoluble fibrin. This fibrin forms the basis of clot formation.

3. What are the two classifications of clotting factors?

Vitamin K-dependent factors and vitamin K-independent factors.

4. How can clotting be inhibited?

The clotting cascade can be inhibited through several pathways. These include:
- The inhibition of the conversion of profactors to active factors, which results in disruption of the clotting cascade.
- The inactivation of activated factors, which results in disruption of the clotting cascade.
- Interference with vitamin K recycling or reduction in vitamin K stores. Because the majority of clotting factors are vitamin K-dependent, reduction of vitamin K levels will result in anticoagulation.
- Interference with platelet activation. This will result in inhibition of the formation of a platelet plug and lack of activation of platelet activated clotting factors.

5. What is an anticoagulant?

An anticoagulant is a drug that disrupts the clotting cascade, thus inhibiting clot formation. It does not affect platelets, nor does it have an appreciable effect on an established clot.

6. Describe an antithrombotic drug.

An antithrombotic drug is one that affects platelets. These drugs decrease platelet aggregation, and affect the activation of platelets, thus decreasing the initiation of the clotting cascade.

7. What is a thrombolytic drug?

A thrombolytic drug is one that actually disrupts an established clot. Unlike an anticoagulant, these drugs are not prophylactic, but actually dissolve the fibrin web that forms the basis of the clot, causing dissolution.

8. Describe a hemostatic drug.

These drugs decrease blood flow and thus blood loss.

9. What is a hemoperfusion agent?

These drugs decrease blood viscosity and increase the flow of blood, resulting in increased tissue perfusion.

ANTICOAGULANT DRUGS

10. What is heparin?

Heparin is a polymer of acidic, sulfated disaccharides, derived from porcine or bovine mucosa. The structure of heparin includes glucosamine sulfate, iduronic acid and sulfated iduronic acid, and N-acetyl glucosamine. The length of the polysaccharide chain determines the properties of the molecule—shorter chains are low molecular weight heparins, and longer chains are high molecular weight heparins. The length of the chain determines the properties of the drug.

11. How is heparin dispensed commercially?

Heparin is normally dispensed as unfractionated heparin, which includes forms of various molecular weights.

12. Discuss the primary mechanism of action of heparin.

Heparin acts to potentiate antithrombin III, an endogenous substance that inhibits the conversion of fibrinogen to fibrin. The drug induces a conformational change in antithrombin III, and binds simultaneously to thrombin and antithrombin III, facilitating the inactivation of thrombin.

13. What are the secondary mechanisms of action of heparin?

The conformational change in antithrombin III induced by heparin allows the molecule to bind to, and inactivate, factors involved in the clotting cascade. Primary factors affected are the activated forms of factor IX ("Christmas factor," or plasma thromboplastin component) and X ("Stuart-Prower factor").

14. How is heparin administered?

Heparin is a proteoglycan and would be destroyed by digestive enzymes. It is thus given by parenteral route.

15. Discuss the types of heparin and their actions.

Heparin and heparin-like compounds are available in a variety of molecular weight fractions. The lower molecular weight heparins are not able to bind both antithrombin III and thrombin simultaneously, which is necessary for the inactivation of thrombin. These drugs, consequently, affect the actions of factors IXa and Xa, rather than thrombin.

16. Describe the possible effect of heparin on bone.

Heparin inhibits the carboxylation of bone proteins, and decreases the activity of vitamin K in osteoblasts. It may increase the rate of bone loss with chronic therapy, through binding to osteoblasts and subsequent decrease in osteoblast activity. Heparin may also inhibit the formation of bone in the fetus.

17. Does heparin affect platelet aggregation?

Not at therapeutic doses. However, in high doses, platelet aggregation is affected and bleeding time is prolonged.

18. Which types of heparin have the greatest effect on platelet aggregation?

The higher molecular weight forms have more antithrombotic activity than the low molecular weight forms.

19. Discuss the protein binding of heparin.

Heparin is highly plasma protein-bound. Because of the negative charge associated with the molecule, it binds to any positively charged protein, including tissue proteins and cytoskeletal/membrane proteins. This results in a somewhat unpredictable anticoagulant effect between patients, as the amount and types of available binding proteins varies with the patient and state of health.

20. Discuss the metabolism of heparins.

Heparins are metabolized within vascular endothelial cells and macrophages This metabolism follows first order kinetics.

21. Discuss the half-life of heparin as a function of metabolism.

Heparin is metabolized according to a saturable pathway. Thus, half-life varies with dose. The half-life within the low therapeutic dose range is approximately 30 minutes. This may increase to as much as 3 hours, with doses in the high therapeutic range. These values may increase in individual patients, in proportion to the degree of plasma protein binding.

22. How is heparin eliminated?

After metabolism (depolymerization), heparins are eliminated through the urine.

23. Discuss the elimination rate of heparin with regard to molecular weight.

The elimination rate of the higher molecular weight forms of heparin is faster than that of lower molecular weight forms. Thus, the duration of action is shorter.

24. Does heparin cross the placental barrier?

No. Due to its large size, it does not cross into the placenta.

25. Discuss the adverse effects of heparin therapy.

The major adverse effect is bleeding. This may range from mild bruising to subarachnoid hemorrhage. Thrombocytopenia is also a common adverse effect, particularly with the use of bovine heparin.

26. Are allergic reactions common with heparin?

Yes. Allergies to meat derived from certain animals may precipitate allergic reactions to heparin derived from the same source (e.g., beef or pork). In addition, allergies to sulfites may precipitate allergic reactions to heparin that is administered as sulfur conjugates.

27. Discuss the actions of heparin on aldosterone.

Heparin is known to inhibit aldosterone synthesis. This is not considered clinically significant. However the effects on aldosterone may lead to hyperkalemia and metabolic abnormalities with long term therapy.

28. Discuss the antidote to heparin overdose.

Protamine sulfate is used. This molecule is highly charged and binds tightly to the heparin molecule, thus inhibiting pharmacological action.

29. What is enoxaparin?

Enoxaparin is a low molecular weight heparin of porcine origin.

30. What is the advantage of therapy with enoxaparin?

Enoxaparin and other low molecular weight heparins (e.g., ardeparin, dalteparin) produce a more predictable anticoagulant response than (unfractionated) heparin. This is a result of increased bioavailability, particularly after subcutaneous injection, longer half-life, and dose-independent clearance.

31. What is the major mechanism of action of dalteparin?

Dalteparin, and other low molecular weight heparins, are more selective inhibitors of factors IXa and Xa than the higher weight heparins, and have less effect on the inhibition of thrombin. This primarily results because their smaller size is not conducive to the concurrent binding of antithrombin III and thrombin.

32. Describe the level of protein binding seen with dalteparin and enoxaparin.

These drugs have much less plasma protein binding activity than do the higher molecular weight (unfractionated) heparins. These drugs also have decreased binding to platelets, and factors IV and V, thus producing less thrombocytopenia.

33. What is danaparin?

Danaparin is a "heparinoid" anticoagulant, a mixture of sulfated glycosamine glycans obtained from porcine mucosa. It has similar properties to heparin, but has more antithrombotic activity and an increased effect on factor Xa.

34. Does protamine sulfate affect the activity of danaparin?

No. This drug does not contain heparin and is not affected by protamine sulfate.

35. Discuss the mechanism of action of warfarin.

Warfarin disrupts the recycling of vitamin K epoxide form to active vitamin K. This results in depletion of available vitamin K stores, and eventually to lack of activation of vitamin K-dependent clotting factors—particularly factors II, VII, IX and X (recall that vitamin K is converted to an inactive epoxide form after interaction with platelet factors, and must be "recycled" back to its active form in the liver [see Figure]).

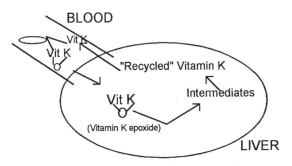

The recycling of vitamin K. Vitamin K interaction with platelet derived clotting factors, conversion to the epoxide form, and hepatic conversion of the epoxide form to vitamin K.

36. Describe the paradox of warfarin actions.

Warfarin, like other vitamin K inhibitors, inhibits the activity of platelet-derived clotting factors (II, VII. IX and X). This results in anticoagulant action. Paradoxically, it also inhibits the synthesis of endogenous proteins with anticoagulant activity such as protein C and protein S.

37. Are the actions of warfarin immediate? Explain.

No. The drug may take up to 4 days to produce a pharmacologic effect. Two things must happen physiologically before the effects of the drug are seen:

- Existing hepatic stores of vitamin K must first be depleted. Inhibition of recycling by the drug will only deplete circulating vitamin K, and the pharmacologic action of the drug will not be seen all the stores of active vitamin K have been exhausted.
- Activated platelet-derived factors must undergo normal catabolism. Factors that are already activated do not depend on the presence of vitamin K, so the effect of the drug is only seen after normal catabolism of activated factors.

38. What percentage of activated clotting factors are reduced by therapeutic doses of warfarin?

Thirty to 50 percent.

39. What is the half-life of warfarin?

Approximately 36 hours.

40. How is warfarin supplied?

This drug is supplied as a racemic mixture of two stereoisomers, the R (D) form and the L (S) form.

41. Describe the differential anticoagulant effects of isomeric warfarin.

The anticoagulant effects of warfarin are stereoselective; the S-isomer of warfarin is 3 to 5 times more potent than the R-isomer.

42. Does the pharmacologic action of warfarin cease upon withdrawal of the drug?

No. There is a recovery time, while hepatic stores of vitamin K are replenished and new, activated clotting factors are synthesized.

43. Discuss the protein binding of warfarin and its ramifications.

Warfarin is heavily plasma protein-bound (> 97 percent). It therefore interacts with other protein-bound drugs (e.g., carbamazepine, phenytoin, and benzodiazepines) in that binding of warfarin to plasma proteins may displace bound drug that is administered as concurrent therapy. Thus, toxicity may result, due to elevated plasma levels, and the clearance rate of the drug may increase to compensate.

44. Is warfarin metabolized?

Yes. The primary route of metabolism is through cytochrome P_{450} to hydroxylated metabolites. Several cytochrome P_{450} isozymes may be involved. Warfarin may also be reduced in the liver to an alcohol ("warfarin alcohol").

45. Do the metabolites of warfarin have pharmacologic activity?

Yes. The reduced metabolites are inactive, but the hydroxylated metabolites do have pharmacologic activity.

46. Discuss the variation in metabolism of warfarin between patients.

Due to genetic variability in cytochrome P_{450} isozymes, some patients may preferentially metabolize either the "R" or "S" form. This results in radical changes in pharmacologic action and interpatient variability.

47. Describe the food interactions that exist with warfarin therapy.

The diet of the patient may not include foods that are sources of vitamin K, such as green leafy vegetables.

48. Describe the drug interactions seen with warfarin.

Several drugs may increase or decrease the activity of warfarin—primarily through similar actions or by the alteration of warfarin metabolism. These include:

- Phenylbutazone and related (sulfapyridine) drugs.The activity of these drugs on platelet action is synergistic with the actions of warfarin. In addition, these drugs increase the pharmacologic effects of warfarin by displacement of protein binding.
- Aspirin and other antiplatelet drugs synergize with the actions of warfarin.
- Barbiturates may increase the metabolism of warfarin through induction of hepatic cytochrome P_{450}.
- Cimetidine, metronidazole and fluconazole affect metabolism of warfarin.
- Some antibiotics (e.g., third generation cephalosporins) affect the populations of vitamin K-producing bacteria in the gut, causing increased amounts of vitamin K to become available. This interferes with the action of warfarin.

49. Does warfarin cross the placenta?

Yes. Warfarin can cause hemorrhagic disorders in the fetus, and can cause abnormal bone formation.

50. Describe the reduced efficacy of warfarin in hyperthyroid patients.

Thyroid hormone increases the catabolism of clotting factors, resulting in an increased rate of synthesis of active clotting factors (recall that the function of vitamin K is primarily in reactivation).

51. Compare and contrast warfarin and heparin with respect to their mechanism of action.

- Heparin acts very quickly to inhibit clot formation, whereas warfarin has a slow onset. Conversely, upon withdrawal of the drug, heparinized patients quickly recover, whereas the withdrawal of warfarin will have no appreciable effect for as much as several days.
- Both drugs have an indirect action on the clotting cascade—heparin must form a complex with antithrombin III in order to produce an effect, and warfarin acts through depletion of vitamin K, which affects specific clotting factors.

52. Discuss the toxicity of warfarin.

The major adverse effect is bleeding. In addition, warfarin can cause necrosis of the skin with initial therapy, particularly with a loading dose.

53. What are the antidotes to warfarin overdose?

Vitamin K and/or whole plasma may be administered to counteract effects.

54. Differentiate the pharmacokinetics of warfarin and heparin.

- Warfarin may be administered orally or parenterally, whereas heparin must be administered by slow infusion (e.g., subcutaneous injection or intravenous [IV] admixture).
- Both drugs are highly plasma protein-bound. However, the binding of heparin is less specific than that of warfarin in that the drug can bind to any positively charged protein, including those on cell membranes.
- Warfarin is metabolized in the liver, whereas heparin is depolymerized in endothelial cells and within macrophages. The elimination of heparin is primarily renal.

55. Describe the mechanism of action of anisindione.

This drug interferes with the synthesis of vitamin K-dependent clotting factors. The mechanism of action is similar to that of warfarin.

56. Discuss the mechanism of action of lepirudin.

This drug is a potent inhibitor of thrombin activity.

57. Describe a lepirudin antagonist.

No antagonists to direct thrombin inhibitors are known.

58. Is dicumarol frequently used as an anticoagulant?

No. It is incompletely absorbed and is irritating to the gastrointestinal tract.

59. Should products containing ginkgo biloba be used in the presence of anticoagulants?

No. Ginkgo products interfere with platelet aggregation and thus make the actions of anticoagulant drugs less predictable.

ANTITHROMBOTIC AGENTS

60. Describe the mechanism of action of aspirin.

Aspirin irreversibly acetylates cyclooxygenase, the rate-limiting enzyme in the arachidonic acid cascade (prostanoid synthesis) (see Figure).

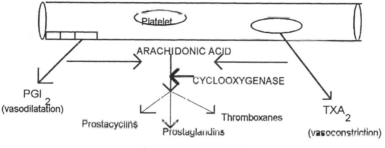

Arachidonic acid pathway.

61. Discuss the effects of aspirin on the platelet.

Aspirin inhibits the aggregation of platelets and also platelet degranulation.

62. Describe the actions of aspirin on the production of platelet thromboxane.

By inhibiting cyclooxygenase (COX-1), aspirin and similar drugs (e.g., indomethacin) inhibit the synthesis of thromboxanes by platelets in a dose-dependent manner. This results in a decrease in platelet aggregation and decreased local vasoconstriction.

63. Describe the effect of aspirin on the vascular endothelium.

The vascular endothelium preferentially produces prostacyclins (e.g., PGI_2) rather than prostaglandins or thromboxanes. Prostacyclins mediate a decrease in platelet aggregation ("stickiness") and local vasodilatation. Aspirin decreases the synthesis of prostacyclins by the vascular endothelium.

64. Why would a net vasodilatation and decreased platelet activation be seen with low-dose aspirin but not high-dose aspirin?

Aspirin irreversibly acetylates cyclooxygenase. Thus, enzyme exposed to the drug is permanently nonfunctional. Also, platelets are not entire cells—they are fragments of megakaryocytes, and thus have no cellular "machinery;" they are not capable of synthesizing new enzyme.

With either low-dose or high-dose aspirin, both endothelial and platelet cyclooxygenase are rendered inactive. Endothelial cells are capable of synthesizing new enzyme, as opposed to platelets. Thus, the inhibition of prostacyclin production is only temporary, while inhibition of platelet thromboxane synthesis is permanent—new platelets must be produced in order for thromboxane to be synthesized. The net effect is vasodilatation with a decrease in platelet aggregation. With high-dose aspirin, both platelet and endothelial cell prostanoid production is inhibited, as new enzyme produced by endothelial cells is rapidly acetylated by circulating levels of drug.

65. Describe the mechanism of action of abciximab.

Abciximab inhibits platelet glycoprotein (GP) IIb/IIIa binding to fibrinogen, as well as von Willebrand's factor and other adhesive molecules. This decreases platelet aggregation ("stickiness").

66. Discuss the duration of action of abciximab.

The pharmacologic action of abciximab is approximately 48 hr. However, the drug remains in the circulation bound to platelets for up to 10 days.

67. Is abciximab used as monotherapy?

Abciximab is generally used in conjunction with aspirin and heparin.

68. Should abciximab be used with oral anticoagulants?

No. Oral anticoagulants are contraindicated. Abciximab should not be administered within 7 days of administration of an oral anticoagulant.

69. Would clopidogrel be effective in a patient with compromised liver function?

No. The drug requires hepatic metabolism in order to be active.

70. Does clopidogrel require therapeutic monitoring?

No.

71. Discuss the mechanism of action of ticlopidine.

Ticlopidine interferes with the ADP-induced binding of fibrinogen to the platelet membrane at specific receptor sites. This interferes with platelet aggregation.

72. Does ticlopidine affect blood viscosity?

Yes, by reducing serum fibrinogen concentrations.

73. Are the actions of ticlopidine reversible?

No. The effects of the drug continue until new platelets are produced (at least 3 days, and up to 2 weeks, are required for platelet activity to return to normal).

THROMBOLYTIC DRUGS

74. What is alteplase?

Alteplase is an enzyme derived from human melanoma. It is a tissue plasminogen activator.

75. Describe the mechanism of action of alteplase.

This enzyme binds to fibrin in an existing clot, and activates the conversion of plasminogen to plasmin. The plasmin then lyses the fibrin. The clot, without its fibrin support, disintegrates.

76. Does alteplase have only a localized action on fibrinogen?

No. It also mediates a decrease in circulating fibrinogen.

77. Should a tissue plasminogen activator be used in the presence of cranial trauma?

No. Bleeding (and increased intracranial pressure) could be exacerbated with cranial trauma, recent cranial surgery (within 6 months), or subarachnoid hemorrhage.

78. Discuss the relationship of reteplase and fibrin.

Reteplase is a "fibrin selective" tissue plasminogen activator (TPA). It is activated by the presence of fibrin. Thus, if no clot is present, the drug is inactive.

79. Describe the mechanism of action of reteplase.

Reteplase is an enzyme that cleaves the Arg-Val bond in plasminogen, converting it to plasmin.

80. Distinguish the action of reteplase and TPA.

Reteplase acts from within the clot, and so must penetrate the clot before it is active. TPA binds to the fibrin matrix on the outside of the clot. Thus, higher clot lysis rates are reported for reteplase than for TPA.

81. Describe the half-life of reteplase.

The drug is redistributed within 15 minutes (the distribution half-life), but is metabolized and eliminated from the body in approximately 3 hours (terminal half-life).

82. Discuss the mechanism of action of streptokinase.

Streptokinase forms an activator complex with plasminogen, which results in the cleavage of the Arg-Val bond in plasminogen, and conversion of plasminogen to plasmin. The activator complex also diffuses into the clot and activates preplasmin-2, a mediator that also lyses fibrin.

83. Describe the tolerance effect to streptokinase.

Repeated or excessive use of the drug can deplete pools of plasminogen, resulting in decreased effect of the drug.

84. What are the adverse effects of thrombolytic agents?

The major adverse effect is bleeding. However, cholesterol microembolization has been reported rarely in patients receiving invasive vascular procedures.

85. What are some homeopathic remedies that may interfere with the action of anticoagulants and antithrombotics?

Ginger, which inhibits thromboxane synthase and decreases the rate of platelet aggregation, may increase bleeding time. Feverfew, which also inhibits platelet activity, should also be avoided.

HEMOSTATIC AND HEMOPERFUSION AGENTS

86. What is morrhuate sodium?

It is a mixture of the sodium salts of fatty acids derived from cod liver oil.

87. Describe the mechanism of action of morrhuate sodium.

This drug is a sclerosing agent. It causes irritation to the vascular wall, causing an inflammatory response and vasoconstriction. This results in hemostasis.

88. Is the use of morrhuate sodium indicated for diabetic patients?

No. Patients with type I diabetes may already have compromised vascular integrity.

89. Describe the use of gelatin (e.g., Gelfoam) as a hemostatic agent.

Gelatin adheres to the surfaces of tissues and forms a barrier, effectively slowing the flow of blood. Once the platelet plug has been formed and the clotting cascade has been initiated, the gelatin is reabsorbed into the body as nonspecific protein.

90. What is pentoxifylline?
It is a hemoperfusion agent structurally related to methylxanthines.

91. Describe the mechanism of action of pentoxifylline.
This drug alters erythrocyte flexibility, allowing erythrocytes to pass more easily through vessels. In addition, it causes a decrease in fibrinogen, and increased fibrinolytic activity. These functions result in a decrease in blood viscosity and an increase in perfusion, particularly through the microcirculation, increasing tissue oxygenation.

92. Does pentoxifylline have a significant first-pass effect?
Yes.

93. Describe the metabolism of pentoxifylline.
The drug is metabolized in the liver and is also taken up into erythrocytes for metabolism.

94. Is the half-life of pentoxifylline constant?
No. The half-life varies with dose.

BIBLIOGRAPHY

1. Aronow WS: Thrombolysis and antithrombotic therapy for coronary artery disease. Clin Geriatr Med 17(1):173–188, 2001.
2. Arosio E, Montesi G, Zannoni M, et al: Comparative efficacy of ketanserin and pentoxiphylline in treatment of Raynaud's phenomenon. Angiology 40(7):633–638, 1989.
3. Billett HH: Direct and indirect antithrombins. Heparins, low molecular weight heparins, heparinoids, and hirudin. Clin Geriatr Med 17(1):15–29, 2001.
4. Bornstein NM: Antiplatelet drugs: how to select them and possibilities of combined treatment. Cerebrovasc Dis 11 Suppl 1:96–99, 2001.
5. Burgmann H, Stauffer F, Hollenstein U, et al: Effect of various pentoxiphylline concentrations on macrophage inflammatory protein 1 alpha production. Antimicrob Agents Chemother 39(2):574–575, 1995.
6. Catella-Lawson F, Crofford LJ: Cyclooxygenase inhibition and thrombogenicity. Am J Med 110(3 Suppl 1):28–32, 2001.
7. Chuang YJ, Swanson R, Raja SM, et al: Heparin enhances the specificity of antithrombin for thrombin and factor Xa independent of the reactive center loop sequence. Evidence for an exosite determinant of factor Xa specificity in heparin-activated antithrombin. J Biol Chem Feb 7, 2001.
8. Colman RW: Role of the light chain of high molecular weight kininogen in adhesion, cell-associated proteolysis and angiogenesis. Biol Chem 382(1):65–70, 2001.
9. Comp PC, Spiro TE, Friedman RJ, et al: Prolonged enoxaparin therapy to prevent venous thromboembolism after primary hip or knee replacement. Bone Joint Surg Am 83-A(3):336–345, 2001.
10. Csete K, Barzo P, Bodosi M, et al: Influence of nitrovasodilators and cyclooxygenase inhibitors on cerebral vasoreactivity in conscious rabbits. Eur J Pharmacol 412(3):301–309, 2001.
11. Fareed J, Hoppensteadt DA, Bick RL: An update on heparins at the beginning of the new millennium. Semin Thromb Hemost 26 Suppl 1:5–21, 2000.
12. Fernandez JS, Sadaniantz A: Use of low-molecular-weight heparin and glycoprotein IIb/IIIa inhibitors in acute coronary syndromes. Med Health R I 84(2):37–43, 2001.
13. Golino P, Ragni M, Cirillo P, et al: Emerging antithrombotic treatments for acute coronary syndromes. Cardiologia 44(11):969–980, 1999.
14. Hardman J, Limbird L, Gilman A (eds): Goodman & Gilman's The Pharmacological Basis of Therapeutics, 10th ed. New York, McGraw-Hill, 2001.
15. Hershenson MB, Schena JA, Lozano PA, et al: Effect of pentoxiphylline on oxygen transport during hypothermia. J Appl Physiol 66(1):96–101, 1989.
16. Juang JH, Kuo CH, Hsu BR: Beneficial effects of pentoxiphylline on islet transplantation. Transplant Proc 32(5):1073–1075, 2000.
17. Kakkar VV, Iyengar SS, De Lorenzo F, et al: Low molecular weight heparin for treatment of acute myocardial infarction (FAMI): Fragmin (dalteparin sodium) in acute myocardial infarction. Indian Heart J 52(5):533–539, 2000.
18. Katzung B: Basic and Clinical Pharmacology, 8th ed. Stamford, CT, Appleton & Lange, 2001.
19. Khosla AA, Chintu C: A pilot study: An open clinical trial of pentoxiphylline in patients with painful sickle cell crises. East Afr Med J 61(11):829–836, 1984.

20. Lethias C, Elefteriou F, Parsiegla G, et al: Identification and characterization of a conformational heparin-binding site involving two fibronectin type III modules of bovine tenascin-X. J Biol Chem Feb 7, 2001.
21. Lj-Saw-Hee FL, Blann AD, Lip GY: Effects of fixed low-dose warfarin, aspirin-warfarin combination therapy, and dose-adjusted warfarin on thrombogenesis in chronic atrial fibrillation. Stroke 31(4):828–833, 2000.
22. Loo BM, Kreuger J, Jalkanen M, et al: Binding of heparin/heparan sulfate to fibroblast growth factor receptor 4. J Biol Chem Feb 7, 2001.
23. Merli GJ: Treatment of deep venous thrombosis and pulmonary embolism with low molecular weight heparin in the geriatric patient population. Clin Geriatr Med 17(1):93–106, 2001.
24. Momi S, Nasimi M, Colucci M, et al: Low molecular weight heparins prevent thrombin-induced thrombo-embolism in mice despite low anti-thrombin activity. Evidence that the inhibition of feedback activation of thrombin generation confers safety advantages over direct thrombin inhibition. Haematologica 86(3):297–302, 2001.
25. Ranganath LR, Beety JM, Wright J, et al: Nutrient regulation of post-heparin lipoprotein lipase activity in obese subjects. Horm Metab Res 33(1):57–61, 2001.
26. Sarafanov AG, Ananyeva NM, Shima M, et al: Cell surface heparan sulfate proteoglycans (HSPGs) participate in factor VIII catabolism mediated by low density lipoprotein receptor-related protein (LRP). J Biol Chem Jan 12, 2001.
27. Shah PK: New antithrombotic drugs of coronary artery disease. J Cardiovasc Pharmacol Ther 1(2):165–176, 1996.
28. Sidelmann JJ, Gram J, Jespersen J, et al: Fibrin clot formation and lysis: Basic mechanisms. Semin Thromb Hemost 26(6):605–618, 2000.
29. Singer DE, Go AS: Antithrombotic therapy in atrial fibrillation. Clin Geriatr Med 17(1):131–147, 2001.
30. Yoon Y, Shim WH, Lee DH, et al: Usefulness of cilostazol versus ticlopidine in coronary artery stenting. Am J Cardiol 84(12):1375–1380, 1999.

19. DRUGS USED IN THE THERAPY OF HYPERLIPIDEMIA

1. How does the body obtain cholesterol?
- Dietary cholesterol may be taken up to form a core lipoprotein (e.g., very-low-density lipoprotein [VLDL] core) and catabolized in the liver to release free cholesterol, which is used in the synthesis of cell membranes and steroid hormones.
- Cholesterol may be synthesized in the liver by a synthetic pathway involving the actions of 3-hydroxy-3-methylglutaryl coenzyme A (HMG-CoA) reductase (see Figure).

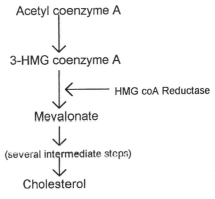

Acetyl coenzyme A

3-HMG coenzyme A

HMG coA Reductase

Mevalonate

(several intermediate steps)

Cholesterol

Major steps in cholesterol biosynthesis.

2. How is the production of low-density lipoproteins (LDL) receptors and HMG-CoA reductase regulated?
The production of both LDL receptors and HMG-CoA reductase is regulated at the level of transcription, by a feedback loop involving levels of intracellular cholesterol.

3. How is cholesterol eliminated from the body?
Elimination of cholesterol occurs mainly by production of bile by the liver. Free cholesterol is eliminated by hepatic secretion into bile, and is also incorporated into bile salts.

4. What are the physiologic effects of niacin?
Niacin increases the clearance of VLDL, and increases levels of high-density lipoproteins (HDL). It also decreases the synthesis of VLDL, which in turn results in lower levels of LDL.

5. Does niacin have an effect on the synthesis or reabsorption of bile salts?
No.

6. What is the dose-limiting side effect of niacin?
Niacin causes peripheral vasodilation, resulting in flushing of the skin and lower pelvic area. This effect radically decreases patient compliance.

7. Describe the cholesterol-lowering effects of niacinamide.
Niacinamide was formulated to be a form of niacin that does not cause flushing of the skin. However, it has little effect on lowering cholesterol.

8. Is niacin useful in a patient with hypertriglyceridemia?
Yes. It lowers triglycerides through the reduction of hepatic biosynthesis of VLDL.

9. For which types of hyperlipidemia is niacin useful?
Niacin is useful in the therapy of all types of hyperlipidemia.

10. Can niacin cause orthostatic hypotension?
Yes, particularly in patients with low blood pressure.

11. Discuss the gastrointestinal effects of niacin.
Niacin may cause diarrhea and gastrointestinal (GI) discomfort, including nausea and vomiting.

12. What are the effects of niacin on liver function?
Niacin may cause hepatotoxicity with prolonged therapy. This is usually manifested as nausea and vomiting, with altered liver enzyme profile.

13. Discuss the events that potentiate the liver toxicity of niacin.
Liver toxicity is seen most often with use of the sustained release formulations. Concurrent therapy with an HMG-CoA reductase inhibitor (e.g., a statin) also results in increased incidence of hepatotoxicity.

14. Why might niacin therapy be contraindicated in a type II diabetic patient?
Niacin promotes glucose intolerance, particularly among patients who have high insulin resistance.

15. Explain the contraindication to niacin therapy in patients with gout.
Elevated uric acid level is a common side effect of nicotinic acid therapy. Thus, gout would be exacerbated.

16. What is eicosapentaenoic acid (EPA)?
EPA is a vasodilatory prostanoid found in fish oil.

17. Describe the beneficial actions of eicosapentaenoic acid (EPA) on lipid related incidence (e.g., stroke, angina and myocardial infarction [MI]).
This substance has been shown to reduce the incidence of stroke and infarction, due to its vasodilatory actions. In animals, it has been shown to alter the lipid profile of cardiac myocytes and reduce the production of inositol triphosphate (a vasoconstrictor substance).

BILE-BINDING RESINS

18. What are the bile-binding resins currently in use?
Gemfibrozil, colestipol, and colesevelam.

19. Describe a bile-binding resin.
These drugs are non-absorbable, charged polymers which bind ionically charged bile salts in the intestinal lumen.

20. Discuss the mechanism of action of bile-binding resins.
These drugs bind bile salts (which are cholesterol-based) in the small intestine, preventing their reabsorption. This disruption of the enterohepatic recycling of bile salts forces the liver to use exogenous cholesterol stores for the synthesis of new bile salts. This results in a cascade effect: the decrease in hepatic cholesterol triggers an increase in LDL receptor expression, which results in removal of increased amounts of LDL from the blood (see Figure).

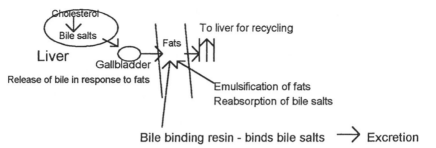

Actions of bile binding resins in the reduction of total cholesterol.

21. Describe the changes in lipid profile seen with bile-binding resin therapy.

These drugs affect mainly LDL—as bile salts are depleted, the hepatic enzyme cholesterol 7-alpha-hydroxylase, is up regulated, which increases the conversion of cholesterol to bile acids. The cholesterol used in production of bile acids is obtained mainly fromLDL, by cleavage of triglycerides from the cholesterol core. Thus, LDL levels decrease, triglycerides increase, and levels of HDL are unaffected.

22. Would bile-binding resins be effective in conjunction with a low fat diet?

These drugs would be less effective with such a diet, because digested fats trigger the release of cholecystokinin, which acts to facilitate contraction of the gall bladder and subsequent release of bile. Without the presence of fats in the diet, less bile acids are released and subsequently bound and excreted by the drug.

23. Describe the effect of bile binding resins on triglyceride levels.

These drugs increase triglyceride levels, particularly in patients with preexisting hyper-triglyceridemia.

24. What are the disadvantages of therapy with bile-binding resins?

These drugs cause GI distress, and have low patient compliance, due to lack of palatability. These drugs may also cause liver toxicity.

25. Discuss drug interactions with bile-binding resins.

These drugs may interfere with absorption of orally administered drugs. In particular, drugs that are lipid soluble (e.g., central nervous system [CNS] drugs such as anticonvulsants and anti-depressants) could be bound by the drug and excreted, rather than absorbed.

26. Which class of antilipemic drugs would be indicated for a patient with hypertriglyceridemia?

The fibric acid derivatives (e.g., gemfibrozil and clofibrate) are most effective in lowering triglyceride levels.

27. Describe the pharmacokinetics and dynamics of the fibric acid derivatives.

These drugs are highly protein-bound (> 95 percent), and are metabolized, undergoing enterohepatic recirculation. Elimination is primarily renal.

HMG-COA REDUCTASE INHIBITORS

28. Describe the mechanism of action of HMG-CoA reductase inhibitors (e.g., simvastatin, atorvastatin).

These drugs inhibit HMG coenzyme A reductase, which is essential for the conversion of 3HMG coenzyme A to mevalonate, a precursor of cholesterol (see Figure at Question 1). This inhibition is dose-dependent. The formation of HDL is decreased, resulting in a decrease in formation of sclerotic plaques.

29. Discuss the effect of statins (e.g., pravastatin, lovastatin) on carotid artery intima media thickness.

This class of drugs has been shown to significantly reduce intima media thickness with long-term therapy. Incidence of stroke, cardiovascular events, and mortality are correspondingly decreased.

30. Discuss the adverse effects of HMG-CoA inhibitors.

Adverse effects tend to be mild GI effects—dyspepsia, constipation and flatulence. More serious effects, such as renal tubular obstruction, rhabdomyolysis and myopathy, have been reported. These are most likely to occur with concurrent therapy of other drugs that inhibit the metabolism of the drug (e.g., systemic anti-fungals or macrolide antibiotics) or with consumption of grapefruit. Elevated liver enzymes (e.g., transaminase) may also be present.

31. Discuss the interactions of calcium channel blockers with HMG-CoA reductase inhibitors.

Verapamil and diltiazem may inhibit the metabolism of these drugs, due to an inhibition of CYP_{3A4} metabolism and reduction of first pass metabolism.

32. Why is grapefruit and its juice contraindicated when on statin therapy?

Grapefruit enzymes interfere with the metabolism of the drug and should be avoided.

33. Describe the effect of pravastatin on HDL levels.

Pravastatin has been shown to increase levels of HDLC in patients with heterozygous familial and nonfamilial primary hypercholesterolemia and mixed dyslipidemia, as well as Frederickson Types 2a and 2b.

BIBLIOGRAPHY

1. Arntz H, Agrawal R, Wunderlich W, et al: Beneficial effects of pravastatin (+/-cholestyramine/niacin) initiated immediately after a coronary event (the randomized lipid-coronary artery disease). Am J Cardiol 86(12):1293–1298, 2000.
2. Davis M, Atwal AS, Nair DR, et al: The effect of short-term lipid lowering with atorvastatin on carotid artery intima media thickness in patients with peripheral vascular disease: A pilot study. Curr Med Res Opin 16(3):198–204, 2000.
3. Despres J, Lemieux I, Dagenais G, et al: HDL-cholesterol as a marker of coronary heart disease risk: The Quebec cardiovascular study. Atherosclerosis 153(2):263–272, 2000.
4. Hardman J, Limbird L, Gilman A: Goodman & Gilman's The Pharmacological Basis of Therapeutics, 10th ed. McGraw-Hill Publishers, 2001.
5. Katzung B: Basic and Clinical Pharmacology, 8th ed. Appleton & Lange, 2001.
6. Nair SS, Leitch J, Garg ML: Suppression of inositol phosphate release by cardiac myocytes isolated from fish oil-fed pigs. Mol Cell Biochem 215(1–2):57–64, 2000.
7. Tonkin AM, Colquhoun D, Emberson J, et al: Effects of pravastatin in 3260 patients with unstable angina: results from the LIPID study. Lancet 2:356(9245):1871–1875, 2000.
8. Waters DD, Azar RR: Should intensive cholesterol lowering play a role in the management of acute coronary syndromes? Am J Cardiol 86(8 Suppl 2):35–42, 2000.

WEBSITES:
Clinical Pharmacology 2000: http://cp.gsm.com
Medline plus: http://medlineplus.nlm.nih.gov/medlineplus/
Medscape Multispecialty Journal Room: http://pharmacotherapy.medscape.com/Home/Topics/multispecialty/directories/dir-MULT.JournalRoom.html
Medscape Pharmacotherapy News (cardiology):
http://cardiology.medscape.com/home/topics/pharmacotherapy/directories/dir-PHAR.News.html

20. DRUGS USED IN THE THERAPY OF GOUT

1. Briefly explain the physiology of gout.

Gout is a condition in which excess plasma urate precipitates in joints, forming uric acid crystals. These crystals precipitate an inflammatory response, which involves the migration of neutrophils into the affected area, and release of inflammatory mediators.

2. What types of drugs are effective in the treatment of gout?

The major emphasis in drug therapy is on suppression of the inflammatory response, particularly during an acute attack. Thus, anti-inflammatory drugs such as corticosteroids and nonsteroidal anti-inflammatory drugs, or drugs which affect neutrophil function are used. Basic therapy might include drugs which decrease serum urate, either through interfering with its production, or by enhancing its elimination.

3. Explain the primary mechanism of action of allopurinol.

Allopurinol decreases the formation of uric acid, by inhibiting xanthine oxidase, a key enzyme in the catabolism of oxypurines (hypoxanthine and xanthine) to uric acid. The rate of formation of uric acid is therefore decreased in a dose-dependent manner.

4. What are the secondary mechanisms of action of allopurinol?

Allopurinol facilitates the incorporation of xanthine and hypoxanthine into nucleic acids, lowering the substrates for catabolism. In addition, the decrease in xanthine metabolism facilitates a negative feedback on purine synthesis.

5. How quickly are reductions in serum uric acid seen with allopurinol therapy?

Reductions are seen in 24 to 48 hours.

6. What is the half-life of allopurinol?

The half-life of the parent drug is 1 to 3 hours, and that of the metabolite is 18 to 30 hours.

7. Discuss the pharmacokinetics of allopurinol.

The drug is highly bioavailable (> 90 percent, taken orally). It is metabolized by the liver to oxypurinol, and eliminated via the urine.

8. Does allopurinol have active metabolites?

Yes. The metabolite, oxypurinol, is responsible for the majority of the pharmacologic actions of the drug.

9. Is allopurinol a good choice for a patient with renal calculi?

Yes. The drug is not a uricosuric agent, and thus does not promote additional formation of calculi.

10. Discuss the adverse effects of allopurinol.

The most common adverse effects are gastrointestinal (GI) effects such as dyspepsia, gastritis, diarrhea, and abdominal pain. Also common are dermatologic effects, which range from urticaria and maculopapular rash to serious dermatological effects such as exfoliative dermatitis and Stevens-Johnson syndrome.

11. Are hematologic effects seen with allopurinol therapy?

Yes. Leukopenia, granulocytopenia, and fatal bone marrow suppression have been reported, particularly in patients under therapy with a myelosuppressive drug (e.g., cancer chemotherapeutics).

12. Discuss the mechanism of action of probenecid.

Probenecid is a uricosuric agent. It acts at the luminal side of the renal tubular cell to decrease tubular reabsorption of uric acid. It may also increase secretion of uric acid into the urine, via the organic acid secretory system.

13. Describe the interactions of probenecid with drugs such as isoniazid and aspirin.

Probenecid acts at the luminal side of the renal tubular cell. Thus, it must use the organic acid secretory system to enter the lumen of the tubule, because it is not filtered. Drugs such as aspirin and isoniazid (as well as most β-lactam antibiotics, and a host of other drugs that are organic acids) also use the organic acid secretory system for transport into the nephron, in their elimination. Thus, there is competition for transport, which may result in a decrease in drug elimination and subsequent increase in plasma levels of the concurrent drug, as well as a decrease in the efficacy of probenecid.

14. Discuss the pharmacokinetics of probenecid.

The drug is approximately 100 percent absorbed, and highly plasma protein-bound (particularly to albumin). It is metabolized by the liver, forming active metabolites. The drug and metabolites are eliminated by the kidney.

15. What is the disposition of urinary probenecid?

As the parent drug and metabolite enter the urine, the parent drug is almost completely reabsorbed in the proximal tubule. Only a small amount of metabolite is reabsorbed.

16. Can probenecid be used with methotrexate therapy?

No. Methotrexate increases serum uric acid, and concurrent therapy with probenecid results in increased uricosuria. The levels of methotrexate may also be increased, through competition with probenecid for the organic acid secretory system. The probability of methotrexate-induced uric acid neuropathy is increased by the administration of probenecid.

17. Discuss the use of colchicine in the therapy of gout.

Colchicine is used for therapy of acute attacks only. It is not used as prophylactic therapy.

18. Describe the mechanism of action of colchicine.

This drug is an inhibitor of microtubule assembly. It therefore inhibits cell division (spindle formation), cellular movement, and transport of substances within a cell (gel-sol transformations, through microtubule dissolution and reformation). The therapeutic action of the drug lies in the inhibition of microtubule assembly in neutrophils—neutrophil migration into affected areas is inhibited, as is the secretion of inflammatory substances (due to inhibition of gel-sol transformations). Thus, inflammation is reduced.

19. Discuss the toxicity of colchicine.

Due to its effect on microtubule assembly, this drug has the ability to arrest mitotic cells in metaphase. Particularly affected are rapidly dividing cells, such as those in skin, hair and bone marrow. In addition, the activity of secretory cells is diminished, as movement of secretory substances out of a secretory cell is inhibited. This could potentially affect all systems in the body (e.g., endocrine systems and systems heavily regulated by the autonomic nervous system). In short, this drug is extremely toxic if administered improperly, and could result in fatality.

20. Describe the actions of colchicine on neurotransmitter release and homeostasis.

Colchicine disrupts the movement of secretory vesicles within a cell, and thus interferes with chemical neurotransmission. If administered quickly or in elevated dose, the drug interferes with homeostatic mechanisms, particularly those mediated by the autonomic nervous system. Inhibition of medullary regulation of respiration, decreased thalamic control of core temperature, as well as inhibition of peripheral vasodilatation, leading to hypertension, may be seen.

21. Is colchicine administered intravenously?

No. Intravenous administration results in rapidly increased levels of drug and may precipitate alterations in homeostatic mechanisms, depressed respiration, and a hypertensive crisis.

22. Discuss the distribution of colchicine.

Colchicine distributes to major peripheral organs, primarily liver, intestine and spleen. The drug concentrates in leukocytes, to such a degree that it may be found in circulating leukocytes as long as 10 days after administration.

23. Discuss the onset of action of colchicine.

The onset of action is within 12 hours, with the peak anti-inflammatory effect occurring within 24 to 48 hours.

24. What is the major route of elimination of colchicine?

Although colchicine is metabolized, the major route of elimination of conjugated drug is renal.

25. Is colchicine subject to enterohepatic recirculation?

Yes. The drug is metabolized by the liver and may be reabsorbed from the bile.

26. Compare the distribution half-life and therapeutic half-life of colchicine.

The distribution half-life is very short—it is 3 to 5 minutes. Therapeutic half-life may extend up to 21 hours, or longer in a patient with compromised renal function.

27. What is the use of nonsteroidal anti-inflammatory drugs in the therapy of gout?

These drugs inhibit the formation of inflammatory prostanoids, particularly those formed within leukocytes (e.g., leukocytic pyrogen, leukotrienes), which reduces inflammation in affected joints. These drugs also affect the stimulation of unmyelinated pain fibres and decrease articular pain.

28. Discuss the use of corticosteroids in the therapy of gout.

Corticosteroids (e.g., prednisone, cortisone, dexamethasone) stabilize membranes of leukocytes, decreasing the release of inflammatory mediators, as well as chemotaxic factors. This decreases inflammation and also decreases the influx of leukocytes to the affected area, which further decreases inflammatory tendencies.

29. Would opiate analgesics be useful in the therapy of gout?

Yes. Although not of use in a true therapeutic sense, as these drugs are not antiinflammatory, they would be of use in decreasing the sensation of articular pain.

BIBLIOGRAPHY

1. Cicogna AC, Robinson KG, Conrad CH, et al: Direct effects of colchicine on myocardial function: Studies in hypertrophied and failing spontaneously hypertensive rats. Hypertension 33:60–65, 1999.
2. Davis JC: A practical approach to gout. Current management of an "old" disease. Postgrad Med 106:115–116, 1999
3. Fam AG, Dunne SM, Iazzetta J, et al: Efficacy and safety of desensitization to allopurinol following cutaneous reactions. Arthritis Rheum 44(1):231–238, 2001.
4. Freeman DL: Frequent doses of intravenous colchicine can be lethal. N Engl J Med 309:310, 1983
5. Guerrero RO, Guzman AL: Inhibition of xanthine oxidase by Puerto Rican plant extracts. P R Health Sci J 17(4):359–364, 2000.
6. Goldbart A, Press J, Sofer S, et al: Near fatal acute colchicine intoxication in a child. A case report. Eur J Pediatr 159(12):895–897, 2000.
7. Hardman J, Limbird L, Gilman A: Goodman & Gilman's The Pharmacological Basis of Therapeutics, 10th ed. McGraw-Hill Publishers, 2001.

8. Harris M, Bryant LR, Danaher P, et al: Effect of low dose daily aspirin on serum urate levels and urinary excretion in patients receiving probenecid for gouty arthritis. J Rheumatol 27(12):2873–2876, 2000.
9. Hill J: Gout: Its causes, symptoms and treatment. Nurs Times 95:48–50, 1999.
10. Hoeper MM, Hohlfeld JM, Fabel H: Hyperuricaemia in patients with right or left heart failure. Eur Respir J 13(3):682–685, 1999.
11. Kastrop P, Kimmel I, Bancsi L, et al: The effect of colchicine treatment on spermatozoa: A cytogenetic approach. J Assist Reprod Genet: 16(9):504–507, 1999.
12. Katzung B: Basic and Clinical Pharmacology, 8th ed. Appleton & Lange, 2001.
13. Kong LD, Cai Y, Huang WW, et al: Inhibition of xanthine oxidase by some Chinese medicinal plants used to treat gout. J Ethnopharmacol 73(1–2):199–207, 2000.
14. Margalit A, Hauser SD, Isakson PC: Regulation of in vivo prostaglandin biosynthesis by glutathione. Adv Exp Med Biol 469:165–168, 1999.
15. Lilley LL, Guanci R: 'Until diarrhea occurs'? There's a maximum dosage to prevent colchicine toxicity. Am J Nurs 99(4):12, 1999.
16. Melsom RD: Familial hypersensitivity to allopurinol with subsequent desensitization. Rheumatology (Oxford). 38(12):1301, 1999.
17. Mullins ME, Carrico EA, Horowitz BZ: Fatal cardiovascular collapse following acute colchicine ingestion. J Toxicol Clin Toxicol 38(1):51–54, 2000.
18. Mullins ME, Robertson DG, Norton RL: Troponin I as a marker of cardiac toxicity in acute colchicine overdose. Am J Emerg Med 18(6):743–744, 2000.
19. Munns MJ, King RG, Rice GE: Reduction of human recombinant type II phospholipase A2 and prostaglandin F2 alpha release by microtubule depolymerizing agents. Clin Exp Pharmacol Physiol 26(3):230–235, 1999.
20. Owen PL, Johns T: Xanthine oxidase inhibitory activity of northeastern North American plant remedies used for gout. J Ethnopharmacol 64(2):149–160, 1999.
21. Turnheim K, Krivanek P, Oberbauer R: Pharmacokinetics and pharmacodynamics of allopurinol in elderly and young subjects. Br J Clin Pharmacol 48(4):501–509, 1999.
22. van Doornum S, Ryan PF: Clinical manifestations of gout and their management. Med J Aust 172:493–497, 2000.

IV. Diuretics and Antidiuretics

Patricia K. Anthony, Ph.D.

21. DIURETICS

1. Describe the mechanism of action of loop diuretics.
These drugs inhibit the sodium/potassium/2-chloride cotransporter in the ascending limb of the loop of Henle. This results in retention of sodium (and its associated layer of hydration) in the filtrate, resulting in an increased loss of water. These drugs also inhibit medullary concentration of the tubular filtrate.

2. Describe the phenomenon of "medullary washout" caused by loop diuretics.
The renal interstitium normally increases in osmotic concentration from the cortex to the renal papilla, forming a concentration gradient. This facilitates the sequential concentration of urinary filtrate as it moves through the descending loop of Henle. This concentration gradient is maintained by the actions of the vasa recta, which pick up salts from the interstitium surrounding the ascending limb of the loop of Henle, resulting in a passive absorption of water from the interstitium surrounding the descending limb. Because these drugs, by inhibiting sodium and potassium transport, decrease the extrusion of salts into the interstitium at the ascending limb, the vasa recta pick up less salts, and the osmolality of the plasma in the vasa recta is decreased. This results in reabsorption of water from the interstitium at the descending limb, causing it to become saturated with water (less concentrated), or "washed out."

3. What are the effects of medullary washout on diuresis?
Normally, the renal filtrate is concentrated as it moves down the descending loop of Henle, due to the osmotic gradient in the renal interstitium. As the interstitium becomes saturated with water, the concentration gradient disappears and the filtrate becomes less concentrated, due to the retention of water normally reabsorbed into the interstitium. This results in an increase in urine volume and decreased filtrate osmolarity.

4. Describe the effect of loop diuretics on potassium.
Inhibition of the sodium/potssium/2-chloride cotransporter by these drugs results not only in the retention of urinary sodium, but also retention of potassium in the filtrate   potassium which is normally reabsorbed. Thus these drugs cause a dose-dependent fall in serum potassium levels, which may require supplementation, particularly with long-term therapy.

5. Discuss the efficacy of loop diuretics.
These drugs are extremely efficacious. They result in a high volume of urine, and may also lead to dehydration and loss of electrolytes.

6. Explain the excessive potassium loss seen with loop diuretics.
Loop diuretics cause potassium loss by the initial inhibition of the $Na^+/K^+/2Cl^-$ cotransporter. In addition, the abrupt loss in plasma volume, due to the efficacy of these drugs, results in the stimulation of aldosterone secretion, which promotes an additional loss of potassium.

7. Describe the effect of loop diuretics on plasma ionic concentration.

Loop diuretics cause an increase in the elimination of bicarbonate, sodium, hydrogen, magnesium and calcium ions, as well as ammonium and phosphate ions. To some extent, the loss of a particular ion varies with the choice of drug.

8. What effect do loop diuretics have on plasma pH?

These drugs tend to cause systemic alkalosis, due to the increase in hydrogen ion elimination. This effect may be more marked with furosemide, due to its possible effects on the activity of carbonic anhydrase.

9. Discuss the adverse effects of loop diuretics.

Loop diuretics can cause a dose-related, reversible ototoxicity. Hyperuricemia, hypomagnesemia and hyponatremia are also seen.

10. Are loop diuretics plasma protein bound?

Yes. These drugs are greater than 90 percent protein bound.

11. Compare the potency of bumetanide, torsemide, and furosemide.

Bumetanide is the most potent of the three, with five times the potency of torsemide. Torsemide, in turn, has 2 to 4 times the potency of furosemide.

12. Discuss the actions of bumetanide on cyclic adenosine monophosphate (cAMP).

It has been suggested that bumetanide inhibits renal cAMP. This could affect tubule reabsorption.

13. Review the effects of bumetanide, furosemide and torsemide on the chloride channel.

Bumetanide and torsemide both block chloride channels, to varying degrees. This results in a decrease in sodium and chloride reabsorption, and increased diuretic potency, as compared to furosemide, which does not appear to block chloride channels.

14. Compare the dosing intervals of torsemide, bumetanide, and furosemide.

Torsemide has a significantly longer duration of action, and thus is administered once daily, whereas the other loop diuretics are administered twice daily.

15. Does torsemide affect renal blood flow?

No. Neither renal blood flow or glomerular filtration rate (GFR) are affected. This is in contrast to furosemide and bumetanide, both of which increase renal blood flow (RBF).

16. Describe the effects of torsemide on the reabsorption of salts.

Torsemide decreases the reabsorption of sodium and potassium, but also affects bicarbonate and calcium reabsorption. This effect is variable and may be due to the actions of the drug in the inhibition of chloride reabsorption.

17. What is the duration of action of furosemide?

This drug has a duration of approximately 2 to 3 hours. Elimination is dependent on renal function, so compromised renal function would increase the duration of action of the drug.

18. Describe the importance of tubular secretion of furosemide.

Furosemide is secreted into the tubular lumen and acts from the luminal side. Thus, tubular secretion of the drug is necessary for drug action.

19. Discuss the elimination of furosemide.

Ninety percent of plasma furosemide is excreted unchanged in the urine; 10 percent undergoes metabolism.

20. Differentiate the pharmacokinetics of bumetanide and of furosemide.

Bumetanide is more completely absorbed from the GI tract than furosemide (100 percent versus approximately 60 percent) and is also more extensively metabolized than furosemide—only 60 percent of the drug is excreted unchanged in the urine.

21. Describe the interaction between furosemide and gentamycin.

Gentamycin, an aminoglycoside antibiotic, is ototoxic at the level of the eighth cranial nerve. Furosemide causes ototoxicity due to loss of fluid in the inner ear. Thus, the two drugs (or drug classes) act synergistically to produce ototoxicity and the combination should be avoided.

22. What are the ramifications of administration of loop diuretics to a patient with gout?

Loop diuretics exacerbate gout, because these drugs enter the tubule lumen through the organic acid secretory system. Because uric acid utilizes this system for transport into the renal tubule and subsequent elimination, competition exists for the transporter. This results in both increased levels of uric acid and increased plasma drug levels. In the same way, the drug interferes with the tubular secretion of probenecid, which is used in the therapy of gout.

23. Why is ethacrynic acid seldom used in practice?

This drug is less potent than the other loop diuretics on the market, and also causes severe ototoxicity.

24. Describe the mechanism of action of thiazide diuretics.

Thiazides decrease the transport of chloride ion in the early distal tubule. This results in a decrease in sodium and water reabsorption.

25. Discuss the actions of thiazides on GFR.

The increase in sodium load in the distal tubule mediated by these drugs causes feedback inhibition at the level of the glomerulus, which results in a decrease in GFR.

26. Discuss the use of thiazides in patients with compromised renal function.

The decrease in GFR mediated by these drugs may be beneficial to a patient with compromised renal function, as filtrate load would be reduced.

27. Do thiazide diuretics cause potassium loss?

Yes. These drugs cause an indirect increase in aldosterone levels, which results in net potassium loss. In addition, the increased sodium load in the distal tubule of the nephron promotes increased activity of the sodium-potassium exchange mechanism, resulting in additional loss of potassium.

28. Discuss the adverse effects of thiazide diuretics.

Like other diuretics, thiazides can induce hypokalemia, hyponatremia, hypochloremia, hypomagnesemia, hypercalcemia, hyperuricemia, glucose intolerance, dehydration, and changes in the lipid profile. Thiazides may also cause photosensitivity reactions.

29. How are thiazide diuretics eliminated?

Primarily in the urine.

30. Discuss the drug interactions with thiazides.

Drug interactions with these drugs are in part related to their side effects. Thiazides increase fasting blood glucose concentration, and thus interfere with drugs used for type II diabetes, such as diazoxide and sulfonylureas. The hypokalemic effect of the drugs may precipitate toxicity with potassium-sensitive drugs such as digitalis glycosides and corticosteroids (additive depletion of potassium). As a result of the secretion of the drug by the organic acid secretory system, it may also interfere with the elimination of lithium, and decrease the effectiveness of drugs used in the therapy of gout. Bile-binding resins may bind these drugs and reduce absorption, and nonsteroidal anti-inflammatory drugs (NSAIDs) may interfere with the prostaglandin-mediated actions of thiazide diuretics (e.g., vasodilatation).

31. Describe the actions of thiazide diuretics on urinary calcium levels.

Thiazides enhance parathyroid hormone (PTH)-mediated calcium reabsorption from the distal tubule. Thus, urinary calcium is decreased. This characteristic is especially useful in the treatment and prophylaxis of renal calculi.

32. A patient is allergic to sulfa drugs. Are loop diuretics or thiazides a good choice for therapy?

No. These drugs have a sulfonamide structure and cross-sensitivity may precipitate an allergic reaction.

CARBONIC ANHYDRASE INHIBITORS

33. Describe the mechanism of action of acetazolamide.

Acetazolamide inhibits the activity of carbonic anhydrase (CA) in the proximal tubule. This results in a dose-dependent decrease in bicarbonate formation. Because the formation of bicarbonate is accomplished by the enzymatically catalyzed reaction of water and carbon dioxide, the lack of CA results in unreacted water and CO_2 in the lumen. The CO_2 is lipophilic and passes easily through the tubular cell, leaving the water to be eliminated in the urine.

34. Are carbonic anhydrase inhibitors good diuretics? Explain.

No. They are weak diuretics, in part because their action occurs so early in the nephron. The increased amount of water to be diuresed is produced in the earliest tubule of the nephron and thus must pass through the entire nephron before it can be eliminated. There are many segments through which it can be reabsorbed.

35. Discuss the uses of acetazolamide.

This drug is a weak diuretic. In addition, it is useful in the therapy of glaucoma, as it reduces the formation of water in the ocular fluid. It is also useful in the therapy of metabolic alkalosis. Additionally, carbonic anhydrase inhibitors may also be useful in the therapy of hypooxygenation ("mountain sickness"), because they decrease alkalinization of the blood by increased excretion of bicarbonate, and in some types of seizures.

36. Describe the adverse effects of carbonic anhydrase inhibitors.

The alkalinization of the urine caused by these drugs may contribute to an increase in urinary calcium and phosphate, which increases the formation of renal calculi. In addition, the bicarbonate wasting effect can cause hyperchloremic metabolic acidosis and excessive loss of potassium. In large doses, or in renally compromised patients, the drug may cause central nervous system (CNS) effects, such as sedation and paresthesias.

37. Explain the contraindication of acetazolamide in cirrhotic patients.

The increase in urinary pH due to excessive bicarbonate elimination may contribute to the decreased urinary trapping of ammonium ions. This may contribute to hepatic encephalopathy.

POTASSIUM-SPARING DIURETICS

38. Discuss the mechanism of action of amiloride.

Amiloride acts to inhibit sodium-potassium adenosinetriphosphatase (ATPase) in the distal convoluted tubule. This prevents the reabsorption of sodium in exchange for potassium, and results in the retention of potassium, rather than sodium. As sodium is eliminated in the urine, along with its associated layer of hydration, diuresis is produced.

39. Discuss the actions of amiloride in the proximal tubule.

Amiloride acts to inhibit the sodium-hydrogen ion exchanger in the proximal tubule. This results in retention of sodium in the urine, and decreased secretion of acid.

40. Is amiloride a potent diuretic?

No. Potassium-sparing diuretics have only weak diuretic activity and are mainly used as an adjunct to therapy with other drugs that promote the elimination of potassium.

41. Discuss the elimination of amiloride.

Amiloride is eliminated both in the urine and feces. It is primarily eliminated unchanged.

42. Is amiloride plasma protein bound?

To a small extent—about 23 percent of the drug binds to proteins.

43. Discuss the use of amiloride in a digitalized patient.

The use of amiloride may help to keep potassium levels from falling, due to the actions of digitalis glycosides. As the heart is exquisitely sensitive to potassium, use of amiloride may help to prevent the generation of cardiac anomalies due to glycoside therapy.

44. A patient on digoxin therapy is receiving potassium supplementation. Would amiloride therapy be indicated?

No. Potassium-sparing diuretics are contraindicated with potassium supplementation.

45. Describe the mechanism of action of triamterene.

This drug stabilizes membrane potentials in the distal tubule, decreasing the exchange of urinary sodium for serum potassium. Thus, potassium is conserved and sodium/water is eliminated.

46. Is the potassium-sparing effect of triamterene reflected as a constant amount?

No. This drug actually increases the retention of potassium when a large amount of excretion exists, and decreases retention when potassium loss is minimal.

47. Compare the duration of action of triamterene and amiloride.

Triamterene has a shorter duration than amiloride—12 to 16 hours—as compared to 24 hours duration for amiloride.

48. Is triamterene metabolized?

Yes. At least one active metabolite has been characterized.

49. Discuss the mechanism of action of spironolactone.

Spironolactone is a competitive antagonist of aldosterone. It binds to the aldosterone receptor and prevents the induction of protein channels that exchange sodium for potassium in the urinary filtrate in the distal portion of the distal convoluted tubule and collecting ducts. Thus, sodium is excreted and potassium is retained.

50. Is spironolactone useful in any condition requiring a potassium sparing diuretic?

No. This drug is only useful in the presence of elevated levels of aldosterone.

51. What is the use of spironolactone in a diagnostic capacity?

This drug is useful in the diagnosis of primary aldosteronism.

52. Is spironolactone useful as an antihypertensive?

No. It is primarily useful in the therapy of heart failure and ascites, secondary to cirrhosis.

53. Describe the benefits of spironolactone in the therapy of heart failure.

Spironolactone has been shown to decrease mortality and increase the quality of life of patients with severe heart failure, when added to a conventional therapy regimen.

54. Discuss the treatment of edema secondary to renal failure.

In this case, the use of loop diuretics is of choice. Thiazides do not tend to be effective at a low GFR (< 30 mL/min), and both acetazolamide and potassium-sparing drugs can exacerbate existing hyperkalemia.

OSMOTIC DIURETICS

55. Discuss the properties of mannitol that make it useful as an osmotic diuretic.

Mannitol is sugar alcohol that is not metabolized. It is filtered and eliminated by the kidney. The structure contains six hydroxyl groups (see Figure), each of which is capable of binding a water molecule.It is thus hygroscopic.

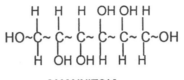

[MANNITOL]

56. Discuss the mechanism of action of mannitol.

The mannitol molecule is capable of binding water in a ratio of greater than six to one. Once bound, the water is carried through the kidney in a nonreabsorbable state. This results in profound diuresis.

57. Explain the actions of osmotic diuretics on the concentration of urine.

The mannitol molecule is not transported across the thin limb of the loop of Henle. Thus, the associated water molecules also cannot pass into the renal interstitium. The countercurrent mechanism is thus disrupted, and, to some extent, results in the dehydration of the renal interstitium.

58. Explain the contraindication of the use of mannitol with heart failure.

Osmotic diuretics cause a rapid expansion of extracellular volume, as water is drawn from the intracellular compartment to the extracellular compartment. This expansion results in an increased preload and increased ventricular filling, which exacerbate the failing heart, and produce pulmonary edema.

59. What adverse effects are common with mannitol therapy?

Headache, nausea, and vomiting, due to increased intracranial pressure, are common. If adequate fluid replacement is not administered, severe dehydration will also result.

BIBLIOGRAPHY

1. Beermann B, Groschinsky-Grind M: Clinical pharmacokinetics of diuretics [review]. Clin Pharmacokinet 5(3):221–245, 1980.
2. Brater DC: Pharmacology of diuretics [review]. Am J Med Sci 319(1):38–50, 2000.
3. Brater DC: The use of diuretics in congestive heart failure [review]. Semin Nephrol 14(5):479–484, 1994.
4. DuBose TD, Good DW: Effects of diuretics on renal acid-base transport [review]. Semin Nephrol 8(3):282–294.
5. Friedman PA: Biochemistry and pharmacology of diuretics [review]. Semin Nephrol 8(3):198–212, 1998.

6. Hardman J, Limbird L, Gilman A: Goodman & Gilman's The Pharmacological Basis of Therapeutics, 10th ed. McGraw-Hill Publishers, 2001.
7. Heidenreich O, Greven J, Heintze K: Molecular actions of diuretics. Klin Wochenschr 60(19):1258–1263, 1982.
8. Herkel U, Pfeiffer N: Update on topical carbonic anhydrase inhibitors. Curr Opin Ophthalmol 12(2):88–93, 2001.
9. Imai M: Effect of bumetanide and furosemide on the thick ascending limb of Henle's loop of rabbits and rats perfused in vitro. Eur J Pharmacol 41(4):409–416, 1977.
10. Johnston PA, Kau ST: The effect of loop of Henle diuretics on the tubuloglomerular feedback mechanism. Methods Find Exp Clin Pharmacol 14(7):523–529.
11. Katzung B: Basic and Clinical Pharmacology, 8th ed. Appleton & Lange, 2001.
12. Kemp G, Kemp D: Diuretics. Am J Nurs 78(6):1006–1010, 1978.
13. Mende CW: Current issues in diuretic therapy [review]. Hosp Pract (Off Ed) 25 Suppl 1:15–21; [discussion 30–31], 1990.
14. Odlind B: Site and mechanism of the action of diuretics [review]. Acta Pharmacol Toxicol (Copenh) 54 Suppl 1:5–15, 1984.
15. Puscas I, Coltau M, Baican M, et al: The inhibitory effect of diuretics on carbonic anhydrases. Res Commun Mol Pathol Pharmacol 105(3):213–236, 1999.
16. Puschett JB: Pharmacological classification and renal actions of diuretics [review]. Cardiology 84 Suppl 2:4–13, 1994.
17. Remmers AR, Beathard GA, Lindley JD, et al: Diuretics. Am Fam Phys 8(4):208–215, 1973.
18. Shirley DG, Walter SJ, Unwin RJ, et al: Contribution of Na+-H+ exchange to sodium reabsorption in the loop of Henle: A microperfusion study in rats. J Physiol 513 (Pt 1):243–249, 1998.
19. Stafford GO: Diuretics [review]. Clin Anesth 10(1):269–281.
20. Steinmetz PR, Koeppen BM: Cellular mechanisms of diuretic action along the nephron [review]. Hosp Pract (Off Ed) 19(9):125–134, 1984.
21. Stier CT, Itskovitz HD: Renal calcium metabolism and diuretics [review]. Annu Rev Pharmacol Toxicol 26:101–116, 1986.
22. Unwin RJ, Walter SJ, Giebisch G, et al: Localization of diuretic effects along the loop of Henle: An in vivo microperfusion study in rats. Clin Sci (Colch) 98(4):481–488, 2000.
23. Wittner M, Di Stefano A, Wangemann P, et al: How do loop diuretics act [review]?Drugs 41 Suppl 3:1–13, 1991.

22. DRUGS USED IN THE THERAPY OF DIABETES INSIPIDUS (DI) AND SIADH

1. Describe the types of DI and their origins.
Diabetes insipidus may be of neurogenic origin, whereby secretion of antidiuretic hormone (ADH) from the hypothalamic/posterior pituitary axis is compromised. This form of DI is readily treatable with pharmacologic agents. DI may also be of nephrogenic origin, where a defect in the ADH receptor or transduction mechanism exists. Pharmacologic treatments for this form of DI are limited, because drugs that increase the activity of ADH are not effective without functioning receptors.

2. Discuss the use of desmopressin (DDAVP) in the therapy of neurogenic DI.
This drug is a vasopressin (ADH) analog, which is longer in duration than endogenous ADH. It binds to, and activates, the ADH receptor, resulting in the opening of channels in the distal tubule and collecting duct, and reabsorption of water.

3. How is desmopressin administered?
This drug is effective orally, and may also be administered intranasally or parenterally.

4. Which of the above formulations of desmopressin would have the slowest onset?
The oral formulation, as absorption is poor and slow, as compared to the intranasal preparation, which is absorbed directly into nasal capillaries, or parenteral administration, which has a high bioavailability and fast onset.

5. Discuss the preferential administration of intranasal desmopressin for the therapy of DI.
When administered intranasally, the drug has a longer duration of action, and fewer adverse effects.

6. Is the oral form of desmopressin used in the therapy of DI?
No. This form is primarily used in the therapy of hemophilia A and Type I von Willebrand's disease.

7. Discuss the effects of desmopressin on intrinsic clotting factors.
This drug increases circulating levels of factor VIII and plasminogen activating factor. This effect is greater than that seen with vasopressin.

8. Does desmopressin affect excretion of sodium and potassium?
No. Serum concentrations of sodium and potassium remain constant, as do the rates of excretion of these ions.

9. Contrast the effects of desmopressin and vasopressin on circulating adrenocorticotropic hormone (ACTH) levels.
In contrast to vasopressin, desmopressin does not increase circulating levels of ACTH or cortisol.

10. Describe the relative vasoconstrictor effects of desmopressin and vasopressin.
Unlike vasopressin, desmopressin has significantly less effect on vascular smooth muscle. Vasoconstriction is less pronounced.

11. Describe the effects of desmopressin on platelet function.
Desmopressin can induce platelet aggregation.

12. How much of an intranasally administered dose is actually absorbed?
Only about 10 to 20 percent.

13. What is the duration of action of desmopressin?
The duration is variable—effects may last from 5 hours to approximately 20 hours. Effects then abruptly disappear.

14. Describe the effect of desmopressin in a patient who is a heavy drinker of coffee or alcoholic beverages.
Both alcohol and caffeine have diuretic activity and would oppose the effects of desmopressin. Thus, therapeutic effects would be lessened.

15. Describe the use of lypressin.
Lypressin is a lysine analog of vasopressin, with little or no vasoactive activity. It is administered intranasally for the treatment of diabetes insipidus.

16. Discuss the interactions of carbamazepine and chlorpropamide with lypressin.
These drugs may potentiate the actions of ADH. Thus, the effects of lypressin are potentiated as well.

17. Compare the actions of vasopressin, lypressin and desmopressin on smooth muscle.
Vasopressin has significant constrictor activity. Lypressin and desmopressin have comparatively little.

18. Explain the mechanism of action of vasopressin.
Vasopressin activates adenylate cyclase, which results in an increase in the production of cyclic adenosine monophosphate (cAMP). This results in enzymatic phosphorylation of channels in the membrane of the collecting tubule cells, allowing water to be reabsorbed from the urine.

19. Describe the actions of vasopressin on cortisol levels.
Vasopressin increases circulating ACTH, which results in increased levels of cortisol.

20. Is vasopressin administered orally?
No. The drug is a peptide, which is degraded by pancreatic enzymes.

21. Does vasopressin have a long half-life?
No. It has a half-life of 10 to 20 minutes.

22. Describe the pharmacokinetics of vasopressin.
This drug is not plasma protein bound and is primarily excreted unchanged in the urine.

23. Discuss the contraindications to the administration of vasopressin.
Due to its vasoactive activity, as well as the rapid increase in extracellular volume produced by the drug, it should be administered with caution in patients with angina, heart failure, coronary artery disease (CAD), thrombosis, or migraines. It is possible that the drug may also exacerbate asthma, as it is a constrictor of smooth muscle.

24. What are the signs of vasopressin-induced water intoxication?
Listlessness, drowsiness, confusion, headache, anuria, and weight gain are symptoms and should be closely monitored.

25. Does vasopressin cause uterine contractions?
Yes. It can affect all smooth muscle. Diarrhea, uterine contractions, and intestinal hyper-motility have all been reported.

26. Are thiazide diuretics useful in the therapy of DI?
Yes, although as yet this use is not FDA approved. The increased sodium load to the distal tubule initiates a negative feedback to the glomerulus and glomerular filtration rate is slowed.

DRUGS USED IN THE THERAPY OF SYNDROME OF INAPPROPRIATE SECRETION OF ANTIDIURETIC HORMONE (SIADH)

27. Describe the use of demeclocycline.
Demeclocycline is a tetracycline antibiotic. Its major clinical use is in the therapy of SIADH.

28. What is the mechanism of action of demeclocycline in the therapy of SIADH?
Demeclocycline inhibits the ADH-induced water reabsorption from the distal convoluted tubule and collecting duct. This induces diuresis.

29. Are actions of demeclocycline immediate?
No. The effects of the drug may not be seen until 5 days after initiation of therapy.

30. Describe the termination of drug action, after demeclocycline withdrawal.
The effects of the drug continue for as long as 6 days after drug withdrawal.

31. Are other tetracyclines useful in the therapy of SIADH?
No. Demeclocycline is the only drug of the class to be effective.

32. Describe the absorption of demeclocycline.
Systemic absorption is inversely proportional to dosage. Like all tetracyclines, divalent ions (e.g., Ca^{++}, Mg^{++}, and Fe^{++}) will chelate the drug in the small intestine and reduce absorption.

33. Describe the distribution of demeclocycline.
This drug is widely distributed in body fluids and in cerebrospinal fluid (CSF). Due to its ability to chelate with divalent ions, it concentrates in tissues high in calcium and iron (e.g., in bony tissues such as teeth and bone, and in the liver).

34. Describe the half-life of demeclocycline.
The half-life is long, due to enterohepatic recycling. Excretion is primarily renal, so the half-life is increased in geriatric or renally compromised patients.

35. Explain the ramifications of concurrent administration of demeclocycline and carba-mazepine or imipramine.
Carbamazepine and tricyclic antidepressants, as well as phenothiazines, opiates, and barbitu-rates can cause hyponatremia, which would be additive with that produced by demeclocycline.

36. Discuss the problems with the administration of demeclocycline post-carbamazepine dosage.
The administration of carbamazepine results in a decrease in the half-life of demeclocycline.

37. Describe the adverse effects seen with demeclocycline.
These include mild central nervous system (CNS) effects, headache, nausea and vomiting. With high intravenous doses, hypotension may be seen, which precipitates a reflex tachycardia. Excessively high doses may induce seizures.

38. Are adverse effects seen with oral demeclocycline?
No appreciable effects are seen.

39. Discuss the use of lithium in the therapy of SIADH.
Lithium decreases the ability of the nephron to concentrate urine, producing a mild nephrogenic diabetes insipidus.

BIBLIOGRAPHY

1. Abrams C: ADH-associated pathologies. Diabetes insipidus and syndrome of inappropriate ADH [review]. MLO Med Lab Obs 32(2):24–28, 30, 32–3; [quiz 36, 38], 2000.
2. Baylis PH: Diabetes insipidus [review]. J R Coll Physicians Lond 32(2):108–111, 1998.
3. Baylis PH, Cheetham T: Diabetes insipidus [review]. Arch Dis Child 79(1):84–89, 1998.
4. Hardman J, Limbird L, Gilman A: Goodman & Gilman's The Pharmacological Basis of Therapeutics, 10th ed. McGraw-Hill Publishers, 2001.
5. Heater DW: If ADH goes out of balance. Diabetes insipidus. RN 62(7):44–46, 1999.
6. Jonat S, Santer R, Schneppenheim R, et al: Effect of DDAVP on nocturnal enuresis in a patient with nephrogenic diabetes insipidus. Arch Dis Child 81(1):57–59, 1999.
7. Katzung B: Basic and Clinical Pharmacology, 8th ed. Appleton & Lange, 2001.
8. Kirchlechner V, Koller DY, Seidl R, et al: Treatment of nephrogenic diabetes insipidus with hydrochlorothiazide and amiloride. Arch Dis Child 80(6):548–552, 1999.
9. Magaldi AJ: New insights into the paradoxical effect of thiazides in diabetes insipidus therapy [review]. Nephrol Dial Transplant 15(12):1903–1905.
10. Negro A, Regolisti G, Perazzoli F, et al: Ifosfamide-induced renal Fanconi syndrome with associated nephrogenic diabetes insipidus in an adult patient. Nephrol Dial Transplant 13(6):1547–1549, 1998.
11. Ray JG: DDAVP use during pregnancy: An analysis of its safety for mother and child [review]. Obstet Gynecol Surv 53(7):450–455, 1998.
12. Siegel AJ, Baldessarini RJ, Klepser MB, et al: Primary and drug-induced disorders of water homeostasis in psychiatric patients: Principles of diagnosis and management [review]. Harv Rev Psychiatry 6(4):190–200, 1998.
13. Stone KA: Lithium-induced nephrogenic diabetes insipidus. J Am Board Fam Pract- 12(1):43–47, 1999.
14. Takemura N: Successful long-term treatment of congenital nephrogenic diabetes insipidus ina dog. J Small Anim Pract 39(12):592–594, 1998.
15. Tetiker T, Sert M, Kocak M: Efficacy of indapamide in central diabetes insipidus. Arch Intern Med 159(17):2085–2087, 1999.

V. Drugs Used In Anesthesia

Patricia K. Anthony, Ph.D., and C. Andrew Powers, Ph.D.

23. GENERAL ANESTHETICS

1. Describe the stages of central nervous system (CNS) depression seen with inhalation anesthetics.
- Stage I: analgesia is present, drowsiness may ensue. No amnesia is present initially, but as depression deepens, amnesia becomes evident.
- Stage II: This is the most perilous stage of anesthesia. In this stage, strong involuntary muscle contractions are present, respiration becomes irregular, and the patient may become delirious. Vomiting and incontinence may also occur. Useful anesthetics produce a swift progression from phase I to phase III, with phase II in limited duration.
- Stage III: This is the phase in which surgical anesthesia is produced. A regular respiration rate resumes in the initial phase of stage III, progressing to a complete lack of respiratory activity as medullary centers are depressed.
- Stage IV: Spontaneous respiration ceases. Inhibition of medullary vasomotor centers leads to circulatory collapse. Circulatory and respiratory support must be maintained, or death rapidly ensues. (See Figure.)

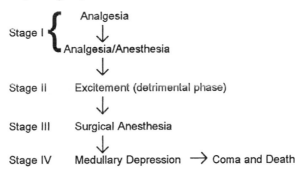

2. Are the physiologic effects of stages I–IV of CNS depression seen only with the onset of anesthesia?
No. The stages are reversed upon withdrawal of the anesthetic.

3. Define "*minimum alveolar concentration*" (MAC) and explain its significance.
The MAC is defined as the lowest alveolar anesthetic gas to air percentage that will yield pharmacologic effects. An anesthetic with a high MAC thus requires a large amount of anesthetic to induce anesthesia, while a drug with a low MAC requires a lower amount to yield the same effect.

4. What is the significance of the blood-gas partition coefficient?
This number gives the lipophilic value of an anesthetic drug. The higher the coefficient, the less miscible it is with water, and the more lipophilic it is. Because the CNS has a large amount of fatty tissue, the more lipophilic a drug is, the faster the drug enters into the CNS, resulting in

faster onset. In the same way, the blood-gas coefficient also predicts the rate of recovery from the anesthetic—the higher the coefficient, the lower the solubility in blood, and the faster the recovery time.

5. Are inhalation anesthetics widely distributed?
    These drugs are carried in the blood, and thus are distributed mainly to richly vascularized organs, such as the heart and liver. Less distribution is seen to poorly vascularized tissues, such as muscle and adipose tissue.

6. How are inhalation anesthetics eliminated?
    In general, these drugs are eliminated via the lung into expired air.

7. Describe the influence of the duration of anesthesia on recovery time.
    With a long duration of anesthesia, the drug accumulates to a greater extent in adipose tissue, muscle and skin. These tissues release the drug more slowly, increasing recovery time. Thus, a drug with a low partition coefficient may have a paradoxically longer recovery time. A short duration of anesthesia will produce a recovery time proportional to the blood-gas coefficient of the drug (e.g., a faster recovery time with a more lipophilic drug).

8. Discuss the actions of inhalation anesthetics on the brain.
    In general, these agents decrease metabolism in the brain. Perfusion is increased, due to vascular effects of the drugs.

9. Which anesthetic is primarily used in pediatric surgery?
    Halothane.

10. Discuss the cardiovascular effects of halothane.
    Halothane decreases cardiac output, decreases mean arterial pressure, and reduces atrial node firing, resulting in a decrease in heart rate.

11. Which anesthetic produces minimal cardiodepression and lacks toxic metabolites?
    Enflurane.

12. Is enflurane a first choice as a pediatric anesthetic?
    No. It can produce seizures when used in children.

13. Which short-acting inhalation anesthetic can produce megaloblastic anemia?
    Nitrous oxide. The extremely lipophilic character of the gas, and its ability to bind to hemoglobin, may result in a decrease in oxygen transport.

14. Discuss the renal toxicity produced by methoxyflurane.
    Methoxyflurane metabolism produces inorganic fluorine, fluoride and oxalic acid. These are excreted through the urine and may cause renal damage.

15. What is the mechanism of action of etomidate?
    This drug facilitates GABA-ergic transmission.

16. Describe the use of etomidate in general anesthesia.
    Etomidate is used in the induction and maintenance of general anesthesia. It is also used as an adjunct to nitrous oxide anesthesia.

17. Discuss the duration of action of etomidate.
    Etomidate has a rapid onset and rapid recovery, and thus has a short duration of action.

18. Is etomidate useful in the anesthesia of cardiac patients?
Yes. It has minimal cardiodepressant or pulmonary depressant effects.

19. What is responsible for the rapid recovery of consciousness after a bolus dose of thiopental?
Rapid redistribution of the drug from the brain into peripheral organs.

20. Compare the actions of thiopental and propofol.
Propofol is a nonbarbiturate anesthetic that induces anesthesia as quickly as thiopental but has a rate of emergence that is 10 times faster.

21. Discuss the action of propofol on emesis.
Propofol is useful in this regard, because it has an antiemetic action.

22. Is propofol plasma protein bound?
Yes (95–99 percent).

23. Describe the metabolism and excretion of propofol.
Propofol is metabolized by cytochrome P_{450} and is glucuronidated. The conjugates are eliminated in the urine.

24. Compare the actions of methohexital and thiopental.
Methohexital is faster acting than thiopental and has a faster recovery time. Its potency is almost twice that of thiopental, and it exhibits a greater amount of postanesthesia excitatory phenomena.

25. Describe the induction of methohexital.
Once in the plasma, methohexital induces sleep within 30 seconds.

BIBLIOGRAPHY

1. Buggy DJ, Nicol B, Rowbotham DJ, et al: Effects of intravenous anesthetic agents on glutamate release: A role for GABA receptor-mediated inhibition. Anesthesiology: 92(4):1067–1073, 2000.
2. George A: Comparison of sevoflurane and propofol. Anaesthesia 55:189–190, 2000.
3. Dougherty TB, Porche VH, Thall PF: Maximum tolerated dose of nalmefene in patients receiving epidural fentanyl and dilute bupivacaine for postoperative analgesia. Anesthesiology 92(4):1010–1016, 2000.
4. Duong TQ, Iadecola C, Kim SG: Effect of hyperoxia, hypercapnia, and hypoxia on cerebral interstitial oxygen tension and cerebral blood flow. Magn Reson Med 45(1):61–70, 2001.
5. Hardman J, Limbird L, Gilman A: Goodman & Gilman's The Pharmacological Basis of Therapeutics, 10ed. McGraw-Hill Publishers, 2001.
6. Iconomou G, Viha A, Vagenakis AG: Transdermal fentanyl in cancer patients with moderate to severe pain: A prospective examination. Anticancer Res 20(6C):4821–4824, 2000.
7. Katzung B: Basic and Clinical Pharmacology, 8th ed. Appleton & Lange, 2001.
8. McNeely JK, Buczulinski B, Rosner DR: Severe neurological impairment in an infant after nitrous oxide anesthesia. Anesthesiology 93(6):1549–1550, 2000.
9. Nunez JL, Juraska JM: Neonatal halothane anesthesia affects cortical morphology. Brain Res Dev Brain Res 124(1-2):121–124, 2000.
10. Renfrew C, Dickson R, Schwab C: Severe hypertension following ephedrine administration in a patient receiving entacapone. Anesthesiology 93(6):1562, 2000
11. Tschaikowsky K, Ritter J, Schroppel K, et al: Volatile anesthetics differentially affect immunostimulated expression of inducible nitric oxide synthase: role of intracellular calcium. Anesthesiology 92(4):1093–1102, 2000.

24. LOCAL ANESTHETICS

1. Describe the general mechanism of local anesthetics.

These drugs bind to sodium channels at the inner surface of the membrane of excitable cells (e.g., neuronal, cardiac) (see Figure). This decreases the entry of sodium into the cell in a dose-dependent manner, resulting in stabilization of the membrane and decreased conduction.

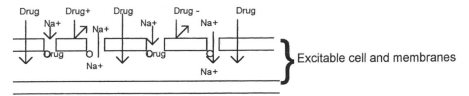

2. Is membrane resting potential changed with use of local anesthetics?

At therapeutic doses, membrane potential is not significantly affected.

3. Relate drug pK_a, physiologic pH and drug efficacy.

The pH of the tissue at the injection site will influence the potency of the drug. In order for the drug to enter the cell and bind to the cytoplasmic side of the sodium channel, it must be in nonionized form (see the Henderson-Hasselbalch equation, Chapter 1, General Pharmacology). The more ionized a drug is, the less potent it is. Thus, dosage must be increased in order to achieve maximal efficacy.

4. Discuss the potency of local anesthetics in an area where inflammation is present.

A drug that is a weak base with a high pK_a (e.g., lidocaine) will be excessively ionized in an acid environment (e.g., with inflammation or infection present) and will require a higher dose to reach minimum efficacy.

5. What are the factors that influence the rate of onset of local anesthetic effects?

In general, the smaller and more lipophilic a drug, the faster the effects will be seen.

6. Describe naturally occurring toxins that may interfere with local anesthetic action.

Toxins that bind to sodium channels and promote sodium flux. Examples of these include tetrodotoxin (puffer fish toxin), and scorpion venom.

7. Discuss the effects of local anesthetics on major organ systems.

These drugs may have profound effects on organ systems—particularly those with excitable tissue, such as the nervous system and heart. The greatest effect is seen in conduction systems with unmyelinated fibers, such as heart, preganglionic autonomic fibers, and pain (type C) fibers.

8. What factors limit the systemic absorption of local anesthetics?

The degree to which a drug binds to tissue proteins, the site of injection (i.e., degree of vascularization of the site), and the characteristics of the individual drug all affect absorption.

9. Why are vasoconstrictor agents often administered with local anesthetic drugs?

Agents such as epinephrine are often co-injected, as they mediate local vasoconstriction. The degree of vasoconstriction limits the amount of drug that enters the blood and is systemically absorbed. This is beneficial in two ways:

1. Limitation of systemic absorption (which influences the proper function of excitable tissues) and

2. If not absorbed into the blood, the drug is concentrated at the site of injection, resulting in increased efficacy.

10. What are the two general classifications of local anesthetic drugs?
Ester-type and amide-type.

11. Discuss the metabolism of ester-type local anesthetics.
These drugs are rapidly metabolized in the blood by plasma pseudocholinesterases.

12. Describe the hypersensitivity reactions seen with local anesthetics.
Hypersensitivity reactions occur with the ester-type of drugs. These drugs are metabolized to paraaminobenzoic acid (PABA) derivatives. Individuals sensitive to PABA may experience allergic reactions to these drugs.

13. Discuss the duration of action of ester-type drugs.
Because metabolism by pseudocholinesterases is very rapid, the half-lives and durations of these drugs are very short.

14. How are the amide-type local anesthetics metabolized?
These drugs are metabolized by hepatic cytochrome P_{450}. The half-lives of these drugs are thus prolonged in patients with liver dysfunction.

15. Are all of the amide-type drugs metabolized at the same rate?
No. Prilocaine is metabolized very quickly, whereas bupivacaine is metabolized slowly. Etidocaine, lidocaine and mepivacaine are intermediate.

16. Discuss the onset and duration of bupivacaine.
This drug has a rapid onset and long duration, as compared to other drugs.

17. Does bupivicaine have similar effects on all sensory nerve fibers?
No. Effects on pain fibers are of longer duration than effects on other sensory fibers. Thus, the analgesic effects are of longer duration than anesthetic effects.

18. Discuss the effects of bupivacaine on muscle relaxation.
The effects on muscle relaxation are dose-dependent. When administered as an epidural or to produce peripheral nerve blockade, use of low-dose bupivacaine will produce partial relaxation. Progressively higher doses produce more effect, and high doses (e.g., use of a 75 percent solution) will produce complete muscle relaxation.

19. Compare the half-life of bupivacaine in adults and in neonates.
The half-life is significantly increased in neonates. In adults, the mean $T\frac{1}{2}$ is approximately 3.5 hours, which increases to 8 hours in the neonate.

20. Does etidocaine produce muscle relaxation that is used in spinal anesthesia?
Etidocaine produces a profound motor blockade and muscle relaxation when used in peridural anesthesia.

21. Compare the actions of lidocaine and mepivacaine.
Lidocaine produces more vasodilatation than mepivacaine. It also has a slower onset and shorter duration of action.

22. Compare the elimination of mepivacaine in adults and in neonates.
Adults are able to both metabolize the drug via cytochrome P_{450} and to excrete unchanged drug via the kidney. Neonates are not able to eliminate unchanged drug. Therefore, the drug must be metabolized. The mean $T^{1/2}$ is therefore substantially increased.

23. What is the relationship between bupivacaine and ropivacaine?
These drugs are stereoisomers. Bupivacaine is the S isomer and ropivacaine the D isomer.

24. What is the advantage of using ropivacaine in a cardiac patient?
Ropivacaine produces less arrhythmogenic activity than bupivacaine. Ropivacaine is also less lipid-soluble and is cleared more rapidly, which may decrease the incidence of adverse effects.

25. Is ropivacaine administered IV?
No. Intravenous administration is to be avoided.

26. Why would prilocaine be a good choice for dental anesthesia?
Because dental anesthesia is often used in conjunction with invasive procedures, this drug would be a good choice as it produces less vasodilatation than other drugs (e.g., lidocaine). However, the drug produces pulp analgesia for only a short duration (10–15 minutes).

BIBLIOGRAPHY

1. Acalovschi I, Cristea T, Margarit S, et al: Tramadol added to lidocaine for intravenous regional anesthesia. Anesth Analg 92(1):209–214, 2001.
2. Challacombe SJ, Hodgson T, Shirlaw PJ: Allergic reactions. Br Dent J 189(10):527, 2000.
3. Debon R, Allaouchiche B, Duflo F, et al: The analgesic effect of sufentanil combined with ropivacaine 0.2% for labor analgesia: A comparison of three sufentanil doses. Anesth Analg 92(1):180–183, 2001.
4. Ezsias A: Local anaesthetics. Br Dent J 189(12):636, 2000.
5. Frawley G, Ragg P, Hack H: Plasma concentrations of bupivacaine after combined spinal epidural anaesthesia in infants and neonates. Paediatr Anaesth 10(6):619–625, 2000.
6. Hansen TG, Ilett KF, Lim SI, et al: Pharmacokinetics and clinical efficacy of long-term epidural ropivacaine infusion in children. Br J Anaesth 85(3):347–353, 2000.
7. Hardman J, Limbird L, Gilman A: Goodman & Gilman's The Pharmacological Basis of Therapeutics, 10th ed. McGraw-Hill Publishers, 2001.
8. Harris R: Sensitivity to local anaesthetic. Aust Dent J 17(5):333–334, 1972.
9. Hesselgard K, Stromblad LG, Reinstrup P: Morphine with or without a local anaesthetic for postoperative intrathecal pain treatment after selective dorsal rhizotomy in children. Paediatr Anaesth 11(1):75–79, 2001.
10. Katzung B: Basic and Clinical Pharmacology, 8th ed. Appleton & Lange, 2001.
11. Kudo K, Hino Y, Ikeda N, et al: Blood concentrations of tetracaine and its metabolite following spinal anesthesia. Forensic Sci Int 116(1):9–14, 2001.
12. Larter M: Local anesthetic complications. Can Forces Dent Serv Bull Fall:47–51, 1983.
13. Lenfant F, Lahet JJ, Vergely C, et al: Lidocaine inhibits potassium efflux and hemolysis in erythrocytes during oxidative stress in vitro. Gen Pharmacol 34(3):193–199, 2000.
14. Librowski T, Filipek B, Czarnecki R: Local anesthetic and antiarrhythmic effect of some imidazolidin-2-one derivatives. Acta Pol Pharm- 57(5):391–396, 2000.
15. Malamed SF: Morbidity, mortality and local anaesthesia. Prim Dent Care 6(1):11–15, 1999.
16. McClellan KJ, Faulds D: Ropivacaine: An update of its use in regional anaesthesia. Drugs 60(5):1065–1093, 2000.
17. Meyer JS, Slotkin TA, Buckley NE, et al: Receptors for abused drugs: development and plasticity. Neurotoxicol Teratol- 22(6):773–784, 2000.
18. Moore PA, Hersh EV: Local anesthesia toxicity review revisited. Pediatr Dent 22(1):7–8, 2000.

VI. *Drugs that Affect Muscle Tissue and Bone*

Patricia K. Anthony, Ph.D.

25. SKELETAL MUSCLE RELAXANTS

1. Explain the action of depolarizing blockers in skeletal muscle relaxation.

These drugs keep muscle constantly in a depolarized state. Thus, since the neuromuscular junction has no opportunity to repolarize, it cannot be stimulated, and no contraction can occur.

2. Is there an antidote for an overdose of a drug such as succinylcholine?

No. Supportive measures must be instituted.

3. Explain the mechanism of action of a nondepolarizing blocker in skeletal muscle relaxation.

These agents act at receptor sites to compete with acetylcholine (ACh). Thus, they are competitive antagonists at the nicotinic receptor.

4. How are muscles affected by a nondepolarizing blockade?

Muscle groups are affected in order of bundle size those associated with finer movements (small bundles) are affected first, followed by limbs, postural muscles (trunk and chest) and finally the diaphragm. These events are dose-related. Recovery upon withdrawal of the drug occurs in reverse order—large muscle groups recover first, followed by muscle groups associated with fine movement (e.g., facial muscles, and muscles of the eye).

5. Discuss the action of centrally-acting skeletal muscle relaxants.

These agents act at the level of the brain stem to initiate muscle relaxation. This may be related to a blockade of afferent pathways, or by a central depression of central nervous system (CNS) function.

6. What are examples of centrally-acting skeletal muscle relaxants?

These agents include baclofen, carisoprodol, chlorzoxazone and cyclobenzaprine.

7. What is the only depolarizing blocker currently approved for use in the United States?

Succinylcholine.

8. What are some nondepolarizing blockers?

Atracurium, doxacurium, pancuronium, pipecuronium, d-tubocurarine, mivacurium, and metocurine are examples of nondepolarizing blockers.

9. Describe drugs that mediate skeletal muscle relaxation directly.

Directly acting agents include dantrolene. In addition, most benzodiazepines (e.g., diazepam, lorazepam), relax skeletal muscle both directly, by potentiation of gamma-aminobutyric acid (GABA) at the level of the muscle, as well as indirectly by CNS effects.

10. Which skeletal muscle relaxants are effective in muscle spasm secondary to cerebral or spinal cord disease?

Directly acting muscle relaxants, such as dantrolene. Centrally acting agents are not effective because they ultimately act at the level of the spinal cord.

11. Describe the mechanism of action of dantrolene.

Dantrolene acts to decrease the release of calcium from the sarcoplasmic reticulum, resulting in decreased excitation-contraction coupling. Thus, contraction of skeletal muscle is impaired.

12. Does dantrolene have significant cardiovascular effects?

No. Smooth muscle and cardiac muscle have little sarcoplasmic reticulum, and are thus not significantly affected by the drug.

13. What is the major adverse effect of dantrolene?

Hepatotoxicity is a dose-limiting factor.

14. Describe the mechanism of action of baclofen.

Baclofen is considered a GABA agonist. The drug thus decreases afferent activity at the level of the spinal cord, resulting in a decrease in the release of glutamic acid and aspartic acid, and decreased activation of α-motor neurons. In addition, the drug mediates some CNS depression, particularly in large doses. This supraspinal action also contributes to muscle relaxation.

15. Discuss the mechanism of action of cyclobenzaprine.

The mechanism of action of cyclobenzaprine is thought to result from an increase in stimulation of central α_2 receptors and subsequent decrease in noradrenergic activity. New evidence, however, suggests that the antagonist actions of the drug at 5-HT$_2$ receptors are responsible for the muscle relaxation effect.

16. Describe the mechanism of action of chlorzoxazone.

Chlorzoxazone appears to increase the activity of calcium-dependent potassium channels, resulting in hypopolarization of spinal and supraspinal neurons. This results in a decrease in firing of α-motor neurons and a decrease in spasm.

17. Describe the effect of chlorzoxazone on the liver.

Chlorzoxazone has a high potential for hepatotoxicity. The incidence of hepatotoxicity increases markedly when the drug is combined with acetaminophen.

DEPOLARIZING SKELETAL MUSCLE BLOCKERS

18. Explain the physiologic response observed with the initial dose of a depolarizing blocker.

Initially, muscle contraction is observed. The reason for this is that the initial dose causes depolarization of skeletal muscle and an initial excitation-contraction coupling, leading to a contraction. After the initial dose, the membrane remains depolarized, and further excitation-contraction couplings do not occur, causing the muscle to be flaccid.

19. Describe the onset and duration of succinylcholine.

This drug has a rapid onset—paralysis occurs within 60 seconds. The duration is correspondingly short—around 5 to 10 minutes.

20. How is succinylcholine eliminated?

Succinylcholine is rapidly eliminated by tissue cholinesterases.

21. Is succinylcholine useful in pediatric patients?

Only in emergency situations, due to a high incidence of cardiac dysrhythmias and reported cardiac arrest seen with the use of the drug in pediatric patients.

NONDEPOLARIZING AGENTS

22. Compare rocuronium and succinylcholine.

The onset of rocuronium is similar to that of succinylcholine, but rocuronium's duration of action is significantly longer.

23. Explain the adverse cardiac effects seen with d-tubocurarine.

This drug has an extremely high potential for induction of histamine release. Thus, vasodilatation results in hypotension. Decreased venous return also results in decreased cardiac output. In addition, the drug blocks nicotinic receptors at sympathetic ganglia.

24. Describe the duration of action of d-tubocurarine.

The initial dose produces effects lasting up to approximately 1.5 hours. Subsequent doses produce a longer duration of action.

25. Does mivacurium decrease cardiovascular function?

The drug has no direct effect on the heart, but can cause substantial histamine release, which may result in hypotension.

26. Explain the effects of pancuronium on the heart.

This drug blocks muscarinic receptors and may cause an increase in heart rate. This effect is minimal at normal doses.

27. Does pancuronium affect nicotinic ganglia?

No.

28. Compare pancuronium and pipecuronium.

Pipecuronium has a long duration of action as compared to pancuronium (up to 2 hours), but is structurally related. It is also 20 to 50 percent more potent than pancuronium and does not produce the adverse cardiovascular effects seen with pancuronium.

29. Compare the potencies of doxacurium and pancuronium.

Doxacurium is 2.5 to 3 times more potent than pancuronium.

30. Which competitive blocker is short-acting?

Mivacurium, with a duration of less than 30 minutes.

31. Describe the duration of action of atracurium.

This drug is considered intermediate-acting, with an elimination half-life of 20 minutes.

32. Describe the interaction between atracurium and general anesthetics.

The potency and duration of the drug is affected by the type of anesthetic used—if either enflurane or isoflurane are used in conjunction with the drug, the potency of atracurium is increased, and the duration of neuromuscular blockade is increased by 35 percent.

BIBLIOGRAPHY

1. Cao Y, Dreixler JC, Roizen JD, et al: Modulation of recombinant small-conductance Ca(2+)-activated K(+) channels by the muscle relaxant chlorzoxazone and structurally related compounds. J Pharmacol Exp Ther 296(3):683–689, 2001.
2. Elenbaas JK: Centrally acting oral skeletal muscle relaxants [review]. Am J Hosp Pharm 37(10):1313–1323, 1980.
3. Frakes MA: Muscle relaxant choices for rapid sequence induction. Air Med J 20(1):20–21, 2001.
4. Hardman J, Limbird L, Gilman A: Goodman & Gilman's The Pharmacological Basis of Therapeutics, 10th ed. McGraw-Hill Publishers, 2001.

5. Gyermek L: Muscle relaxants and 5-HT(3) receptors. Anesth Analg 91(4):1039, 2000.
6. Katzung B: Basic and Clinical Pharmacology, 8th ed. Appleton & Lange, 2001.
7. Kobayashi H, Hasegawa Y, Ono H: Cyclobenzaprine, a centrally acting muscle relaxant, acts on descending serotonergic systems. Eur J Pharmacol 311(1):29–35, 1996.
8. Laurin EG, Sakles JC, Panacek EA, et al: A comparison of succinylcholine and rocuronium for rapid-sequence intubation of emergency department patients. Acad Emerg Med 7(12):1362–1369, 2000.
9. Linden CH, Mitchiner JC, Lindzon RD, et al: Cyclobenzaprine overdosage. J Toxicol Clin Toxicol 20(3):281–288, 1983.
10. Poloyac SM, Perez A, Scheff S, et al: Tissue-specific alterations in the 6-hydroxylation of chlorzoxazone following traumatic brain injury in the rat. Drug Metab Dispos 29(3):296–298, 2001.
11. Singh AK, Devor DC, Gerlach AC, et al: Stimulation of Cl(-) secretion by chlorzoxazone. J Pharmacol Exp Ther 292(2):778–787, 2000.
12. Spiller HA, Winter ML, Mann KV, et al: Five-year multicenter retrospective review of cyclobenzaprine toxicity [review]. J Emerg Med 13(6):781–785, 1995.
13. Stump L: Rapacuronium bromide. J Perianesth Nurs 15(4):258–259, 2000.
14. Waldman HJ: Centrally acting skeletal muscle relaxants and associated drugs [review]. J Pain Symptom Manage 9(7):434–441, 1994.
15. Wang RW, Liu L, Cheng H: Identification of human liver cytochrome P_{450} isoforms involved in the in vitro metabolism of cyclobenzaprine. Drug Metab Dispos: 24(7):786–791, 1996.

26. AGENTS USED IN CONTRACTING SMOOTH MUSCLE

PROSTAGLANDIN ANALOGS

1. What is dinoprostone?

Dinoprostone is a synthetic preparation of naturally occurring prostaglandin E_2.

2. What is the clinical use of dinoprostone?

This drug is used as an abortifacient. It may also be used to cause expulsion of an expired fetus from the uterus.

3. Describe the effects of dinoprostone on the cervix.

Dinoprostone causes relaxation of the cervix and "cervical ripening."

4. How is dinoprostone eliminated?

Drug that enters the circulation is 95 percent metabolized with the first pass through the lung.

5. Describe the contraindications to administration of dinoprostone.

Because this drug contracts smooth muscle, it is contraindicated in patients with vascular disease, diabetes mellitus, hypertension, or asthma.

6. What is misoprostol?

Misoprostol is a prostaglandin analog used in the therapy of ulcers. It is also used as a contractile agent in the induction of labor.

OXYTOCICS

7. Describe the uses of methylergonovine.

This drug is an oxytocic and is used in the therapy of post-partum atony, placental delivery, and to control post-partum bleeding.

8. Does oxytocin produce uterine contractions in the early stages of pregnancy?

Not at therapeutic dosage. Contractions may be initiated with extremely high doses.

9. Describe the use and administration of oxytocin.

This drug is administered by parenteral route for induction of labor and control of post-partum bleeding, or by the intranasal route for induction of milk let-down.

10. Is oxytocin given orally?

No. It is metabolized in the duodenum by pancreatic enzymes (trypsin and chymotrypsin).

11. Is oxytocin administered by intravenous (IV) drip?

No. Administration with large volumes of water can precipitate water intoxication.

12. Discuss the effect of oxytocin on blood pressure.

Oxytocin contracts vascular smooth muscle, which can cause an increase in blood pressure, particularly if administered in a large dose. This is usually preceded by a decrease in pressure.

13. Describe the effect of oxytocin on the blood pressure of a patient anesthetized with an inhalation anesthetic.

In the presence of an inhalation anesthetic, blood pressure can markedly decrease in the presence of oxytocin.

14. Discuss the role of estrogens in the pharmacologic action of oxytocin.

The effects of oxytocin are dependent on adequate levels of serum estrogens. This is caused by an estrogen induction of oxytocin receptors.

15. Describe the duration of uterine response after oxytocin administration.

Uterine contraction persists for approximately one hour after IV injection (2–3 hours after intramuscular (IM) injection).

16. How is oxytocin metabolized?

Oxytocin is metabolized by oxytocinase, which is produced by the placenta and appears to regulate uterine oxytocin. Oxytocinase does not appear to affect plasma oxytocin, which is metabolized by the liver and kidney.

17. Discuss the hypersensitivity reactions to oxytocin.

These reactions can precipitate extremely strong contractions, resulting in uterine rupture or laceration. Severely hypersensitive patients can also go into anaphylactic shock.

18. Discuss the adverse cardiac effects of oxytocin.

Oxytocin can precipitate cardiac arrhythmias, as well as vascular-related effects such as decreased venous return and hypotension, leading to a decrease in cardiac output. Cardiac effects are exacerbated by the use of inhalation anesthetics.

19. Discuss the possible effects of oxytocin on the fetus.

Increased contractile force during delivery can cause trauma to the brain and spinal cord. Direct effects of the drug can include induction of cardiac arrhythmias, jaundice, and retinal hemorrhage.

ERGOT ALKALOIDS

20. Describe the general properties of ergot alkaloids.

In addition to oxytocic activity, these drugs act as partial agonists on alpha-adrenergic receptors, as well as receptors for dopamine and serotonin. They also inhibit norepinephrine reuptake. The degree of each effect varies with the individual drug.

21. Describe the properties of dihydroergotamine.

Dihydroergotamine is a weak serotonin antagonist, with prominent alpha-receptor blocking activity. It is primarily a venoconstrictor.

22. Describe the actions of dihydroergotamine on vessel capacitance.

Dihydroergotamine constricts capacitance vessels more than resistance vessels. Therefore, it increases venous return and decreases venous stasis and pooling.

23. Describe the possible effects of dihydroergotamine on the heart.

Dihydroergotamine can cause coronary vasospasm. This can precipitate serious events, such as angina, myocardial infarction, ventricular tachycardia, ventricular fibrillation, and death. These events are primarily seen with injected dihydroergotamine, rather than the intranasal formulation.

24. What are the general symptoms of ergot toxicity?

Ergot toxicity is characterized by severe peripheral vasoconstriction. In the peripheral circulation this effect is characterized by pain in the extremities, myalgia, numbness and tingling in fingers and toes, cyanosis, and/or cold extremities.

25. Which ergot alkaloids are primarily agonists at the dopamine receptor?

Cabergoline and bromocriptine. These agents are used in the therapy of hyperprolactinemia.

26. Differentiate between cabergoline and bromocriptine in the therapy of hyperprolactinemias.

Cabergoline is more effective than bromocriptine in suppressing prolactin secretion and it is more favorably tolerated. In addition, the long half-life of cabergoline allows for twice-weekly dosing, as compared to multiple daily dosing of bromocriptine.

BIBLIOGRAPHY

1. Antoni FA, Chadio SE: Essential role of magnesium in oxytocin-receptor affinity and ligand specificity. Biochem J 257(2):611–614, 1989.
2. Birlain M: Comparison of low doses of misoprostol with the traditional use of oxytocin for effective cervical ripening and labor induction. Obstet Gynecol 97(4 Suppl 1):S67, 2001.
3. Dussolati G, Cassoni P: The oxytocin/oxytocin receptor system-expect the unexpected [editorial]. Endocrinology 142(4):1377–1379, 2001.
4. Chong YS, Chua S, El-Refaey H, et al: Postpartum intrauterine pressure studies of the uterotonic effect of oral misoprostol and intramuscular syntometrine. BJOG 108(1):41–47, 2001.
5. Colao A, Lombardi G, Annunziato L: Cabergoline. Expert Opin Pharmacother 1(3):555–574, 2000.
6. Gimpl G, Fahrenholz F: The oxytocin receptor system: Structure, function, and regulation. Physiol Rev 81(2):629–683, 2001.
7. Goetzl L, Shipp TD, Cohen A, et al: Oxytocin dose and the risk of uterine rupture in trial of labor after cesarean. Obstet Gynecol 97(3):381–384, 2001.
8. Hardman J, Limbird L, Gilman A: Goodman & Gilman's The Pharmacological Basis of Therapeutics, 10th ed. McGraw-Hill Publishers, 2001.
9. Johnson AE: The regulation of oxytocin receptor binding in the ventromedial hypothalamic nucleus by gonadal steroids. Ann N Y Acad Sci 652:357–373, 1992.
10. Katzung B: Basic and Clinical Pharmacology, 8th ed. Appleton & Lange, 2001.
11. Lau LC, Adaikan PG, Arulkumaran S, et al: Oxytocics reverse the tocolytic effect of glyceryl trinitrate on the human uterus. BJOG 108(2):164–168, 2001.
12. Sanchez-Ramos L, Kaunitz AM: Outpatient cervical ripening with intravaginal misoprostol. Obstet Gynecol 97(2):325–326, 2001.
13. Schmid B, Wong S, Mitchell BF: Transcriptional regulation of oxytocin receptor by interleukin-1beta and interleukin-6. Endocrinology 142(4):1380–1385, 2001.
14. Sherman DJ, Frenkel E, Pansky M, et al: Balloon cervical ripening with extra amniotic infusion of saline or prostaglandin E2: A double-blind, randomized controlled study. Obstet Gynecol 97(3):375–380, 2001.
15. Tsui BC, Stewart B, Fitzmaurice A, et al: Cardiac arrest and myocardial infarction induced by postpartum intravenous ergonovine administration. Anesthesiology 94(2):363–364, 2001.

27. DRUGS THAT AFFECT BONE MINERALIZATION

1. Explain the mechanism of action of biphosphate drugs (e.g., alendronate, risedronate).

These drugs are internalized into osteoclasts, disrupting the cell and inhibiting osteoclast activity (see Figure). Thus, bone resorption is decreased.

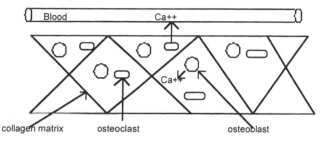

The mineralization of bone. Shown are the bone matrix (collagen/proteoglycan), osteoblasts (bone mineralization), and osteoclasts (bone resorption in response to decreased blood calcium).

2. Discuss the effects of high-dose alendronate.

In high doses, alendronate inhibits bone mineralization.

3. What is the effect of alendronate on calcium salts and the formation of hydroxyapatite?

Alendronate binds to calcium salts and inhibits formation of hydroxyapatite. Thus, both the formation and the dissolution of bone are inhibited.

4. Is the action of alendronate on osteoclasts permanent?

No. Continuous administration of alendronate is necessary to maintain osteoclast suppression.

5. Are the actions of alendronate dependent on estrogen levels?

No. Alendronate has been shown to significantly increase bone mineral density in women with postmenopausal osteoporosis.

6. Does alendronate decrease catabolism of the bone matrix?

Yes. The drug decreases collagen degradation as well as bone resorption.

7. Discuss the bioavailability of alendronate.

The bioavailability is poor (< 1 percent), and may be reduced to zero absorption with the concurrent ingestion of food or high-acidity drinks (e.g., coffee or citrus juice). Because the drug binds to calcium, concurrent administration of divalent cations (e.g., calcium, magnesium) binds the drug in the intestine and decreases availability.

8. Discuss the half-life of alendronate.

The plasma half-life is approximately 6 hours, because the drug is rapidly bound to bone tissue. Elimination half-life is approximately 3 days. Once bound to bone tissue, however, the drug half-life becomes greater than 10 years.

9. What is the therapeutic use of calcitonin?

Calcitonin decreases osteoclast activity and the rate of bone turnover in Paget's disease.

10. Compare calcitonin obtained from salmon to that from human sources.
   Calcitonin obtained from salmon has a significantly higher potency and longer duration of action than that obtained from human thyroid.

11. Does calcitonin affect the peripheral manifestations of Paget's disease?
   Yes. Reductions in hearing deficit, cardiac dysfunction, and neurological deficits have been observed with the administration of calcitonin.

12. Is calcitonin administered orally? Explain.
   No. It is a peptide and is degraded in the GI tract.

13. What is the half-life of calcitonin?
   Administered intranasally or parenterally, the half-life is approximately 40 minutes to an hour.

14. Discuss calcitriol.
   Calcitriol is a highly potent vitamin D_3 analog (see Figure) used in the therapy of secondary hypoparathyroidism and osteomalacia.

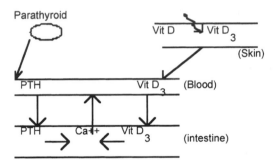

Diagrammatic representation of the role of activated vitamin D and parathyroid hormone in the absorption of calcium.

15. Describe the mechanism of action of calcitriol in the therapy of osteomalacia and osteoporosis.
   Calcitriol promotes renal reabsorption of calcium, and promotes a receptor-mediated increase in intestinal absorption of calcium and phosphorus.

16. Describe the mechanism of action of etidronate.
   Etidronate acts as an endogenous pyrophosphate to inhibit bone resorption.

17. Is etidronate susceptible to enzymatic degradation?
   No. Unlike endogenous pyrophosphates, it is resistant to enzymatic degradation.

18. Describe the use of etidronate in the therapy of Paget's disease.
   Etidronate adsorbs to hydroxyapatite crystals, preventing both their growth and dissolution.

19. What is the pharmacologic action of estrogen agonists in the therapy of osteoporosis?
   Estrogen and related anabolic steroids increase bone density, primarily by increasing bone matrix.

20. What is lasofoxifene?
   Lasofoxifene is a partial agonist at estrogen receptors, which has been shown to increase bone density.

21. Why is the administration of a partial estrogen receptor agonist beneficial?

A partial estrogen receptor agonist better mimics normal physiological milieu. Reduced incidence of adverse effects can also result, because of the antagonist component of the drug.

22. Do partial estrogen agonists such as lasofoxifene promote cancer of the breast or uterus?

These agents have a fairly low potential to promote estrogen-dependent cancers, due to their antagonist component.

23. What is raloxifene?

Raloxifene is a selective estrogen receptor modulator of the benzothiophene class.

24. Describe the receptor selectivity of raloxifene.

This drug is selective for stimulation of estrogen receptors in bone, but acts as an antagonist at estrogen receptors in reproductive tissue (e.g., mammary and uterine).

25. Discuss the bioavailability of raloxifene.

The absolute bioavailability is very low (around 1 percent), which results from the rapid glucuronidation of the drug.

26. Describe risedronate.

Risedronate is a drug of the pyridinyl bisphosphonate class that has potent antiresorptive activity.

27. Contrast the antiresorptive action of risedronate with that of other bisphosphonates.

Risedronate has more potent antiresorptive activity than etidronate, clodronate, pamidronate, or alendronate.

28. What are the therapeutic uses of risedronate?

Risedronate is approved for the therapy of Paget's disease, as well as for the therapy of both postmenopausal and corticosteroid-induced osteoporosis.

29. Does risedronate affect bone mineralization?

No. It primarily affects osteoclast function.

30. What effect does risedronate have on osteoclasts that is unique to the drug?

Risedronate causes apoptosis of osteoclasts.

31. Differentiate between tamoxifen and raloxifene in the therapy of osteoporosis.

Both of these drugs have differential effects on the alpha- and beta-subtypes of estrogen receptor. Both mediate a decrease in bone resorption, and decrease estrogen stimulation of breast tissue. Tamoxifen, unlike raloxifene, stimulates endometrial tissue, and can promote or exacerbate uterine cancer.

32. Are estrogens used in the treatment of osteoporosis?

No. Estrogen therapy is mainly used prophylactically.

BIBLIOGRAPHY

1. Alkhenizan A, Almarri S, Evans MF: Alendronate and male osteoporosis. Can Fam Physician 47:509–510, 2001.
2. Baran D: Osteoporosis. Efficacy and safety of a bisphosphonate dosed once weekly. Geriatrics 56(3):28–32, 2001.
3. Bergstrom JD, Bostedor RG, Masarachia PJ, et al: Alendronate is a specific, nanomolar inhibitor of farnesyl diphosphate synthase. Arch Biochem Biophys 373(1):231–241, 2000.

4. Compston JE: Sex steroids and bone [review]. Physiol Rev 81(1):419–447, 2001. Review
5. Crandall C: Gender differences in osteoporosis treatment: A review of clinical research. J Gend Specif Med 3(8):42–46, 2000.
6. Gallagher JC: Role of estrogens in the management of postmenopausal bone loss. Rheum Dis Clin North Am 27(1):143–162, 2001.
7. Hardman J, Limbird L, Gilman A: Goodman & Gilman's The Pharmacological Basis of Therapeutics, 10th ed. McGraw-Hill Publishers, 2001.
8. Katzung B: Basic and Clinical Pharmacology, 8th ed. Appleton & Lange, 2001.
9. Lane JM, Khan SN, O'Connor WJ, et al: Bisphosphonate therapy in fibrous dysplasia. Clin Orthop (382):6–12, 2001.
10. Miller MM, Franklin KB: Theoretical basis for the benefit of postmenopausal estrogen substitution [review]. Exp Gerontol 34(5):587–604, 1999.
11. Mincey BA, Moraghan TJ, Perez EA: Prevention and treatment of osteoporosis in women with breast cancer [review]. Mayo Clin Proc 75(8):821–829, 2000.
12. Morales-Piga A: Tiludronate. A new treatment for an old ailment: Paget's disease of bone. Expert Opin Pharmacother 1(1):157–170, 1999.
13. Oura S, Tanino H, Yoshimasu T, et al: Bisphosphonate therapy for bone metastases from breast cancer: Clinical results and a new therapeutic approach. Breast Cancer 7(4):307–310, 2000.
14. Reid IR: Preventing glucocorticoid-induced osteoporosis. Z Rheumatol 59 Suppl 2:II/97–II/102, 2000.
15. Scheiber MD, Rebar RW: Isoflavones and postmenopausal bone health: A viable alternative to estrogen therapy [review]? Menopause 6(3):233–241, 1999.
16. Scott JA, Da Camara CC, Early JE: Raloxifene: A selective estrogen receptor modulator [review]. Am Fam Physician 60(4):1131–1139, 1999.
17. Sewell K, Schein JR: Osteoporosis therapies for rheumatoid arthritis patients: Minimizing gastrointestinal side effects. Semin Arthritis Rheum 30(4):288–297, 2001.
18. South-Paul JE: Osteoporosis: Part II. Nonpharmacologic and pharmacologic treatment. Am Fam Physician 63(6):1121–1128, 2001.
19. Watts NB: Treatment of osteoporosis with bisphosphonates. Rheum Dis Clin North Am 27(1):197–214, 2001.
20. Wimalawansa SJ: Prevention and treatment of osteoporosis: Efficacy of combination of hormone replacement therapy with other antiresorptive agents [review]. J Clin Densitom 3(2):187–201, 2000.
21. Yilmaz L, Ozoran K, Gunduz OH, et al: Alendronate in rheumatoid arthritis patients treated with methotrexate and glucocorticoids. Rheumatol Int 20(2):65–69, 2001.

VII. The Therapy of Pain and Inflammation

Patricia K. Anthony, Ph.D., C. Andrew Powers, Ph.D., and Arvind Kashap, Ph.D.

28. NONSTEROIDAL PAIN RELIEVERS

1. Discuss the mechanism of action of nonsteroidal anti-inflammatory drugs (*NSAIDs*).
These drugs decrease both pain and inflammation by the inhibition of the prostaglandin synthesis cascade. These drugs primarily inhibit the actions of cyclooxygenase.

2. Is acetaminophen (Tylenol) a true NSAID?
No. This drug has no anti-inflammatory properties.

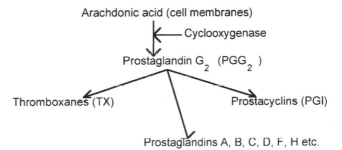

Schematic representation of the prostaglandin synthesis cascade.

3. Discuss the difference between cyclooxygenase-1 and -2 (COX-1 and COX-2).
COX-1 is expressed in all tissues and regulates the conversion of arachidonic acid to prostaglandin G_2 (PGG_2), which is the first step in prostanoid synthesis. The COX-2 isozyme is selectively expressed—it appears in renal, bone, brain, and reproductive tissues, as well as in some tumor types. The COX-2 enzyme is inducible by various mediators of inflammation (e.g., interleukins and superoxide radicals), whereas the COX-1 isomer is expressed constitutively.

4. Which nonsteroidal antiinflammatory agents are specific for inhibition of COX-1?
Indomethacin, piroxicam, and aspirin.

5. Discuss the inhibitory specificity of ibuprofen, naproxen, and diclofenac on cyclooxygenase.
These agents are nonspecific, and affect both isoforms of the enzyme.

6. Which NSAIDS are specific for the inhibition of COX-2?
Celecoxib and rofecoxib. Meloxicam, nabumetone, and etodolac have some COX-2 specificity, but still have a potent effect on COX-1.

7. Describe the actions of agents that act as simple competitors to cyclooxygenase.
These agents act as competitive inhibitors that bind and dissociate from the enzyme. They include ibuprofen, naproxen, piroxicam, and sulindac.

8. Describe the actions of agents considered to be "time-dependent" cyclooxygenase inhibitors.

These agents cause a conformational change in the COX enzymes, resulting in robust binding, which deteriorates over time. They are thus longer-acting than the simple competitors, and include diclofenac, flubiprofen, indomethacin, and meclofenamate.

9. Which nonsteroidal agent produces irreversible inactivation of cyclooxygenase?

Aspirin. This agent irreversibly acetylates the enzyme, rendering it inactive.

10. How do NSAIDs lower fever?

These agents decrease the synthesis of prostaglandin E_2 (PGE$_2$), which acts to "reset" the hypothalamic thermoregulatory mechanisms at increased temperature.

11. Explain how acetaminophen lowers fever.

Acetaminophen acts directly on the hypothalamic regulatory centers, resulting in a decreased temperature "set-point."

12. Discuss the metabolism of acetaminophen.

Acetaminophen is metabolized by the hepatic cytochrome P_{450} system and, in large part, is subsequently glucuronidated. Sulfated metabolites are also produced, as is the toxic metabolite N-acetylbenzoquinone.

13. Discuss the hepatotoxicity of acetaminophen.

The hepatotoxicity of acetaminophen results from the production of the minor metabolite N-acetylbenzoquinone. In small, occasional doses (such as with occasional headache), the drug does not produce significant hepatotoxicity, because this metabolite is produced in only small quantities, and is rapidly inactivated by hepatic-reduced glutathione. However, with frequent or large doses, more of the toxic metabolite is produced, and the reduced glutathione present is not sufficient to inactivate all of the toxic metabolite produced. Thus, toxicity results.

14. Discuss aspirin "allergy."

This phenomenon is not a true allergy, nor is it specifically caused by aspirin. It is the result of decreased synthesis of bronchodilatory prostanoids in the lung. In susceptible individuals, prostaglandin synthesis inhibitors may inhibit the synthesis not only of inflammatory prostanoids, but also of those prostanoids that contribute to patent airways. Thus, sensitivity to prostaglandin synthesis inhibitors can precipitate bronchoconstriction and blockade of airways. These events can arise from increased dosing of NSAIDs, increased frequency of dosage, or concurrent administration of more than one drug (e.g., naproxen with ibuprofen).

15. Do all NSAIDs have the same potency with regard to specific effects (e.g., platelet inhibition)?

No. The individual agents vary significantly in tissue specificity.

16. Describe the possible effects of cyclooxygenase inhibitors on kidney function.

Prostacyclins (PGI$_2$) mediate vasodilatation and also stimulate the secretion of renin. Thus, they increase renal blood flow. Inhibition of prostacyclin synthesis by high doses of NSAIDs, therefore, can be detrimental to kidney function.

17. What adverse renal effects are seen with the administration of NSAIDs?

NSAIDs are associated with sodium and potassium retention, acute renal failure, interstitial nephritis, and analgesic nephropathy.

18. Discuss the effects of NSAIDs on parturition and labor.

Prostaglandins increase smooth muscle contraction in the uterus. Administration of NSAIDs thus can adversely affect parturition and labor.

19. Describe the beneficial effect of using ibuprofen in a patient with angina.

Ibuprofen causes a lysosomal membrane stabilizing effect. This may help to protect myocardial integrity during ischemia.

20. Describe the mechanism of action of NSAIDS in the reduction of algesia.

Prostaglandins sensitize pain receptors. Inhibition of the prostaglandin synthesis cascade thus results in a decrease in receptor sensitivity.

21. Acute alcohol intake may produce potentially dangerous drug interactions with which nonsteroidal anti-inflammatory drug?

Aspirin.

22. Discuss the absorption of aspirin.

Aspirin is acetylsalicylic acid. It is therefore absorbed in the acid milieu of the stomach.

23. Describe how aspirin is utilized.

Aspirin is absorbed through the gastric epithelium and subsequently deacetylated to salicylic acid, which is the active form.

24. Is aspirin bound to plasma proteins?

Yes. It binds to (and acetylates) serum albumin.

25. Discuss the metabolism and elimination of aspirin.

Aspirin is rapidly glucuronidated in the liver to form a polar metabolite. This glucuronidated form is excreted through the urine.

26. Does aspirin utilize the renal organic acid secretory system (OASS)?

Yes. Thus, it competes with other organic acids for secretion and elimination.

27. Describe the effect of aspirin in gout.

Aspirin exacerbates gout, by competing with uric acid for secretion by the OASS. Competition for sites on the OASS also decreases the efficacy of therapeutic agents for gout (e.g., probenecid), which must mediate their actions from the luminal side of kidney tubules.

28. Discuss the action of aspirin on the platelet.

Aspirin irreversibly acetylates platelet cyclooxygenase, rendering it inactive. Thus, thromboxane A_2 is no longer formed, decreasing platelet adhesion.

29. Are the actions of aspirin on the platelet reversible, with time?

No. Since the platelet is not an actual cell, it does not have the ability to synthesize new enzyme. Thus, the effects on the platelet are permanent, and new platelets that contain active enzyme must be synthesized.

30. Why does aspirin have the potential to cause gastric ulcers?

The gastric epithelium produces a cytoprotective prostanoid that protects the cells from acid damage. Since aspirin is absorbed directly across the gastric epithelium, synthesis of this prostanoid is inhibited in a dose-dependent manner. This renders the cells vulnerable to acid damage and, with repeated dosage, can promote ulcers.

31. Compare high-dose and low-dose aspirin in the therapy of angina.

In low doses, aspirin inhibits platelet function and mediates vasodilatation, both of which are beneficial in angina. In doses that are analgesic, however, the drug inhibits the formation of vasodilatory prostacyclins, which decreases oxygen delivery to the heart and thus exacerbates the condition.

32. Discuss the anti-inflammatory effects of naproxen.

Naproxen and naproxen sodium are good anti-inflammatory agents. However, anti-inflammatory effects are not immediate, but are manifested with repeated dosage.

33. Compare the potencies of ibuprofen and ketoprofen.

Ketoprofen has significantly greater potency than ibuprofen, allowing lower doses to be utilized.

34. Describe the metabolism and elimination of ibuprofen.

Ibuprofen is metabolized in the liver, through the cytochrome P_{450} system. It undergoes glucuronidation, and the glucuronidated metabolite is excreted through the urine.

35. Are propionic acid derivatives (e.g., ketoprofen) plasma protein-bound?

These drugs are highly protein-bound, existing up to 99 percent protein-bound in the plasma.

36. Compare naproxen and naproxen sodium.

The sodium salt is more rapidly absorbed, and peak plasma concentrations occur in a shorter length of time.

37. Describe the metabolism and elimination of naproxen and naproxen sodium.

These drugs are metabolized by hepatic enzymes and excreted through the urine. Approximately 30 percent of a dose is metabolized in the liver to 6-desmethylnaproxen. The remainder is excreted unchanged or as glucuronidated metabolites.

38. Describe sulindac.

Sulindac is a biologically active pro-drug. Upon absorption, the drug is oxidized, forming a sulfide metabolite, which is the active form of the drug.

39. Explain the long half-life of sulindac.

The sulfide metabolite is excreted through the bile and is subject to enterohepatic recirculation.

40. Is sulindac likely to promote ulcer formation?

No. Because the drug is not active when absorbed, no inhibition of epithelial prostaglandins is likely to occur.

41. Discuss nabumetone.

Nabumetone is a pro-drug. Once absorbed, it is converted to a drug chemically similar to naproxen. Because it is absorbed in an inactive form, it produces less adverse gastrointestinal (GI) effects than naproxen or naproxen sodium.

42. Describe diclofenac.

Diclofenac is an anti-inflammatory drug that is available as a sodium salt (sustained acting) or potassium salt (rapid acting). The potassium salt is used in the therapy of dysmenorrhea. Diclofenac sodium is used in the therapy of inflammatory conditions such as osteoarthritis, and is available as an ocular formulation for postsurgical cataract removal.

43. Describe the absorption of diclofenac.

Diclofenac is best absorbed in the presence of food. Administration in the fasting state results in erratic absorption.

44. What is the advantage of piroxicam administration?

Piroxicam has a long half-life, which allows once-daily dosing.

45. Describe the use of indomethacin in premature neonates.

Indomethacin is used to accelerate closure of patent ductus arteriosus.

46. Is the plasma concentration of indomethacin steady?

No. Elimination of the drug is biphasic, resulting from enterohepatic recycling. The parent drug has a half-life of approximately 1 hour, but the half-life of the metabolite is significantly longer, ranging from 3 to 11 hours.

47. Discuss the elimination of indomethacin.

Approximately 30 percent of urinary drug excretion occurs as indomethacin and its glucuronide. The remainder is excreted through the bile.

48. Does celecoxib have adverse effects on the gastric mucosa?

Adverse effects (e.g., ulcer promotion) are limited, because products of the COX-1 enzyme primarily cause the cytoprotective effects, and the drug is selective for the COX-2 isoform.

49. Do COX-2 inhibitors (e.g., celecoxib and rofecoxib) inhibit platelet function?

No. This effect is mediated by the COX-1 isoform.

50. Discuss the adverse effects of rofecoxib and celecoxib.

Celecoxib may cause significant detrimental effects to intestinal mucosa. The effects of rofecoxib appear to be less than those of celecoxib.

51. Describe the potential positive effect of COX-2 inhibitors on colorectal cancer.

Expression of COX-2 by colorectal cancers has been associated with decreased survival rate. Thus, the administration of drugs such as celecoxib and rofecoxib can potentially be useful in the prevention and/or therapy of such tumors.

52. What is the mechanism of action of gold?

Gold-containing drugs appear to inhibit macrophage activity and inflammatory response.

BIBLIOGRAPHY

1. Bertin P: Current use of analgesics for rheumatological pain. Eur J Pain 4 Suppl A:9–13, 2000.
2. Brown WA, Skinner SA, Malcontenti-Wilson C, et al: Nonsteroidal anti-inflammatory drugs with activity against either cyclooxygenase 1 or cyclooxygenase 2 inhibit colorectal cancer in a DMH rodent model by inducing apoptosis and inhibiting cell proliferation. Gut 48(5):660–666, 2001.
3. Dannhardt G, Kiefer W: Cyclooxygenase inhibitors-current status and future prospects. Eur J Med Chem 36(2):109–126, 2001.
4. Hardman J, Limbird L, Gilman A: Goodman & Gilman's The Pharmacological Basis of Therapeutics, 10th ed. McGraw-Hill Publishers, 2001.
5. Hankey GJ: Current oral antiplatelet agents to prevent atherothrombosis. Cerebrovasc Dis. 11 Suppl S2:11–17, 2001.
6. Katzung B: Basic and Clinical Pharmacology, 8th ed. Appleton & Lange, 2001.
7. Isbister G, Whyte I, Dawson A: Pediatric acetaminophen poisoning. Arch Pediatr Adolesc Med 155(3):417–419, 2001.
8. Lapane KL, Spooner JJ, Pettitt D: The effect of nonsteroidal anti-inflammatory drugs on the use of gastroprotective medication in people with arthritis. Am J Manag Care. 7(4):402–408, 2001.
9. Li M, Wu X, Xu XC Induction of apoptosis in colon cancer cells by cyclooxygenase-2 inhibitor NS398 through a cytochrome c-dependent pathway. Clin Cancer Res. 7(4):1010–1016, 2001.
10. Maddrey WC, Maurath CJ, Verburg KM, et al: The hepatic safety and tolerability of the novel cyclooxygenase-2 inhibitor celecoxib. Am J Ther 7(3):153–158, 2000.
11. Maxim R: Atrial fibrillation and anticoagulation. Med Health R I 84(3):96–97, 2001.
12. Ostensen M, Villiger PM: Nonsteroidal anti-inflammatory drugs in systemic lupus erythematosus. Lupus 10(3):135–9, 2001.
13. Pavelka K: Treatment of pain in osteoarthritis. Eur J Pain 4 Suppl A:23–30, 2000.
14. Silva VM, Chen C, Hennig GE, et al: Changes in susceptibility to acetaminophen-induced liver injury by the organic anion indocyanine green. Food Chem Toxicol 39(3):271–278, 2001.

15. Sztajnkrycer MJ, Bond GR: Chronic acetaminophen overdosing in children: Risk assessment and management. Curr Opin Pediatr 13(2):177–182, 2001.
16. Verburg KM, Maziasz TJ, Weiner E, et al: Cox-2-specific inhibitors: Definition of a new therapeutic concept. Am J Ther 8(1):49–64, 2001.
17. Whelton A, Maurath CJ, Verburg KM, et al: Renal safety and tolerability of celecoxib, a novel cyclooxygenase-2 inhibitor. Am J Ther 7(3):159–175, 2000.

29. STEROIDS AND IMMUNOSUPPRESSANT AGENTS

1. Briefly describe the actions of glucocorticoids on inflammation.

Glucocorticoids interfere with macrophage action, decrease capillary permeability, and decrease the activity of local mediators (see Figure).

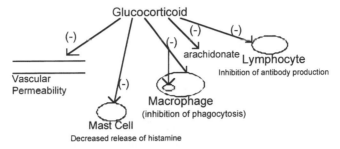

Diagrammatic representation of the membrane-stabilizing effects of glucocorticoids.

2. Describe the action of glucocorticoids on lysosomes.

Glucocorticoids stabilize lysosomal membranes, resulting in an inhibition of lysosomal action and, thus, an inhibition of phagocytic activity.

3. Explain the actions of glucocorticoids on leukocytic function.

Glucocorticoids inhibit the release of leukocytic acid hydrolases, and also inhibit the adhesion of leukocytes to the vascular endothelium.

4. Do corticosteroids affect histamine levels? Explain.

Yes. These drugs stabilize the mast cell membrane and prevent the release of histamine.

5. Explain the actions of corticosteroids on the immune system.

Corticosteroids stabilize lymphocytic membranes, reducing the production of immunoglobulins and their compliment. Lymphocyte production is also inhibited, producing lymphocytopenia.

6. What is the effect of exogenous steroid administration on the adrenal gland?

Exogenously administered glucocorticoids produce a negative feedback inhibition on the production of adrenocorticotropic hormone (ACTH) from the anterior pituitary. This results in a decrease in stimulation of the adrenal cortex and a decrease in the production of cortisol and aldosterone.

7. Discuss the ramifications of prolonged corticosteroid therapy.

The major effect of prolonged therapy is adrenal atrophy. In addition, corticosteroids, which have a similar structure to reproductive steroids (e.g., estrogen and testosterone), can feed back on the production of reproductive steroids. This can result in decreased sperm maturation, in particular, and infertility.

8. Are the reproductive effects of prolonged corticosteroid therapy reversible?

Yes. With time, the adrenal cortex will regenerate and production of viable gametes will resume.

9. Why should corticosteroid therapy be tapered?

As discussed previously, prolonged therapy, in particular, will cause adrenal atrophy. The degree of atrophy is dose-dependent, and, therefore, administration of progressively smaller doses over time will allow the adrenal cortex to regenerate, while supplementing endogenous cortisol levels.

10. Do glucocorticoids exhibit mineralocorticoid activity?

Yes. The degree of mineralocorticoid activity (e.g., sodium retention and edema) varies with the drug.

11. Which corticosteroids are short-acting?

Hydrocortisone and prednisone.

12. Describe the adverse effects of glucocorticoid therapy.

In addition to the suppression of the hypophysial-pituitary axis and adrenal atrophy, these drugs can cause a variety of adverse effects, including osteoporosis, pancreatitis, steroid-induced diabetes mellitus, cataracts, glaucoma, psychosis, oral candidiasis and other opportunistic infections, immunosuppression, infertility, weight gain, and skin atrophy. Severe edema may also be produced, particularly in the face, depending on the degree of mineralocorticoid activity.

13. Is fludrocortisone a pure glucocorticoid?

No. This drug possesses a high degree of mineralocorticoid activity.

14. Rank the potencies of hydrocortisone, prednisone, and betamethasone.

Hydrocortisone has relatively low potency. In contrast, betamethasone has very high potency. Prednisone is intermediate.

15. What property of corticosteroid chemical structure confers high potency?

In general, fluorinated corticosteroids are highly potent.

16. Discuss the potency and duration of action of dexamethasone.

Dexamethasone has approximately 10 times the potency of cortisol. It is extremely long acting.

17. Which property of dexamethasone makes it useful in the therapy and prophylaxis of cerebral edema?

Dexamethasone crosses easily into the central nervous system (CNS), in contrast to most other steroids. In addition, it is a potent and long-acting corticosteroid.

18. What is alclometasone?

Alclometasone is a low potency steroid that is used topically for dermatitis.

19. Discuss amcinonide.

This drug is a highly potent fluorinated corticosteroid, which is used topically.

20. Discuss the use of beclomethasone.

Beclomethasone is a highly potent inhaled steroid used in the therapy of asthma and upper respiratory infections.

21. Compare the potencies of beclomethasone and cortisone.

Beclomethasone possesses roughly 5000 times the potency of cortisone.

22. Which corticosteroid is considered to have the greatest potency?

Clobetasol. It is used topically and for short-term therapy only.

23. What is clocortolone?
Clocortolone pivalate is a topical, medium-potency, synthetic fluorinated corticosteroid.

24. Why is cortisone useful in patients with adrenocortical insufficiency?
This drug has potent mineralocorticoid activity as well as glucocorticoid activity.

25. Contrast desonide and desoximetasone.
These drugs are both topical glucocorticoids. However, desonide has relatively low potency, whereas desoximetasone is a high-potency drug.

26. Why is fluorometholone used as an ophthalmic?
This drug is one of the few corticosteroids that has a decreased potential for mediation of increased intraocular pressure. In addition, it has a low potential for systemic absorption.

27. How are ophthalmic corticosteroids distributed?
These drugs are absorbed through the aqueous humor and distributed into surrounding tissues.

28. Compare the elimination of ophthalmic and systemic corticosteroids.
Ophthalmic corticosteroids are metabolized in surrounding tissues. As a result, the duration of action is longer, because they are eliminated more slowly than systemic steroids, which are metabolized in the liver and eliminated through the bile or urine.

29. Do corticosteroids affect the prostaglandin synthesis cascade?
Yes. The membrane-stabilization effect of these drugs decreases the release of arachidonic acid from the cell membrane. Thus, the production of all prostanoids may be affected in a dose-dependent manner.

30. Explain the action of chloroquine on the immune system.
Chloroquine is an antimalarial agent which affects erythema nodosum leprosum.

31. Explain the action of dapsone and rifampin on the immune system.
These drugs have anti-complement activity.

32. What is the effect of chloroquine on lysosomal enzyme production?
This drug inhibits the production of lysosomal enzymes.

33. Discuss the use of chloroquine in lepra reaction.
It inhibits immune complex formation.

34. Does multidrug therapy exhibit anticomplement activity?
Yes. Multidrug therapy exhibits anticomplement activity via the complement activation cascade.

BIBLIOGRAPHY

1. Andreae J, Tripmacher R, Weltrich R, et al: Effect of glucocorticoid therapy on glucocorticoid receptors in children with autoimmune diseases. Pediatr Res 49(1):130–135, 2001.
2. Gamper N, Huber SM, Badawi K, et al: Cell volume-sensitive sodium channels upregulated by glucocorticoids in U937 macrophages. Pflugers Arch 441(2-3):281–286, 2000.
3. Hardman J, Limbird L, Gilman A: Goodman & Gilman's The Pharmacological Basis of Therapeutics, 10th ed. McGraw-Hill Publishers, 2001.
4. Graziani G, Santostasi S, Angelini C, et al: Corticosteroids in cholesterol emboli syndrome. Nephron 87(4):371–373, 2001.
5. Haynes LE, Griffiths MR, Hyde RE, et al: Dexamethasone induces limited apoptosis and extensive sublethal damage to specific subregions of the striatum and hippocampus: Implications for mood disorders. Neuroscience 104(1):57–69, 2001.

6. Katzung B: Basic and Clinical Pharmacology, 8th ed. Appleton & Lange, 2001.
7. Mussot-Chia C, Flechet ML, Napolitano M, et al: Methylprednisolone-induced acute generalized exan-thematous pustulosis. Ann Dermatol Venereol 128(3):241–243, 2001.
8. Peskova H, Kalina P: Inhaled corticosteroids and glaucoma. Ophthalmology 108(5):837, 2001.
9. Raimer SS: The safe use of topical corticosteroids in children. Pediatr Ann 30(4):225–229, 2001.
10. Yosipovitch G, Hoon TS, Leok GC: Suggested rationale for prevention and treatment of glucocorticoid-induced bone loss in dermatologic patients [review]. Arch Dermatol 137(4):477–481, 2001.

30. DRUGS USED IN THE THERAPY OF ASTHMA

1. Discuss the pharmacologic agents that can be useful in the therapy of asthma.

Effective agents may include glucocorticoids, anticholinergic agents, leukotriene-receptor antagonists, and β_2-adrenergic receptor agonists. Methylxanthines, such as theophylline, are also useful.

2. Are antihistamines useful in the therapy of asthma?

No. Histamine is only one of several inflammatory mediators involved, and plays a secondary role.

3. Describe the postulated role of corticosteroids in the therapy of asthma.

Corticosteroids can decrease inflammatory responses in the lung by several mechanisms. These include the inhibition of synthesis of inflammatory prostanoids, induction of β_2-adrenergic receptors, and the inhibition of histamine release through stabilization of mast cells.

4. What is flunisolide?

Flunisolide is an extremely potent synthetic fluorinated glucocorticoid. It is administered by metered dose inhaler.

5. Is flunisolide useful during an acute asthma attack?

No. The drug has no bronchodilatory properties.

6. Is inhaled flunisolide absorbed?

Yes. Inhaled drug that comes in contact with oral mucosa can be swallowed or absorbed into underlying vessels.

7. Does flunisolide have active metabolites?

Yes.

8. Describe budesonide.

Budesonide is a potent corticosteroid agent used in the therapy of asthma. It is a glucocorticoid, but has potent mineralocorticoid activity.

9. Describe the primary actions of a β_2-adrenergic agonist in the therapy of asthma.

These agents relax smooth muscle, thereby mediating bronchodilatation.

10. What is salmeterol?

Salmeterol is an agonist at the adrenergic β_2 receptor.

11. Is salmeterol useful in acute asthma attacks?

No. The onset of this drug is very slow.

12. What is an advantage of salmeterol therapy over therapy with other agents?

Salmeterol has a long duration of action, which allows for twice-daily dosing. In addition, because of its long duration of action, the drug is useful in preventing late phase bronchoconstriction, whereas shorter acting agents can require additional dosing.

13. Which property of the salmeterol molecule effects its extended action?

The molecule has a lipophilic side chain, which binds to the cell membrane surrounding the receptor and prevents degradation of the molecule, while allowing maximum stimulation of the receptor.

14. Compare salmeterol and albuterol.

Salmeterol has an onset of action roughly twice that of albuterol, making it less useful in an acute asthma attack. However, the duration of action is also double that of albuterol, making it more useful in late-phase therapy.

15. Discuss the pharmacokinetics of salmeterol.

Salmeterol is highly plasma protein-bound (up to 98 percent). It is metabolized by hepatic microsomal enzymes; hydroxylated; and excreted through the bile.

16. Describe the mechanism of action of montelukast and zafirlukast.

Montelukast inhibits the actions of leukotriene D_4 (LTD$_4$) at the CysLT$_1$ receptor. This results in a decrease in sensitivity to antigen challenge, and decreased bronchoconstriction.

17. Do LTD$_4$-antagonists mediate bronchodilatation?

To a certain degree. However, these agents antagonize only bronchoconstriction due to the actions of LTD$_4$. Thus, the degree of dilatation produced is proportionate to the activity of this mediator.

18. How is montelukast administered?

Orally. It can be administered without regard to food.

19. Describe the distribution of montelukast.

This drug has a very small volume of distribution. It is highly protein-bound (> 99 percent).

20. How is montelukast eliminated from the body?

Montelukast is metabolized by the hepatic cytochrome P_{450} system (CYP $_{3A4}$ and CYP $_{2C9}$). Metabolites are excreted in the bile and eliminated through the feces.

21. Is montelukast useful in an acute asthma attack?

Not as monotherapy. It may be used as an adjunct medication, but is not useful in mediating bronchodilatation.

22. Is zafirlukast useful in combination therapy?

Yes. It is often useful in combination with inhaled corticosteroids or beta-agonists.

23. Does zafirlukast exhibit anti-inflammatory properties?

Yes.

24. Describe the receptor selectivity of zafirlukast.

Zafirlukast inhibits the binding of leukotrienes D_4 and E_4.

25. Is zafirlukast bronchodilatory?

Yes. It is a mild bronchodilator.

26. Compare the bronchodilator response of zafirlukast to that of albuterol.

The onset of action of zafirlukast is much slower and the bronchodilatation is less pronounced than with a β_2 agonist such as albuterol.

27. Compare the actions of zafirlukast and montelukast on hepatic cytochrome P_{450}.

Zafirlukast inhibits the activity of cytochrome isozymes CYP 3A4 and CYP 2C9, resulting in the interruption of metabolism of other drugs metabolized by this pathway. Montelukast has no effect on the activity or level of these isozymes and thus has less potential for drug interaction.

28. Describe the mechanism of action of methylxanthines (e.g., theophylline, diphylline).

These drugs inhibit the actions of cellular phosphodiesterase, resulting in increased levels of cyclic adenosine monophosphate (cAMP). The actions are tissue-specific and mimic (or potentiate) the effects of sympathetic beta agonists. Other bronchodilatory actions may also be present, but as yet are undefined.

29. Discuss the actions of methylxanthines on bronchiolar smooth muscle.

These agents relax smooth muscle, resulting in bronchodilatation.

30. Compare the relative potencies of theophylline and caffeine.

Theophylline is significantly more potent than caffeine. Its actions are peripheral.

31. What is the advantage of therapy with theophylline over caffeine in the therapy of asthma?

Theophylline is more potent and thus a smaller dose can be used. In addition, theophylline does not cross the blood-brain barrier in as significant amounts as does caffeine, resulting in less central nervous system (CNS) effects.

32. How are methylxanthines eliminated?

These dugs are metabolized by the cytochrome P_{450} system, and the metabolites are excreted primarily through the urine.

BIBLIOGRAPHY

1. Bagley J, Sawada T, Wu Y, et al: A critical role for interleukin 4 in activating alloreactive CD4 T cells. Nat Immunol 1(3):257–261, 2000.
2. Bellamy D: New drugs and asthma care. Community Nurse 2(2):25–26, 1996.
3. Di Lorenzo G, Esposito Pellitteri M, Drago A, et al: Effects of in vitro treatment with fluticasone propionate on natural killer and lymphokine-induced killer activity in asthmatic and healthy individuals. Allergy 56(4):323–327, 2001.
4. Duschl A: Inhibiting the IL-4 receptor: Why, how, and for whom? Eur Cytokine Netw 11(3):521–522, 2000.
5. Ferguson GT Update on pharmacologic therapy for chronic obstructive pulmonary disease [review]. Clin Chest Med 21(4):723–738, 2000.
6. Forbes HJ: Practical management of asthma [review]. Lippincott's Prim Care Pract 1(2):207–216, 1997.
7. Fujita K, Kasayama S, Hashimoto J, et al: Inhaled corticosteroids reduce bone mineral density in early postmenopausal but not premenopausal asthmatic women. J Bone Miner Res 16(4):782–787, 2001.
8. Hardman J, Limbird L, Gilman A: Goodman & Gilman's The Pharmacological Basis of Therapeutics, 10th ed. McGraw-Hill Publishers, 2001.
9. Katzung B: Basic and Clinical Pharmacology, 8th ed. Appleton & Lange, 2001.
10. Leff AR: Regulation of leukotrienes in the management of asthma: Biology and clinical therapy [review]. Annu Rev Med 52:1–14, 2001.
11. Long K, Long R: A closer look at therapy for chronic asthma. Nurse Pract Forum 3(4):192–193, 1992.
12. McCrory DC, Brown C, Gelfand SE, et al: Management of acute exacerbations of COPD: A summary and appraisal of published evidence. Chest 119(4):1190–1209, 2001.
13. Oga T, Nishimura K, Tsukino M, et al: Changes in indices of airway hyperresponsiveness during one year of treatment with inhaled corticosteroids in patients with asthma. J Asthma 38(2):133–139, 2001.
14. Paton J: Managing asthma in the under twos [review]. Practitioner 240(1567):576–578, 580, 582, passim, 1996.
15. Pongracic JA: Asthma medications and how to use them [review]. Curr Opin Pulm Med 6(1):55-58, 2000. Review.
16. Redington AE, Meng QH, Springall DR, et al: Increased expression of inducible nitric oxide synthase and cyclo-oxygenase-2 in the airway epithelium of asthmatic subjects and regulation by corticosteroid treatment. Thorax 56(5):351–357, 2001.
17. Wijnhoven HA, Kriegsman DM, Hesselink AE, et al: Determinants of different dimensions of disease severity in asthma and COPD: Pulmonary function and health-related quality of life. Chest 119(4):1034–1042, 2001.
18. Williams DM: Clinical considerations in the use of inhaled corticosteroids for asthma. Pharmacotherapy 21(3 Pt 2):38S–48S, 2001.

19. Williams PV: Management of asthma [review]. Clin Symp 49(3):1–32, 1997.
20. Wilson AM, Dempsey OJ, Sims EJ, et al: Evaluation of salmeterol or montelukast as second-line therapy for asthma not controlled with inhaled corticosteroids. Chest 119(4):1021–1026, 2001.
21. Worcester L: A closer look at therapy for chronic asthma. Nurse Pract Forum 4(1):8, 1993.
22. Zhu J, Zou L, Zhu S, et al: Cytotoxic T lymphocyte-associated antigen 4 (CTLA-4) blockade enhances incidence and severity of experimental autoimmune neuritis in resistant mice. J Neuroimmunol 115(1–2):111–117, 2001.
23. Zurlinden J: New treatments for asthma. Nurs Spectr (Wash D C) 7(10):10, 1997.

31. ANTIHISTAMINES

1. Describe the mechanism of action of antihistamines.

These drugs bind to the H_1 receptor and prevent the activation of the receptor by histamine.

2. What are the general actions of antihistamines?

These drugs decrease histamine-induced vasodilatation, edema, and secretion. They may also act at the level of the central nervous system (CNS) to inhibit the reticular activating system.

3. Are antihistamines indicated for therapy of sinus infections?

No. These drugs decrease secretion, causing discharged fluid to have increased viscosity and remain in the sinus cavities for a longer period of time. Since one physiologic purpose of the drainage is to remove bacteria and toxins from the sinus cavities, administration of antihistamines allows the accumulation of these bacteria and may precipitate the onset of a bacterial infection.

4. Do antihistamines affect the actions of the autonomic nervous system?

Yes. These drugs tend to have anticholinergic activity.

5. Describe the adverse CNS effect that can be seen with antihistamine therapy.

Effects on the CNS can include drowsiness, sedation, dizziness, fatigue, lassitude, confusion, and anorexia.

6. What adverse cardiovascular effects can be seen with antihistamine therapy?

Cardiac effects can include postural hypotension and palpitations.

7. A patient on carbamazepine therapy is taking antihistamines for a cold. What activity in particular should the patient avoid?

The patient should avoid exposure to direct sunlight, because both drugs cause photosensitivity.

8. Why are antihistamines contraindicated in a patient taking a monoamine oxidase (MAO) inhibitor?

The anticholinergic effects of the antihistamines can synergize with the increased sympathetic activity mediated by the drug, and a hypertensive crisis or other cardiovascular event can result.

9. Which antihistamines are structurally related to phenothiazine antipsychotics and are used for motion sickness?

Promethazine and meclizine.

10. Which antihistamines inhibit the release of histamine from the mast cell?

Cromolyn and nedocromil.

11. Which antihistamine is similar in structure to a butyrophenone antipsychotic and has the potential to produce torsades de pointes?

Terfenadine. The potential of this drug to cause ventricular arrhythmias and death has precipitated its removal from the U.S. market.

12. Which antihistamine is the active metabolite of terfenadine?

Fexofenadine.

13. Does fexofenadine have proarrhythmogenic properties?
No.

14. Why are fexofenadine and terfenadine nonsedating?
These drugs are charged at physiologic pH and do not cross the blood-brain barrier in significant amounts.

15. Which ethylenediamine-type H$_1$ blocker is used in combination with pentazocine for drug abuse treatment?
Tripelennamine. In combination with pentazocine, it is used as a substitute for heroin.

16. Discuss loratadine.
Loratadine is an oral H$_1$-receptor blocker which is administered once daily. It crosses the blood-brain barrier poorly and, therefore, is nonsedating.

17. Does loratadine affect the autonomic nervous system?
Yes. It produces a weak blockade of both muscarinic receptors and adrenergic α_1 receptors.

18. Does loratadine cause cardiac arrhythmias?
No. This drug does not produce torsades de pointes.

19. Discuss the metabolism and elimination of loratadine.
Loratadine has a high first-pass effect and is rapidly metabolized by the liver into descarboethoxyloratadine, which has weak activity. Elimination is through the bile. Elimination may be prolonged in the elderly or in patients with liver disease.

20. Which antihistamines are included in the ethanolamine class of drugs?
Diphenhydramine, carbinoxamine, clemastine, dimenhydrinate, doxylamine, and phenyltoloxamine.

21. What is the relationship between dimenhydrinate and diphenhydramine (DPH)?
Dimenhydrinate is a salt of diphenhydramine.

22. What are the uses of diphenhydramine?
This drug is used to decrease sleep latency, and in the therapy of minor allergic reactions. It is also used topically for treatment of insect bites, urticaria, minor burns, and abrasions.

23. What are the uses of dimenhydrinate?
This drug is used orally as an antiemetic, for prevention of motion sickness.

24. What is cyproheptadine?
Cyproheptadine is an H$_1$ antagonist of the piperidine type.

25. Discuss the actions of cyproheptadine that can make the drug useful in the management of vascular headaches.
This drug antagonizes serotonin receptors.

26. Explain the effect of cyproheptadine on appetite.
Cyproheptadine stimulates appetite, through actions on serotonin receptors in the ventrolateral hypothalamus.

27. Describe the actions of cyproheptadine with long-term administration.
This drug exhibits tolerance. Thus, with high-dose or long-term administration, effects are attenuated.

28. Discuss clemastine.

Clemastine is structurally related to diphenhydramine and dimenhydrinate. It has a long duration of action as compared to other agents. It is extensively metabolized by hepatic microzymes.

29. Describe the actions of cetirizine.

Cetirizine has a very high affinity for the H_1 receptor. In addition to antagonism of histamine, it also appears to decrease the infiltration of inflammatory cells triggered by the histamine response.

30. Does cetirizine cross the blood-brain barrier?

Only in small amounts. It thus causes minimal sedation.

31. Is cetirizine suitable for a patient with compromised liver function?

Yes, because the drug is not significantly metabolized.

32. Describe the actions of cetirizine in a patient with decreased renal function.

Decreased renal function significantly prolongs the half-life of the drug, and can result in overdosage unless a change in dosage regimen is instituted.

33. What problems would be seen with administration of chlorpheniramine maleate to the elderly?

Because this drug is both extensively metabolized and excreted unchanged in the urine, the half-life is substantially increased.

34. Describe the actions of azelastine on the mast cell.

In addition to antagonism of histamine receptors, azelastine blocks histamine release from the mast cell.

BIBLIOGRAPHY

1. Baroody F, Proud D, Kagey-Sobotka A, et al: The effects of H1 antihistamines on the early allergic response. Ann Allergy 63(6 Pt 2):551–555, 1989.
2. Campbell AM, Bousquet J: Anti-allergic activity of H1 blockers [review]. Int Arch Allergy Immunol 101(3):308–310, 1993.
3. De Vos C: H1-receptor antagonists: Effects on leukocytes, myth or reality [review]? Clin Exp Allergy 29 Suppl 3:60–63, 1999.
4. Du Buske LM: Clinical comparison of histamine H1-receptor antagonist drugs [review]. J Allergy Clin Immunol 98(6 Pt 3):S307–S318, 1996.
5. Hardman J, Limbird L, Gilman A: Goodman & Gilman's The Pharmacological Basis of Therapeutics, 10th ed. McGraw-Hill Publishers, 2001.
6. Hendeles L: Cetirizine: A new antihistamine with minimal sedation [no abstract available]. Pharmacotherapy 16(5):967–968, 1996.
7. Howarth PH: Histamine and asthma: An appraisal based on specific H1-receptor antagonism [review]. Clin Exp Allergy 20 Suppl 2:31–41, 1990.
8. Katzung B: Basic and Clinical Pharmacology, 8th ed. Appleton & Lange, 2001.
9. Macaulay DB: Antihistamines in the management of allergic conditions [no abstract available]. Practitioner 196(176):775–780, 1966.
10. Negro-Alvarez JM, Funes E, Garcia-Canovas A, et al: Antiallergic properties of antihistamines [review]. Allergol Immunopathol (Madr) 24(4):177–183, 1996.
11. Pien LC: Appropriate use of second-generation antihistamines [review]. Cleve Clin J Med 67(5):372–380, 2000.
12. Simons FE: The antiallergic effects of antihistamines (H1-receptor antagonists). J Allergy Clin Immunol 90(4 Pt 2):705–715, 1992.
13. Simons FE, Simons KJ: The pharmacology and use of H1-receptor-antagonist drugs [review]. N Engl J Med 330(23):1663–1670, 1994.

VIII. Drugs that Affect the Gastrointestinal System

Patricia K. Anthony, Ph.D.

32. DRUGS THAT AFFECT GASTRIC ACID SECRETION

1. Describe four ways in which the upper gastrointestinal (GI) system can be protected from stomach acid.
- A decrease in the production of stomach acid (e.g., use of a proton-pump inhibitor)
- A decrease in the secretion of stomach acid (e.g., use of an H_2 blocker)
- Neutralization of secreted stomach acid (e.g., use of an antacid)
- Use of a cytoprotective drug (e.g., misoprostol) or luminal protectant (e.g., sucralfate)

2. Discuss the potential danger of the use of H_2 blockers or antacids.
Reabsorbed gastric acid contributes to the overall physiologic pH. Thus, the overuse or misuse of these drugs can decrease gastric acid to the extent that the patient becomes alkalotic.

PROTON-PUMP INHIBITORS

3. What is the mechanism of action of omeprazole?
Omeprazole binds irreversibly to the H+/K+ adenosinetriphosphatase (ATPase) (proton pump) on the secretory surface of the parietal cell membrane. The secretion of hydrogen ions into the gastric lumen is thus inhibited in a dose-dependent manner, decreasing the production of gastric acid.

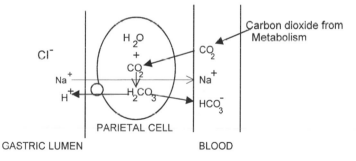

Diagrammatic representation of the production of stomach acid. Carbon dioxide from metabolic processes is converted to carbonic acid under the influence of carbonic anhydrase. Carbonic acid and sodium chloride dissociate, hydrogen ion is actively pumped across the parietal cell membrane and associates with free chloride ion. The remaining sodium and bicarbonate ions combine and remain in the plasma to be utilized in the acid-base buffering system.

4. Does omeprazole block stimulus-induced acid secretion (e.g., stress-related)?
Yes. The drug inhibits both basal and stimulus-induced secretion.

5. Describe the absorption of omeprazole.
The drug is converted to an ionized form by the presence of acid (low pH). Thus, it is absorbed in the duodenum.

6. Does omeprazole have a significant first-pass effect?

Yes. 60–70 percent of the drug is metabolized on the first pass through the liver. Bioavailability is thus higher in persons with compromised liver function.

7. Describe the onset and duration of omeprazole.

The onset of the drug is fairly rapid—approximately 1 hour. The effects of the drug typically persist over 3 days or more.

8. Is omeprazole significantly plasma protein-bound?

Yes. The drug is over 95 percent bound to plasma proteins.

9. Discuss the elimination of omeprazole.

Omeprazole is extensively metabolized to inactive metabolites, and excretion is primarily renal (80 percent), with some elimination through the bile.

10. What pharmacologic attribute does omeprazole have that may make the drug particularly useful in the therapy of gastric ulcers?

This drug has demonstrated significant in vitro activity against *Helicobacter pylori* (*H. pylori*).

11. Does omeprazole affect gastrin levels?

Yes. The drug causes elevated levels of gastrin. However, this change is reversed upon discontinuation of therapy.

12. Describe the actions of omeprazole on cytochrome P_{450}.

Omeprazole inhibits the actions of cytochrome P_{450}, which may result in drug interactions.

13. Is omeprazole likely to cause systemic alkalosis?

Systemic alkalosis caused by an excessive decrease in gastric acid production is unlikely, because the drug must be activated by an acid environment within the parietal cell. Thus, the conversion of the drug to the active form is related to the amount of carbonic acid available.

14. What is esomeprazole?

Esomeprazole is the S-isomer of omeprazole.

15. Discuss the advantage of esomeprazole over omeprazole in ulcer therapy.

The potency of esomeprazole against *Helicobacter pylori* is significantly greater than that of omeprazole.

HISTAMINE-RECEPTOR ANTAGONISTS

16. Describe the actions of H_2 antagonists.

These drugs inhibit the release of gastric acid, via antagonism of the histamine$_2$ receptor.

17. Explain why the efficacy of H_2 antagonists is less than that of proton-pump inhibitors.

Multiple stimuli for the release of gastric acid exist, so blockade of the histamine receptor only decreases secretion to the extent that other stimuli are present or absent. Proton-pump inhibitors act at the last step of gastric acid synthesis and thus are not subject to the effects of other mediators.

18. Describe the action of cimetidine.

Cimetidine inhibits the release of gastric acid, via the inhibition of the histamine (H_2) receptor.

19. Contrast the potencies of cimetidine, ranitidine and famotidine.

Famotidine has been shown to be as much as 100 times as potent as cimetidine. Ranitidine is somewhat less potent than famotidine but is more potent than cimetidine.

20. Describe the effect of cimetidine on cytochrome P_{450}.

Cimetidine inhibits the actions of cytochrome P_{450}.

21. Discuss the relative effects of cimetidine, ranitidine and famotidine on cytochrome P_{450}.

Cimetidine is the most potent of the three. Ranitidine has substantially less inhibitory action, and famotidine has negligible effect on the enzyme.

22. Explain the possible effects of cimetidine on the male reproductive system.

Cimetidine has weak antiandrogenic activity, which can affect the male reproductive system with frequent or prolonged use.

23. Why might famotidine be especially useful in ulcer prophylaxis?

This drug appears to have cytoprotective properties.

24. Discuss the duration of action of famotidine in the renally impaired patient.

Famotidine is primarily eliminated by the kidney, so the elimination half-life is significantly prolonged with renal impairment.

ANTACIDS

25. What types of antacids are commercially available?

Calcium carbonate, magnesium carbonate, and sodium bicarbonate are commonly used. Aluminum hydroxide is still found in some preparations, but has become less popular, as a result of the possible role of aluminum in the etiology of Alzheimer's disease.

26. What is the benefit of using sodium bicarbonate as an antacid?

This chemical acts very rapidly to neutralize stomach acid, as compared to other antacids.

27. Explain the potential danger of the administration of sodium bicarbonate as an antacid.

Sodium bicarbonate is easily absorbed, and can cause systemic alkalosis.

28. Discuss "calcium rebound" with respect to antacids.

Recall that calcium is a factor in the stimulation of the release of gastric acid. Thus, a calcium-containing antacid will first neutralize stomach acid, bringing the pH up, but the calcium may then produce a "rebound" effect by stimulating release of additional acid.

29. Describe an advantage of using magnesium-containing antacids.

These compounds are not absorbed well, as compared to other antacids, making them longer-lasting and decreasing the possibility of alkalosis.

30. Is a magnesium-containing antacid a drug of choice for a patient with osteomalacia?

No. The presence of magnesium can inhibit the absorption of calcium from the gut.

31. What negative gastrointestinal effect may be seen with magnesium-containing antacids?

These agents may cause diarrhea.

32. Discuss the relative potency, efficacy and duration of the available antacids.

• Potency: Aluminum antacids are the most potent, because they carry three negatively charged groups. Magnesium antacids are next in line, because they carry two groups, followed

by calcium antacids, which are decreased in efficacy resulting from the production of calcium rebound. Sodium bicarbonate is the least potent.
- Onset and duration of action: Sodium bicarbonate acts very quickly, but its effects are short-lived. Aluminum antacids are the slowest in onset, but have a long duration. Calcium and magnesium antacids are intermediate, with magnesium antacids being somewhat longer in duration and slower in onset than calcium antacids.

CYTOPROTECTIVE AND HORMONAL AGENTS

33. What is misoprostol?
Misoprostol is a synthetic, oral prostaglandin E_1 analog, which acts as a cytoprotective agent for the gastric epithelium.

34. Discuss the actions of misoprostol.
This drug exhibits a cytoprotective effect, increases gastric mucosal secretions, and may also decrease the time of gastric emptying. In addition, it may also decrease the secretion of gastric acid and pepsin, in a dose-dependent manner.

35. Is the addition of an H_2 blocker appropriate with misoprostol therapy?
Yes. Misoprostol does not affect histamine-mediated release. Therefore, the two drugs would have a synergistic action.

36. Is misoprostol appropriate for existing ulcers or for prophylaxis?
Both. The drug is very effective as a prophylactic, but is also very useful in protecting an existing ulcerated epithelium from further damage, due to its mucus-producing effects.

37. Is the administration of misoprostol appropriate for a pregnant woman?
No. Misoprostol contracts smooth muscle, and thus causes uterine contractions. Its secondary use is actually as an abortifacient.

38. Describe the metabolism of misoprostol.
The drug undergoes extensive first-pass metabolism, to form an active metabolite, misoprostol acid. This metabolism appears to occur within the parietal cell. The metabolite is then further degraded within local tissues.

39. Describe the onset of action of misoprostol.
Inhibition of gastric acid secretion occurs approximately 30 minutes following a single oral dose, reaching a maximum effect within 60 to 90 minutes.

40. What is sucralfate?
Sucralfate is an adhesive carbohydrate polymer that adheres to damaged gastric endothelium and affords protection from further damage, allowing the tissue to heal.

41. Discuss the beneficial effects of bismuth subsalicylate ("Pepto Bismol") in the prophylaxis and therapy of ulcers.
This drug coats the gastric epithelium, decreasing acid damage and irritation. It is also protective against ulcer formation, in combination with a drug such as metronidazole.

42. Describe the benefits of octreotide over H_2 antagonists and proton-pump inhibitors in the therapy of Zollinger-Ellison syndrome.
Octreotide inhibits gastrin secretion, whereas drugs such as cimetidine and omeprazole increase it. Octreotide is also extremely costly, making combination therapy with these agents of maximum benefit.

BIBLIOGRAPHY

1. De Flora S, Picciotto A: Mutagenicity of cimetidine in nitrite-enriched human gastric juice. Carcinogenesis 1(11):925–930, 1980.
2. Ezeamuzie CI, Philips E: Histamine H(2) receptors mediate the inhibitory effect of histamine on human eosinophil degranulation. Br J Pharmacol 131(3):482–488, 2000.
3. Fisher AA, Le Couteur DG: Nephrotoxicity and hepatotoxicity of histamine H2 receptor antagonists [review]. Drug Saf 24(1):39–57, 2001.
4. Freeman HJ: Therapy for ulcers and erosions associated with nonsteroidal anti-inflammatory drugs [review]. Can J Gastroenterol 12(8):537–539, 1989.
5. Graham DY: Famotidine to prevent peptic ulcer caused by NSAIDs. N Engl J Med 335(17):1322, [discussion 1322–1323], 1996.
6. Hardman J, Limbird L, Gilman A: Goodman & Gilman's The Pharmacological Basis of Therapeutics, 10th ed. McGraw-Hill Publishers, 2001.
7. Hawkey CJ, Yeomans ND: The treatment and prophylaxis of nonsteroidal anti-inflammatory drug (NSAID)-associated ulcers and erosions. Can J Gastroenterol 13(4):291, 295, 1999.
8. Isaacs P: Misoprostol and NSAID ulcers. Am J Gastroenterol 91(2):187–188, 1996.
9. Katzung B: Basic and Clinical Pharmacology, 8th ed. Appleton & Lange, 2001.
10. Langman MJ: Treating ulcers in patients receiving anti-arthritic drugs. Q J Med 73(272):1089–1091, 1989.
11. Langman MJ: Omeprazole in the treatment of ulcers induced by NSAIDs. Gut 43(6):744–746, 1998.
12. McLaughlin SA, McKinney PE: Antacid-induced hypermagnesemia in a patient with normal renal function and bowel obstruction. Ann Pharmacother 32(3):312–315, 1998.
13. Sitsen JM, Maris FA, Timmer CJ: Concomitant use of mirtazapine and cimetidine: A drug-drug interaction study in healthy male subjects. Eur J Clin Pharmacol 56(5):389–394, 2000.
14. Shuster J: Cimetidine and hot flashes. Nursing 30(2):68, 2000.
15. Takahashi K, Tanaka S, Ichikawa A: Effect of cimetidine on intratumoral cytokine expression in an experimental tumor. Biochem Biophys Res Commun 281(5):1113–1119, 2001.
16. Yeomans ND: Approaches to healing and prophylaxis of nonsteroidal anti-inflammatory drug-associated ulcers. Am J Med 110(1A):24S–28S, 2001.

33. DRUGS THAT AFFECT THE BOWEL

ANTIDIARRHEALS

1. What is a common characteristic of opiates used as antidiarrheals?

Opiates used as antidiarrheals generally do not cross the blood-brain barrier well. They therefore produce peripheral effects, such as slowing of the bowel, but central effects (e.g., euphoria and addiction) are not manifested at therapeutic doses.

2. Describe how opiates decrease peristalsis.

Opiates act directly at the level of the smooth muscle of the bowel, causing relaxation and decreased peristalsis.

3. Why is atropine added to preparations containing opiates used as antidiarrheals?

Atropine is added to discourage abuse—in large quantities these opiate drugs can still produce euphoria and addiction, but, if these quantities include atropine, the patient also gets uncomfortable effects such as tachycardia, dry mouth, and urinary retention. In smaller amounts (i.e., with therapeutic dosage of the drug), atropine also serves to block the parasympathetic effects produced by the opiate (e.g., miosis and increased peristalsis).

4. At therapeutic dosage, are the effects of atropine evident with opiate-atropine combination antidiarrheals?

In adults, the effects of atropine are negligible or nonexistent. In children, however, atropine-like effects may become evident at therapeutic dosage.

5. What is difenoxin?

Difenoxin is an opiate, structurally similar to meperidine. It is used as an antidiarrheal.

6. Describe the properties of diphenoxylate.

Diphenoxylate is a meperidine-like opiate that has minimal euphoric or physically addictive properties.

7. Can addiction result with high-dose diphenoxylate therapy?

Yes. Administration of an opiate antagonist to a patient on high-dose therapy will precipitate symptoms of opiate withdrawal.

8. Describe the onset of action and duration of diphenoxylate.

The onset of action usually occurs within 45 minutes to 1 hour, and the effects of the drug persist for up to four hours.

9. Does the metabolism of diphenoxylate produce active metabolites?

Yes. Diphenoxylate is metabolized by the liver to diphenoxylic acid, which has therapeutic action.

10. How is diphenoxylate eliminated?

Primarily through the bile and feces. A small amount may be eliminated through the urine.

11. Which opiate antidiarrheal is useful in inflammatory bowel disease?

Loperamide.

12. Contrast loperamide and diphenoxylate.
   The potencies of the two drugs are comparable. However, loperamide has a substantially lower ability to cross the blood-brain barrier. Loperamide thus has a much lower abuse potential.

13. Contrast the controlled substance classifications of loperamide and diphenoxylate.
   Diphenoxylate is classified as a C-V, whereas loperamide is not controlled at all—it is sold over-the-counter.

14. Does loperamide have an effect on fluid and electrolyte secretion in the bowel?
   Yes. The drug appears to block fluid and electrolyte secretion, decreasing electrolyte loss and contributing to a more desiccated (formed) stool.

15. What is octreotide?
   Octreotide is an analog of somatostatin.

16. Describe the uses of octreotide.
   Approved uses for the drug include the control of diarrhea associated with vasoactive intestinal peptide tumors and metastatic carcinoid tumors. Other uses include the control of diarrhea associated with AIDS and with pituitary tumors.

17. How is octreotide administered?
   This drug is administered by intramuscular injection. Injection by the intravenous or subcutaneous routes requires the acetate form of the drug.

18. Describe the pharmacokinetics of octreotide.
   The half-life of the drug is 1.7 hours. It is rapidly distributed, and is about 60 percent protein-bound. The duration of action varies between patients, up to a maximum of 12 hours. Elimination is primarily via the urine.

19. Describe the mechanism of action of attapulgite.
   Attapulgite is a diatomaceous earth, a clay that binds irritants in the bowel, reducing secretions.

20. Describe the actions of bismuth subsalicylate ("Pepto Bismol") as an antidiarrheal.
   This drug coats the intestinal epithelium, decreasing irritation.

LAXATIVES

21. What are the two major classifications of laxatives?
   Irritant laxatives, which cause an increase in secretions through irritation of the intestinal epithelium, and stool softeners, which lubricate the stool or incorporate compliant material into the stool.

22. What are the two major irritant laxatives in use?
   Phenolphthalein and bisacodyl.

23. Name a "natural" irritant laxative.
   Senna.

24. Describe two lubricating stool softeners.
   Mineral oil, which oils the stool, and docusate. Docusate is primarily marketed as docusate sodium, but the potassium and calcium forms are also available.

BIBLIOGRAPHY

1. Amir I, Sharma R, Bauman WA, et al: Bowel care for individuals with spinal cord injury: Comparison of four approaches. J Spinal Cord Med 21(1):21–24, 1998.
2. Artymowicz RJ, Childs AL, Paolini L: Phenolphthalein-induced toxic epidermal necrolysis. Ann Pharmacother 31(10):1157–1159, 1997.
3. Crouch MA, Restino MS, Cruz JM, et al: Octreotide acetate in refractory bone marrow transplant-associated diarrhea. Ann Pharmacother 30(4):331–336, 1996.
4. Ericsson CD: Travelers' diarrhea. Epidemiology, prevention, and self-treatment. Infect Dis Clin North Am 12(2):285–303, 1998.
5. Fiedler LM, George J, Sachar DB, et al: Treatment responses in collagenous colitis. Am J Gastroenterol 96(3):818–821, 2001.
6. Hardman J, Limbird L, Gilman A: Goodman & Gilman's The Pharmacological Basis of Therapeutics, 10th ed. McGraw-Hill Publishers, 2001.
7. Katzung B: Basic and Clinical Pharmacology, 8th ed. Appleton & Lange, 2001.
8. Mboya SA, Bhargava HN: Adsorption and desorption of loperamide hydrochloride by activated attapulgites. Am J Health Syst Pharm 52(24):2816–2818, 1995.
9. McRorie JW, Daggy BP, Morel JG, et al: Psyllium is superior to docusate sodium for treatment of chronic constipation. Aliment Pharmacol Ther 12(5):491–497, 1998.
10. Thorpe DM: Management of opioid-induced constipation. Curr Pain Headache Rep 5(3):237–240, 2001.
11. Zaid MR, Hasan M, Khan AA: Attapulgite in the treatment of acute diarrhoea: A double-blind placebo-controlled study. J Diarrhoeal Dis Res 13(1):44–46, 1995.

34. ANTIHELMINTICS

1. Discuss the mechanism of action of albendazole.
Albendazole inhibits microtubule formation, which disrupts cellular function. This results in an inability of the parasite to survive and reproduce.

2. What is the major use of albendazole?
Albendazole is used in the therapy of tapeworm infestations.

3. Discuss the use of albendazole in pregnancy.
Albendazole inhibits cellular division and thus is contraindicated in pregnancy. To avoid serious complications, the drug must be discontinued at least 1 month before conception.

4. Which antihelmintic may be used in a pregnant patient?
Thiabendazole.

5. Discuss the mechanism of action of thiabendazole.
Like mebendazole and albendazole, thiabendazole disrupts the assembly of microtubules. This results in the formation of aberrant spindles and disrupts cellular replication.

6. Does thiabendazole have the same mechanism of action as colchicine?
No. Both drugs disrupt microtubule assembly. However, thiabendazole appears to specifically depolymerize a sub-population of stable, acetylated microtubules, which are not affected by colchicine.

7. What is the side effect of mebendazole and thiabendazole on skeletal muscle?
Both drugs cause low-level muscle pain and tenderness.

8. Describe the absorption of mebendazole.
This drug is poorly absorbed (5–10 percent), and undergoes a first-pass effect in the liver.

9. What is the half-life of mebendazole?
The $T\frac{1}{2}$ is approximately 1 hour.

10. Discuss the adverse effects of mebendazole.
This drug has few systemic effects because it is poorly absorbed. The adverse effects are related to the gastrointestinal (GI) system and include GI distress and abdominal pain, as well as diarrhea.

11. Why is mebendazole embryotoxic?
It has an affinity for mammalian tubulin, as well as prokaryotic tubulin. Disruption of microspindle formation during gestation results in significant birth defects, and/or loss of fetal life, depending on the stage of pregnancy at which the drug was taken.

12. Is flubendazole embryotoxic?
No. It was developed to have specificity for nematode tubulin.

13. What is the drug of choice for elephantiasis?
Diethylcarbamazine.

14. Discuss the mechanism of action of diethylcarbamazine.
This drug sensitizes microfilariae to the effects of the reticuloendothelial system, making them "targets" of the reticuloendothelial system.

15. Is diethylcarbamazine effective against adult parasites?
No. Its action is primarily against the developing parasites (microfilariae).

16. Which organisms respond to diethylcarbamazine treatment?
This drug is effective against *w. bancrofti* and *w. malayi*, unlike other antihelmintic agents.

17. Why might the plasma half-life of diethylcarbamazine increase with concurrent administration of acetazolamide?
This drug is reabsorbed in an alkaline kidney. Thus, if the urine is basic, the half-life increases. Recall that acetazolamide administration results in the excretion of bicarbonate and alkaline urine. The plasma half-life of diethylcarbamazine is increased, as a result of the alkalinization of the urine and increased reabsorption.

18. Which antihelmintic is used to eliminate whipworm?
Oxantel pamoate.

19. Discuss the use of pyrantel pamoate.
Pyrantel pamoate is a broad-spectrum antihelmintic. It is useful in the eradication of a wide variety of nematodes. Due to its broad-spectrum action, it is considered a drug of second choice in nematode infections.

20. What is the mechanism of action of pyrantel pamoate?
This drug binds to nicotinic receptors at the neuromuscular junction (endplate) in the nematode. This produces paralysis of the organism, which is subsequently expelled from the body.

21. Is pyrantel pamoate well absorbed?
No. Its actions are in the intestine.

22. Discuss the side effects of pyrantel pamoate.
As a result of its lack of absorption, the drug has few adverse effects.

23. What is ivermectin?
Ivermectin is a macrocytic lactone produced by bacteria (*s. avermitilis*).

24. Describe the mechanism of action of ivermectin.
This drug potentiates the release and also the binding of gamma-aminobutyric acid (GABA) at the immature nematodal neuromuscular junction. This leads to paralysis of the parasite and subsequent expulsion.

25. Is ivermectin effective against adult parasites?
No. It is effective only against microfilariae.

26. Does ivermectin affect human neurotransmission?
No, because the drug does not cross into the brain.

27. Describe the adverse effects of ivermectin.
Adverse effects include swelling of the face and legs and dizziness.

28. Contrast diethylcarbamate and ivermectin with respect to the Mazzotti reaction.
Ivermectin does not cause this phenomenon. This is in direct contrast to diethylcarbamate, which has the potential for a strong Mazzotti reaction.

29. Which drugs are useful for tapeworm infections?
Metrifonate and praziquantel. Mebendazole and related drugs can also be used.

30. Which antihelmintic is an organophosphate, used for infections of *S. haematobium*?
Metrifonate.

31. Which antihelmintic drug uncouples parasitic oxidative phosphorylation?
Praziquantel.

BIBLIOGRAPHY

1. Albanese G, Venturi C, Galbiati G: Treatment of larva migrans cutanea (creeping eruption): A comparison between albendazole and traditional therapy. Int J Dermatol 40(1):67–71, 2001.
2. Delescluse C, Ledirac N, Li R, et al: Induction of cytochrome P_{450} 1A1 gene expression, oxidative stress, and genotoxicity by carbaryl and thiabendazole in transfected human HepG2 and lymphoblastoid cells. Biochem Pharmacol 61(4):399–407, 2001.
3. Hardman J, Limbird L, Gilman A: Goodman & Gilman's The Pharmacological Basis of Therapeutics, 10th ed. McGraw-Hill Publishers, 2001.
4. Katzung B: Basic and Clinical Pharmacology, 8th ed. Appleton & Lange, 2001.
5. Pisano C, Battistoni A, Antoccia A, et al: Changes in microtubule organization after exposure to a benzimidazole derivative in Chinese hamster cells. Mutagenesis 15(6):507–515, 2000.
6. Sarcina M, Mullineaux CW: Effects of tubulin assembly inhibitors on cell division in prokaryotes in vivo. FEMS Microbiol Lett 191(1):25–29, 2000.
7. Schaffel R, Nucci M, Portugal R, et al: Thiabendazole for the treatment of strongyloidiasis in patients with hematologic malignancies. Clin Infect Dis 31(3):821–822, 2000.
8. Tan HH, Goh CL: Parasitic skin infections in the elderly: recognition and drug treatment. Drugs Aging 18(3):165–176, 2001.
9. Watt G, Saisorn S, Jongsakul K, et al: Blinded, placebo-controlled trial of antiparasitic drugs for trichinosis myositis. J Infect Dis 182(1):371–374, 2000.

IX. Drugs that Affect the Endocrine System

Patricia. K. Anthony, Ph.D., and C. Andrew Powers, Ph.D.

35. DRUGS USED IN THE THERAPY OF DIABETES MELLITUS

1. Describe type I diabetes and its therapy.

Type I diabetes is characterized by a lack of insulin. Thus, therapy for this condition is daily insulin therapy.

2. What types of insulin are commercially available?

Commercially available insulin may be derived from the pancreas of the pig or the cow.

In addition, human insulin is now available. It is derived from bacterial sources (cloned insulin). (*Note:* Bovine insulin has been removed from the U.S. market because of concerns about spongiform encephalopathies ["mad cow disease"].)

3. Describe insulin complexes and their uses.

Insulin is typically complexed with zinc and/or protamine, a charged protein. This complexing allows the hormone to be slowly dissociated from the complex, making the preparation longer-acting.

4. What is U-100 insulin?

This is normal, uncomplexed insulin. It is termed U-100 because it contains 100 units of insulin per milliliter.

5. What is the plasma half-life of U-100 insulin?

Approximately 9 minutes.

6. What is lente insulin?

Lente insulin is U-100 insulin complexed with zinc. It is intermediate-acting.

7. Describe NPH insulin.

NPH insulin is neutral protamine hagedorn insulin. It is complexed with protamine and is intermediate-acting.

8. What is ultralente insulin?

Insulin complexed with zinc and protamine. This form of insulin has a slower onset and long duration.

9. Explain why ultralente insulin has a slow onset and long duration.

The insulin complex must first be degraded, because free insulin is the active form. Thus, the protein-protein interactions and also the zinc complexes must be disrupted. Because these interactions take time to disrupt, there is a lag time before the free insulin is released, resulting in slower onset. Because the complexed form allows more insulin to be administered per dose, the duration is long, because free insulin is released constantly upon disruption of the protein/zinc interactions.

Questions 10 to 12 refer to the following table that lists three insulin preparations and their pharmacodynamic parameters:

	ONSET OF ACTION	PEAK OF ACTION	DURATION OF ACTION
Insulin #1	30–60 min	2–4 hours	6–8 hours
Insulin #2	1–2 hours	5–7 hours	13–18 hours
Insulin #3	2–4 hours	8–10 hours	18–30 hours

10. Which insulin is regular (U-100) insulin?

Insulin #1, because the onset of action is fastest, and it is of the shortest duration. Uncomplexed insulin acts rapidly, and, because it is a free peptide, it is rapidly degraded.

11. Identify the neutral protamine-complexed insulin (NPH insulin).

Insulin #2, because this insulin has an intermediate onset and duration, consistent with disruption of a protein-insulin complex.

12. Which of the above insulin preparations is ultralente insulin?

Insulin #3, because it has the slowest onset and longest duration.

13. Should complexed forms of insulin (e.g., NPH, lente, or ultralente) be used in emergency situations (e.g., the therapy of diabetic coma)?

No. The onset of action is too slow.

14. Compare insulin lispro and insulin glargine with regular insulin.

Insulin lispro has a shorter duration of action than regular insulin, and is fast-acting, producing a faster glucose-lowering effect, with subcutaneous injection. The substitution of arginine with lysine ("glargine" insulin) results in a longer duration of action.

15. Discuss insulin aspart.

Insulin aspart results from a substitution of proline with aspartate in the insulin molecule. This results in a fast-acting form of insulin.

16. Differentiate the pharmacodynamics of intravenous injection of regular insulin and insulin lispro or insulin aspart.

Administered intravenously, insulin lispro and insulin aspart show pharmacodynamic parameters similar to regular insulin. This is in contrast to administration by the subcutaneous route.

17. Which type of insulin is commonly used for insulin therapy in patients who wear external SC insulin infusion pumps?

Insulin lispro.

18. Which type of insulin allows for once-daily dosing?

Insulin glargine. The glucose-lowering effects of this form do not peak, thus mimicking the patient's basal secretion of insulin.

19. In patients with Type I diabetes, what benefits are associated with strict control of blood glucose levels using multiple daily insulin injections or insulin infusion pumps?

Simulation of basal secretion of insulin using an infusion pump or multiple daily injections can result in decreased vascular complications in patients of all ages. In addition, a more consistent administration of insulin can result in a lower risk of brain damage in pediatric patients.

20. Discuss the adverse effects of insulin.

The major adverse effect is, predictably, hypoglycemia. In addition, patients may have food allergies that can cause reactions to insulins of animal origin (i.e., an allergy to pork may limit the use of porcine insulin, etc.). Patients may also develop abnormalities in fat deposition with repeated injections at the same site (lipodystrophy).

21. What is the result of the administering propranolol with insulin?

Beta-receptor antagonists mask the symptoms of hypoglycemia (e.g., tachycardia, diaphoresis), and thus mask the symptoms of insulin overdose. This could lead to insulin shock.

22. Discuss the development of exogenous insulin resistance.

This occurs to the greatest extent with the use of animal insulins. The body views the insulin as a foreign substance and the patient develops antibodies to the insulin.

TYPE II (ADULT ONSET) DIABETES

23. Discuss type II diabetes.

In type II (adult onset, non–insulin-dependent diabetes mellitus [NIDDM]), the problem lies at the level of the receptor rather than the islet cell. Typically, these patients produce insulin, but the receptors are either desensitized or are associated with a defective transduction mechanism.

24. Describe nonpharmacologic therapies for non–insulin-dependent diabetes.

Since this condition is often caused by hyperinsulinemia associated with obesity, the first course of action is to restrict the diet. A reduction in carbohydrates, in particular, will elicit less insulin repines and eventually mediate an upregulation and/or resensitization of receptors.

25. Discuss pharmacologic therapies for NIDDM.

Pharmacologic therapies include drugs that elicit an increase in insulin secretion in order to maximally stimulate desensitized receptors (e.g., sulfonylureas), and drugs that alter glucose utilization or production (e.g., biguanides, troglitazone), or alter the breakdown of carbohydrates (e.g., acarbose).

26. Is administration of insulin useful in the control of blood glucose in NIDDM?

This depends on the etiology. If the condition is caused by overstimulation of receptors, insulin administration can be useful. If there were a genetic defect in receptor transduction, administration of insulin would not produce benefit in control of blood glucose.

27. Discuss the mechanism of action of sulfonylureas.

These agents are believed to trigger the release of insulin by the blockade of ATP-sensitive potassium-channel receptors on the pancreatic cell. This blockade results in a decrease in potassium conductance and subsequent depolarization of the cell membrane, stimulating calcium ion influx and release of insulin.

28. Which drugs are considered first-generation sulfonylureas?

Tolbutamide, tolazamide and chlorpropamide. (See Table below.)

DRUG	DURATION OF ACTION	HALF-LIFE	PRODUCTION OF METABOLITES
Tolbutamide	Short (6–8h)	< 1 h	No
Acetohexamide	Intermediate (12–18 h)	1.5 h	Yes
Glyburide	Intermediate (10–16 h)	10 h	No
Glipizide	Intermediate (24 h)	4 h	No
Chlorpropamide	Long (> 40 h)	36 h	No
Tolazamide	Long (> 20 h)	7 h	Yes

29. Which drugs are considered second-generation sulfonylureas?
Glyburide and glipizide.

30. Compare the first- and second-generation sulfonylureas.
The first generation drugs are significantly decreased in potency, as compared to second-generation drugs. In addition, plasma protein-binding is much greater with first-generation drugs, so drug interactions are more likely to occur.

31. Do sulfonamides decrease insulin resistance?
No. The possible exception is glimepiride, which may have a direct effect on mobilization of glucose transporters and lowering of insulin resistance.

32. Describe the action of phenylbutazone on the actions of sulfonylureas.
Phenylbutazone increases the potency of sulfonylureas as it displaces these drugs from plasma protein-binding sites. Thus, lower dosage is required.

33. Describe the interactions of a drug such as isoproterenol with sulfonylureas.
Beta-receptor agonists act to increase plasma glucose. Thus, they antagonize the actions of sulfonylureas.

34. Discuss the possible effects of sulfonylureas on the heart.
These drugs affect potassium conductance, not only in islet cells, but also in coronary arteries and the myocardium. Therefore, they can exacerbate ischemic damage in the compromised heart, as a result of a reduced ability to relax cardiac and vascular smooth muscle.

35. What results from concurrent therapy with chlorpropamide and warfarin?
These drugs compete for binding sites on plasma proteins. Thus, the dosages of the drugs would need to be adjusted.

36. Describe the effect of ethanol consumption on the actions of sulfonylureas.
Ethanol induces hepatic metabolic enzymes and can, therefore, interfere with the actions of sulfonylureas by increasing the rate of metabolism.

37. Describe the mechanism of action of biguanide antidiabetic agents.
Biguanides (e.g., metformin, phenformin) enhance the metabolism of glucose by peripheral tissues. In addition, these drugs can inhibit hepatic gluconeogenesis and increase the rate of glycolysis.

38. Does metformin lower fasting or postprandial glucose levels?
The drug lowers both fasting and postprandial levels, as a result of decreased hepatic gluconeogenesis.

39. What effect does metformin have on the serum lipid profile?
These agents have beneficial effects because they lower serum triglycerides and increase levels of serum high-density lipoproteins (HDL).

40. Compare the hypoglycemic effects of biguanides and sulfonylureas.
Sulfonylureas can promote hypoglycemia, because they increase the production of insulin. Biguanides do not affect insulin levels, but simply promote glucose utilization by tissues. They therefore do not promote hypoglycemia.

41. Are biguanides and sulfonylureas used in concurrent therapy?
Yes. The mechanisms of action are dissimilar, so the therapeutic effects are synergistic without increased risk of adverse effects.

42. What is acarbose?

Acarbose is an alpha-glucosidase inhibitor that slows the breakdown of complex carbohydrates in the intestine. Thus, increases in postprandial serum glucose are inhibited, resulting in both a decrease in insulin requirement and a decrease in insulin receptor stimulation.

43. Discuss the treatment of hypoglycemia produced by acarbose.

If hypoglycemia occurs, either oral or intravenous glucose must be administered. Oral sucrose will not be metabolized as a result of the actions of the drug.

44. What is the effect of acarbose on liver enzymes?

Elevation of liver enzymes occurs at high therapeutic doses.

45. What is the action of troglitazone?

This drug lowers insulin resistance in muscle and adipose tissue, reducing the need for insulin.

46. Are the actions of troglitazone immediate?

No. The drug acts at the level of the nucleus to alter transcription of RNA. It thus may take up to 1 to 3 months to be effective.

47. Is troglitazone used as monotherapy?

Troglitazone is effective as monotherapy only at 600 mg doses and above. Monotherapy is most useful in very obese patients, or patients with renal decompensation.

48. Discuss the adverse effects of troglitazone.

Adverse effects include weight gain, anemia, fluid retention, and rare idiosyncratic hepatic necrosis.

49. Do patients on troglitazone therapy require blood work?

Yes. Monthly assessment of liver function is required as a result of the possibility of hepatic necrosis.

BIBLIOGRAPHY

1. Bell DS: Hypertension and antihypertensive therapy as risk factors for type 2 diabetes mellitus. N Engl J Med 343(8):580, 2000.
2. Berne C: Diabetes mellitus-a more solid ground for treatment. J Intern Med 249(5):391–393, 2001.
3. Bhattacharyya A, Brown S, Hughes S, et al: Insulin lispro and regular insulin in pregnancy. QJM 94(5):255–260, 2001.
4. Hardman J, Limbird L, Gilman A: Goodman & Gilman's The Pharmacological Basis of Therapeutics, 10th ed. McGraw-Hill Publishers, 2001.
5. Junge M, Tsokos M, Puschel K: Suicide by insulin injection in combination with beta-blocker application. Forensic Sci Int 113(1–3):457–460, 2000.
6. Katzung B: Basic and Clinical Pharmacology, 8th ed. Appleton & Lange, 2001.
7. Legtenberg RJ, Houston RJ, Oeseburg B, et al: Effects of sulfonylurea derivatives on ischemia-induced loss of function in the isolated rat heart. Eur J Pharmacol 419(1):85–92, 2001.
8. Luna B, Feinglos MN: Oral agents in the management of type 2 diabetes mellitus. Am Fam Physician 63(9):1747–1756, 2001.
9. McCall AL: Clinical review of glimepiride. Expert Opin Pharmacother 2(4):699–713, 2001.
10. Moller AM, Jensen NM, Pildal J, et al: Studies of genetic variability of the glucose transporter 2 promoter in patients with type 2 diabetes mellitus. J Clin Endocrinol Metab 86(5):2181–2186, 2001.
11. Reasner CA, Defronzo RA: Treatment of type 2 diabetes mellitus: A rational approach based on its pathophysiology. Am Fam Physician 63(9):1687–1688, 1691–1692, 1694, 2001.
12. Wolffenbuttel BH, Sels JP, Huijberts MS: Rosiglitazone. Expert Opin Pharmacother 2(3):467–478, 2001.

36. DRUGS THAT AFFECT THE THYROID GLAND

1. What are the symptoms of hyperthyroidism?

Increased metabolism, increased heat production, weight loss, protrusion of the eyes (exophthalmia), and an increase in bone and muscle turnover are the major symptoms. In addition, increased levels of thyroid hormone have detrimental effects on cardiac muscle and cardiac conduction, as well as on vascular smooth muscle function.

2. Explain the detrimental actions of increased levels of thyroid hormone on the heart.

Thyroid hormone L-triiodothyronine (T_3) sensitizes the myocardium to the effects of catecholamines. This can facilitate the production of cardiac arrhythmias.

3. Which of the antithyroid drugs inhibits the proteolysis of thyroglobulin stored in the thyroid gland?

Sodium iodide.

4. Discuss the use of iodide in the treatment of hyperthyroidism.

Iodide decreases the release of thyroid hormone and also decreases the synthesis of iodinated tyrosine and thyronine residues.

5. Discuss the use of iodine (e.g., Lugol's solution) in the surgical removal or reduction of thyroid mass.

Iodine is are primarily used to induce a euthyroid state before surgery. It increases vascularity and increase the density of the thyroid gland, which decreases postoperative complications.

6. Is the use of iodides contraindicated in pregnancy?

Long-term therapy is contraindicated, because iodides will cross the placenta and into breast milk, causing hypothyroidism (goiter) in the fetus and neonate. Short, intensive therapy for thyrotoxic crisis may be utilized without adverse effects to the fetus.

7. What is iodism?

This condition presents as a consequence of iodide or iodine administration. Its symptoms resemble a low-level upper respiratory infection—burning of the mouth and throat, swollen submaxillary glands, and painful teeth and gums. A metallic taste may also be present, caused by the metallic nature of iodine.

8. Which drugs are included in the thioureylene class of antithyroid drugs?

This class includes methimazole, carbimazole, and propothiouracil (PTU). The general mechanism and effects of these drugs are similar.

9. Discuss the therapeutic properties of methimazole.

Methimazole acts as a substrate for thyroid peroxidase, an enzyme that acts as a catalyst in the iodination of thyroglobulin. Thus, there is a dose-dependent competition between the drug and thyroglobulin for iodination. The iodination of thyroglobulin is thus decreased, resulting in a reduced production of thyroid hormone.

10. Describe the effects of methimazole on thyroglobulin levels.

Recall that the iodination of thyroglobulin is random, with some tyrosyl residues monoiodinated, diiodinated or iodinated to form reverse T_3. These ineffective residues may be recycled back to thyroglobulin and reiodinated. Methimazole inhibits this process by inhibiting the coupling of iodotyrosyl residues, as well as inhibiting the oxidation of iodide ions.

11. Does methimazole affect the action of circulating T_3 and L-thyroxine (T_4)?

No.

12. How is methimazole eliminated?

Once the drug is iodinated, it is degraded within the thyroid gland. Circulating methimazole is metabolized in the liver and excreted renally.

13. Describe the distribution of methimazole.

This drug is not significantly protein-bound. Distribution is limited because the drug is actively concentrated within the thyroid gland.

14. Compare the elimination half-life of methimazole and its duration of action.

The elimination half-life of the drug is relatively short—around 5 hours. This is primarily caused by the uptake of the drug by thyroid follicular cells. This is also the reason for the relatively extended therapeutic half-life of the drug (> 40 hours)—once concentrated within follicular cells, it acts as an iodination substrate before degradation within the follicle.

15. Compare the actions of carbimazole and methimazole.

Carbimazole is a precursor to methimazole. It is rapidly converted to methimazole upon absorption, and thus has the same properties.

16. Which antithyroid medication inhibits both iodine organification, and the conversion of T_4 (thyroxine) to T_3 (triiodothyronine)?

Propothiouracil.

17. Discuss the mechanism of action of propothiouracil (PTU).

Like methimazole, PTU acts as a substrate for thyroid peroxidase, and thus inhibits the iodination of thyroglobulin. In addition, the drug inhibits the conversion of T_3 to T_4 in the periphery.

18. Are the actions of exogenously administered thyroid affected by PTU?

No. Thus, exogenous thyroid preparations may be administered in case of overdose.

19. Compare the pharmacodynamics of propothiouracil and methimazole.

Propothiouracil has a shorter duration of action and has significantly less transfer across the placenta and into breast milk than methimazole.

20. Why is PTU a safer drug for administration in pregnancy?

The drug is highly protein-bound and is also significantly ionized at physiologic pH. Thus, the drug does not cross the fetal-placental barrier well.

21. Discuss the adverse effects of the thiourelyene drugs.

Allergic reactions (e.g., skin rash) are relatively common. In addition, serum sickness syndrome, jaundice, hypoprothrombinemia, thrombocytopenia, polyarteritis, and lupus erythematosus can occur.

22. Describe the therapeutic actions of radioactive iodine (^{131}I).

Radiolabeled iodine is taken up into follicular cells and concentrated. As the isotope decays, it destroys surrounding tissue by beta and gamma emissions, reducing thyroid mass and activity.

23. Does ^{131}I treatment of adults increase the risk of developing thyroid cancer?

No.

24. What potential adverse effects can be expected with long-term use of ^{131}I therapy for the treatment of hyperthyroidism?

^{131}I treatment results in a high incidence of hypothyroidism years after its use.

25. Discuss the interactions of thyroid hormone, iodide, and antithyroid drugs with radioactive iodine therapy.

These agents all compete with the radiolabeled iodine for uptake into the thyroid. Thus, the efficacy of the therapy is reduced by these drugs, and potential adverse effects may increase.

26. What are the adverse effects associated with radiolabeled iodine therapy?

This therapy can produce urticaria and skin rashes. In addition, there can be potentially serious adverse effects, including bone marrow depression, acute leukemia, and blood dyscrasias. Symptoms of radiation sickness as well as cardiovascular complications (e.g., angina, sinus tachycardia) can also occur.

TREATMENT OF MYXEDEMA

27. Discuss thyroid hormone replacement.

Replacement therapy may be T_3, T_4 or a combination of the two. Administration of triiodothyronine results in fast onset and a short duration of action, while administration of thyroxine, which is the bound form, requires activation and thus results in a slower onset and longer duration. Thus, the most widely prescribed replacement is a combination of the two in a ratio of approximately 1:4 (T_3:T_4), which roughly mimics the endogenous concentrations of the two hormones.

28. Compare the potencies of liothyronine and thyroxine.

Liothyronine (triiodothyronine or T_3) has approximately three times the potency of thyroxine (T_4).

29. Compare the onset and duration of action of liothyronine and thyroxine.

Thyroxine is bound to thyroid-binding globulin in the plasma, and is converted to triiodothyronine in the periphery. Thus, it has a slower onset and longer duration of action. Liothyronine, in contrast, is not bound and does not require conversion. Thus, it has a faster onset and shorter duration.

30. Describe the adverse effects of thyroid hormone replacement.

Adverse effects essentially mimic the symptoms of hyperthyroidism—excessive weight loss, tachycardia, cardiac arrhythmias, and restlessness. These occur very rarely with therapeutic dosage.

31. Discuss the relationship of thyroid levels and digoxin clearance.

Digoxin clearance is decreased with hypothyroidism. Thus, thyroid replacement will minimize the occurrence of toxicity caused by decreased clearance.

32. Describe the effects of oral contraceptive use on thyroid replacement therapy.

Estrogens can induce the synthesis of thyroid-binding globulin, resulting in an increase in bound T_4. Thus, the therapeutic efficacy of the thyroid replacement is reduced.

33. What effect would a high-fiber diet, or the ingestion of bile-binding resins or antacids, have on thyroid hormone replacement therapy?

The effects are decreased absorption of thyroxine from the GI tract, either through binding of the hormone or changes in pH.

34. Why is desiccated thyroid no longer used as a therapeutic agent?

The amounts and proportions of thyroxine and triiodothyronine are too variable in natural thyroid tissue. Thus, the dosage and potency could not be accurately monitored.

BIBLIOGRAPHY

1. Bunevicius R, Prange AJ: Mental improvement after replacement therapy with thyroxine plus triiodothyronine: Relationship to cause of hypothyroidism. Int J Neuropsychopharmacol 3(2):167–174, 2000.
2. Cornejo P, Tapia G, Puntarulo S, et al: Iron-induced changes in nitric oxide and superoxide radical generation in rat liver after lindane or thyroid hormone treatment. Toxicol Lett 119(2):87–93, 2001.
3. Didonna D, D'Alessandro G, De Michele A, et al: Thyrotoxic periodic paralysis in a Caucasian man in treatment for Graves' disease. Panminerva Med 42(4):293–294, 2000.
4. Glinoer D, de Nayer P, Bex M: Effects of l-thyroxine administration, TSH-receptor antibodies and smoking on the risk of recurrence in Graves' hyperthyroidism treated with antithyroid drugs: A double-blind prospective randomized study. Eur J Endocrinol 144(5):475–483, 2001.
5. Hardman J, Limbird L, Gilman A: Goodman & Gilman's The Pharmacological Basis of Therapeutics, 10th ed. McGraw-Hill Publishers, 2001.
6. Katzung B: Basic and Clinical Pharmacology, 8th ed. Appleton & Lange, 2001.
7. Martocchia A, Labbadia G, Paoletti V, et al: Hashimoto's disease during interferon-alpha therapy in a patient with pre-treatment negative anti-thyroid autoantibodies and with the specific genetic susceptibility to the thyroid disease. Neuroendocrinol Lett 22(1):49–52, 2001.
8. Munte TF, Radamm C, Johannes S, et al: Alterations of cognitive functions induced by exogenous application of thyroid hormones in healthy men: A double-blind cross-over study using event-related brain potentials. Thyroid 11(4):385–391, 2001.
9. Phoojaroenchanachai M, Sriussadaporn S, Peerapatdit T, et al: Effect of maternal hyperthyroidism during late pregnancy on the risk of neonatal low birth weight. Clin Endocrinol (Oxf) 54(3):365–370, 2001.
10. Seven R, Gelisgen R, Seven A, et al: Influence of propylthiouracil treatment on oxidative stress and nitric oxide in Basedow disease patients. J Toxicol Environ Health A 62(7):495–503, 2001.
11. Vaisman M, Spina LD, Eksterman LF, et al: Comparative bioavailability of two oral L-thyroxine formulations after multiple dose administration in patients with hypothyroidism and its relation with therapeutic endpoints and dissolution profiles. Arzneimittelforschung 51(3):246–252, 2001.

37. DRUGS THAT AFFECT THE REPRODUCTIVE SYSTEM

1. What is the major estrogen produced in the human?
Estradiol.

2. How is estradiol metabolized?
Estradiol is metabolized into estrone and estriol (E_3) in the liver.

3. Why is estradiol not administered orally?
It has a high rate of first-pass metabolism in the liver.

4. Describe the adverse effects of the metabolic products of estradiol metabolism.
There are a number of adverse effects seen with estrogen therapy that are due to first-pass metabolic products. These include an increase in the production of clotting factors and increased synthesis of angiotensinogen.

5. How are estrogens eliminated?
Estrogens undergo glucuronide and sulfate conjugation to a variety of minor metabolites that are excreted primarily in the urine.

6. What is the physiologic significance of the estrogen-induced increase in the synthesis of angiotensinogen?
Increased levels of angiotensinogen caused by estrogens may result in an increase in the activity of the renin-angiotensin system and increased angiotensin II production. Thus, hypertension is seen.

7. How can the adverse effects of estrogens be avoided?
Adverse effects, such as those described previously, can be avoided by changes in the route of administration. Vaginal, parenteral or transdermal administration minimizes the first-pass effect seen with oral administration.

8. Compare the potencies of estradiol, estriol, and estrone.
Estriol and estrone have a much lower affinity for the estrogen receptor, and thus are less potent than estradiol.

9. What is the pharmacologic purpose of the alterations in estrogen structure?
Estrogens are conjugated to increase oral effectiveness.

10. What are some examples of nonsteroidal estrogenic drugs?
Diestriol, diethylstilbestrol (DES), benestriol, methestrol, hexestrol and chlorotrianisene are all nonsteroidal estrogenic drugs.

11. Discuss the protein binding of estrogens.
Estrogens, particularly estradiol, primarily bind to α_1 globulin. Binding to albumin is also seen.

12. Describe the mechanism of action of estradiol.
Estradiol binds to a nuclear receptor on DNA. This results in destabilization of support protein structure, and exposes the estrogen response element (ERE). The receptor-hormone complex

then binds to the ERE, and transcription is increased, ultimately resulting in increased protein synthesis.

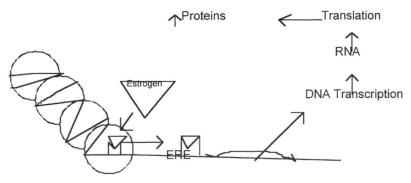

Schematic representation of the actions of estrogens.

13. List the major physiologically important proteins that are induced by estrogens.
These proteins include transcortin, thyroid-binding globulin, transferrin, angiotensinogen, and fibrinogen.

14. What are the effects of estrogens on the lipid profile?
Estrogens increase high-density lipoproteins (HDL) and triglycerides, and decrease low-density lipoproteins (LDL) and total cholesterol.

15. Describe the actions of estrogens on the endometrium.
Estrogens stimulate endometrial hyperplasia.

16. Characterize the effect of estrogens on bone mobilization.
Estrogens inhibit the actions of parathyroid hormone, resulting in decreased bone mobilization.

17. Could an uncontrolled diabetic female show a delayed onset of ketoacidosis? Explain.
Yes, particularly during the pre-ovulatory stages of the menstrual cycle, when estrogen levels are high. This results from the inhibition of lipid oxidation by estrogens, which results in a decreased production of ketones.

18. Describe the effect of estrogens on the actions of progesterone.
Estrogens induce progesterone receptors, which allows for a greater physiologic action of progesterone.

19. Why do estrogens cause retention of sodium and water?
Estrogens increase capillary fenestration, causing edema. The resulting decrease in blood volume results in increased secretion of aldosterone and ADH, resulting in the retention of sodium and water.

20. Describe the effects of estrogens on the sympathetic control of smooth muscle.
Estrogens enhance the actions of the sympathetic nervous system on smooth muscle.

21. Discuss the adverse effects of estrogen therapy.
Estrogens can cause nausea, breast tenderness, and hyperpigmentation. They can also cause or exacerbate migraine headaches, hypertension (due to an increased level of renin substrate), and cholestasis.

22. What effect might estrogen administration have on reproductive cancers?

Many reproductive cancers are estrogen-dependent. Thus, administration of estrogen may promote tumor formation or increase the rate of tumor growth.

23. What are conjugated estrogens?

Conjugated estrogens are traditionally a mixture of the water-soluble salts of sulfate esters from estrogenic compounds such as estrone, equilin and 17 alpha-dihydro equilin.

24. Compare the naturally and synthetically derived conjugated estrogens.

Natural conjugated estrogens are derived from equine urine. The proportions and concentrations of the various estrogens are unpredictable. The synthetic conjugated products are derived from plants (e.g., soy, yams) and contain a more clearly defined population of estrogens in proportions that are also more clearly defined. The two preparations appear equipotent with regard to physiologic effects.

25. Which potent estrogen analog is given parenterally (SC) to induce pubertal changes in girls with hypogonadotropic hypogonadism?

Estradiol valerate.

26. Which orally active estrogen is a common component of preparations used to treat postmenopausal symptoms?

Estrone sulfate.

27. What is the advantage of esterification of estradiol (e.g., estradiol cypionate)?

Esterification for intramuscular administration significantly increases the parenteral duration of action compared to aqueous estradiol formulations.

28. What is tamoxifen?

An antagonist at the estrogen receptor.

29. Tamoxifen decreases the risk of which type of cancer?

Breast cancer.

30. What is norethindrone?

Norethindrone is a progestin with weak androgenic and estrogenic activity.

31. Why is norethindrone added to the estrogen regimen for treatment of menopause?

Estrogen significantly increases the risk of endometrial carcinoma in women with an intact uterus. The addition of norethindrone substantially reduces this risk.

32. What effect is seen on the estrogen-induced changes on the lipid profile, with the addition of a progestin to the regimen?

HDL cholesterol can be reduced, because progestins attenuate some of the positive effects of estrogens on HDL cholesterol. However, estrogen-induced benefits on LDL cholesterol are retained.

33. What is the mechanism of action of norethindrone?

Norethindrone diffuses freely into target cells (e.g., the female reproductive tract, the mammary gland, the hypothalamus, and the pituitary) and binds to the progesterone receptor.

34. Compare the receptor binding of norethindrone and norgestimate.

Norethindrone binds primarily to progesterone receptors, while norgestimate binds to androgenic receptors as well.

35. Describe the activity of norgestimate.

Norgestimate is inactive as administered. It is a pro-drug and is metabolized extensively on first pass by hydrolysis, reduction, and hydroxylation in the gastrointestinal (GI) tract and/or in the liver to 17-deacetyl norgestimate. This is the active form of the drug.

36. Describe the actions of testosterone at the cellular level.

Testosterone stimulates RNA polymerase, increasing production of proteins.

37. Describe the effects of androgen administration on the symptoms of menopause.

The addition of androgens to estrogen replacement therapy appears to improve fatigue, decrease hot-flashes, and increase libido.

38. Androgens with an alkyl group (ethinyl- or methyl-) added to carbon-17 of the steroid nucleus are likely to have which property relative to natural testosterone?

These agents have improved oral bioavailability.

39. Describe the actions of methyltestosterone on the lipid profile.

Methyltestosterone appears to decrease total cholesterol. It appears to decrease HDL as well as apolipoprotein A-I.

40. Describe the metabolism of methyltestosterone.

Methyltestosterone is metabolized in the liver via the same pathways as testosterone and is converted to 5alpha-dihydrotestosterone and its glucuronide and sulfate conjugates.

41. Which androgenic drug is likely to be useful for management of hereditary angioneurotic edema?

Danazol.

CONTRACEPTION

42. Describe the mechanism of action of estrogens as oral contraceptives.

At therapeutic levels, estrogens create a negative feedback on both luteinizing hormone (LH) and follicle-stimulating hormone (FSH) release. This results in both a lack of follicular development and inhibition of secondary maturation and ovulation (see Figure, top of next page).

43. Which potent, orally-active estrogen analog is widely used in oral contraceptives?

Ethinyl estradiol. This drug may also be used as postcoital contraception.

44. Which estrogen may be used as a postcoital contraceptive?

Ethinyl estradiol.

45. Describe the actions of androgens on the female reproductive cycle.

Administration of androgens results in feedback inhibition at the level of the hypothalamus. Hypothalamic release of gonadotropin releasing hormone (GnRH) is inhibited, resulting in decreases in the levels of both LH and FSH. This results in lack of follicular development, and inhibition of ovulation (see Figure, top of next page).

46. What is the mechanism of action of progestins (e.g., levonorgestrel) in contraception?

Progestins suppress the mid-cycle surge of LH, preventing secondary maturation of the follicle, and ovulation.

47. Describe the uses of levonorgestrel in contraception.

It is used for contraception in subdermal implants, IUDs, or as an oral postcoital emergency contraceptive.

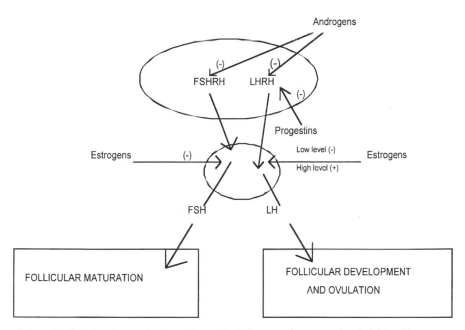

Schematic of the female reproductive cycle and the influences of exogenously administered hormones.

48. Does levonorgestrel need to be administered immediately after coitus?
No. The drug is effective if taken within 72 hours.

BIBLIOGRAPHY

1. Audet MC, Moreau M, Koltun WD, et al: Evaluation of contraceptive efficacy and cycle control of a transdermal contraceptive patch vs an oral contraceptive: a randomized controlled trial. JAMA 285(18):2347–2354, 2001.
2. Bonanni B, Guerrieri-Gonzaga A, Rotmensz N, et al: Hormonal therapy and chemoprevention. Breast J 6(5):317–323, 2000.
3. Girolami A, Tormene D, Simioni P, et al: Long-term use of oral contraceptive therapy in women with the prothrombin 20210 g-a polymorphism without thrombotic complications: A study of 13 women (12 heterozygotes and 1 homozygote). Thromb Res 102(3):205–210, 2001.
4. Greaves M, Preston FE: Rebuttal to: Oral contraceptives and venous thromboembolism. Thromb Haemost 85(5):932–934, [discussion 934-936], 2001.
5. Hardman J, Limbird L, Gilman A: Goodman & Gilman's The Pharmacological Basis of Therapeutics, 10th ed. McGraw-Hill Publishers, 2001.
6. Katzung, B: Basic and Clinical Pharmacology, 8th ed. Appleton & Lange, 2001.
7. Lynch NJ, De Vito G, Nimmo MA: Low dosage monophasic oral contraceptive use and intermittent exercise performance and metabolism in humans. Eur J Appl Physiol 84(4):296–301, 2001.
8. Maltoni M, Nanni O, Scarpi E, et al: High-dose progestins for the treatment of cancer anorexia-cachexia syndrome: a systematic review of randomised clinical trials. Ann Oncol 12(3):289–300, 2001.
9. Mulatero P, Rabbia F, di Cella SM, et al: Angiotensin-converting enzyme and angiotensinogen gene polymorphisms are non-randomly distributed in oral contraceptive-induced hypertension. J Hypertens 19(4):713–719, 2001.
10. Ness RB, Grisso JA, Vergona R, et al: Oral contraceptives, other methods of contraception, and risk reduction for ovarian cancer. Epidemiology 12(3):307–312, 2001.
11. Prifti S, Mall P, Strowitzki T, et al: Synthetic estrogens-mediated activation of JNK intracellular signaling molecule. Gynecol Endocrinol 15(2):135–141, 2001.
12. Shuba YM, Degtiar VE, Osipenko VN, et al: Testosterone-mediated modulation of HERG blockade by proarrhythmic agents (1). Biochem Pharmacol 62(1):41–49, 2001.
13. Silberstein SD: Headache and female hormones: What you need to know. Curr Opin Neurol 14(3): 323–333, 2001.

14. Yovel G, Shakhar K, Ben-Eliyahu S: The effects of sex, menstrual cycle, and oral contraceptives on the number and activity of natural killer cells. Gynecol Oncol 81(2):254–262, 2001.

15. Wilcox AJ, Dunson DB, Weinberg CR, et al: Likelihood of conception with a single act of intercourse: Providing benchmark rates for assessment of post-coital contraceptives. Contraception 63(4):211–215, 2001.

X. Antibiotics and Anti-infectives

Patricia K. Anthony, Ph.D., and Rebecca Thoms, R.N., N.P.

38. GENERAL PRINCIPLES OF ANTIBIOTIC THERAPY

1. Describe a true antibiotic.

A true antibiotic is derived from a natural source (e.g., bacteria). It is an agent that reduces organism proliferation or function (i.e., bacteriostatic or bactericidal), resulting in organism death.

2. Describe a bacteriostatic drug.

A bacteriostatic drug interferes with bacterial cell function and impairs the ability of the bacteria to reproduce. Thus, the bacterial population is gradually reduced, as the organisms gradually die out and are not replaced.

3. Does a bacteriostatic drug kill the cell directly?

No. This type of drug is not directly toxic to the cell.

4. List possible mechanisms of action for a bacteriostatic drug.

These drugs include those that inhibit bacterial replication, inhibit protein synthesis, or inhibit bacterial cell metabolism.

5. Describe a bactericidal drug

A bactericidal drug kills the bacteria directly, by eliminating a necessary means of survival (e.g., disruption of the cell wall).

6. List possible mechanisms of action for a bactericidal drug.

This type of drug can inhibit cell wall formation, cause fenestrations in the cell wall, or inhibit nutrient absorption.

7. Describe the general uses of an antibiotic.

Antibiotics may be used as prophylaxis for anticipated bacterial infections (e.g., secondary infections or procedures in which accumulated pyogenic bacteria are released) or surgical infections. They are also used to treat existing bacterial infections.

8. Why must an antibiotic, particularly a bacteriostatic antibiotic, be taken by the patient beyond the point where improvement in the symptoms of infection is seen?

The drug may only be inhibiting the ability of the bacterial cell to function and reproduce. This inactivation of organisms contributes to symptomatic improvement, but the organisms are still viable, and will return to an active state upon withdrawal of the drug. The plasma levels of drug must be kept at therapeutic levels until the bacterial population has been reduced to a subclinical level.

9. Define the "PAE" of an antibiotic.

PAE stands for "post antibiotic effect." This is a measure of the continued destruction of bacteria after the drug has been withdrawn.

10. Which classes of antibiotics have the highest PAE?
Aminoglycosides, fluoroquinolones, and imipenem.

11. Describe the consequences of antibiotic administration when no bacterial infection is present.
Unnecessary administration of antibiotics can result in a superinfection.

12. Discuss the etiology of superinfections caused by antibiotics.
Antibiotics preferentially affect certain populations of bacteria. Since intestinal flora exist in a state of controlled growth as a result of a competition for nutrients and growth area, preferential elimination of a certain population of bacteria allows proliferation of the remaining strains of bacteria. Because many of these bacteria are potentially virulent, the increased number may be sufficient to result in a potentially serious infection that is superimposed on the existing infection.

13. Describe the pharmacokinetics of an antibiotic that might be useful in a urinary infection.
The most useful antibiotic is one that is eliminated in an active form by the kidney.

14. Describe the pharmacokinetic properties of an antibiotic that would be useful in an intestinal infection (e.g., inflammatory bowel disease).
To be effective in the bowel, this antibiotic should be poorly absorbed. This allows the drug to maintain maximum contact with the affected area.

15. Why is the development of superinfections most prevalent with oral antibiotics?
Antibiotics taken orally have maximum contact with intestinal flora, in a concentrated state, in contrast to intravenously administered antibiotics.

16. Are antibiotics effective against viral infections?
No. However, they are useful in the treatment of secondary bacterial infections.

17. Describe bacterial resistance.
Resistance to antibiotics occurs when bacteria evolve to combat the mechanism of action of the drug.

18. What are the three types of bacterial resistance?
Intrinsic resistance, mutational resistance, and plasmid-mediated resistance.

19. Describe intrinsic resistance.
An organism may evolve to produce an enzyme that degrades the drug (e.g., β-lactamase). This type of resistance is intrinsic to the organism.

20. Describe mutational resistance.
An organism may evolve to form structural mutations that impede the drug's actions.

21. List examples of mutational resistance.
  • synthesis of altered binding proteins (e.g., penicillin binding proteins) resulting in lack of association of the drug with the organism
  • altered ribosomal composition
  • altered conformation of topoisomerases
  • alternate pathways of folic acid synthesis and activation (i.e., not involving dihydrofolate reductase)
  • mutations that result in decreased uptake or an increase in expulsion of the drug

22. Discuss plasmid-based resistance.

This phenomenon involveş the passing of mutational resistance information from one organism to another. Altered DNA, which confers resistance, is packaged into a plasmid, which can then be transferred to other organisms.

BIBLIOGRAPHY

1. Aguilar L, Garcia-Rey G, Gimenez MJ: Antibiotic pressure, development of resistance in Streptococcus pneumoniae and clinical failure: A not-so-vicius [sic] circle for some antibiotics. Rev Esp Quimioter 14(1):17–21, 2001.
2. Baptist EC, Abdel-Rahman S: Recommendations for dosing antibiotics. Pediatr Infect Dis J 20(3):324–325, 2001.
3. Bryan L.E: General mechanisms of resistance to antibiotics. J. Antimicrobial Chemotherapy 22 (suppl. A):1, 1988
4. Crichlow GV, Nukaga M, Doppalapudi VR, et al: Inhibition of class c beta-lactamases: Structure of a reaction intermediate with a cephem sulfone. Biochemistry ;40(21):6233–6239, 2001.
5. Hardman J, Limbird L, Gilman A: Goodman & Gilman's The Pharmacological Basis of Therapeutics, 10th ed. McGraw-Hill Publishers, 2001.
6. Hujer AM, Hujer KM, Bonomo RA: Mutagenesis of amino acid residues in the SHV-1 beta-lactamase the premier role of Gly238Ser in penicillin and cephalosporin resistance. Biochim Biophys Acta 1547(1)37–50, 2001.
7. Jedrzejas MJ: Pneumococcal virulence factors: Structure and function. Microbiol Mol Biol Rev 65(2):187–207, 2001.
8. Katzung B: Basic and Clinical Pharmacology, 8th ed. Appleton & Lange, 2001.

39. PENICILLINS AND DERIVATIVES

1. Discuss the mechanism of action of penicillins.

Penicillins inhibit the cross-linking of muramic acid in the bacterial cell wall. This results in a lack of structural integrity and eventual cell lysis.

2. What determines the activity of a particular penicillin against a particular strain of bacteria?

The degree of activity against a particular organism depends on the ability of the drug to gain access to specific penicillin-binding proteins (PBPs). Since different bacteria contain different numbers of PBPs that perform different functions, the efficacy of a given drug depends on the ability of that drug to locate and bind PBPs that govern key functions (e.g., membrane integrity).

3. Why are penicillins more effective against gram-positive organisms than gram-negative organisms?

The structure of the bacterial cell wall in gram-negative organisms contains only a layer of peptidoglycans attached to the inner membrane, and leaves the PBPs relatively exposed. In a gram-negative organism, the drug must enter through pores (Porin) in order to reach the inner space between the double membrane and attach to PBPs (see Figure).

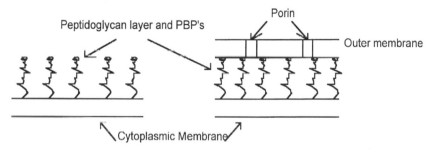

Gram positive bacteria   Gram negative bacteria

The cell wall structures of gram-positive and gram-negative bacteria are diagrammed. Note the relative ease with which the drug may reach the penicillin binding proteins in gram-positive organisms.

4. Describe the gram-negative organisms that are susceptible to penicillins.

Gram-negative organisms readily affected by penicillins include *N. meningitidis*, *Pasteurella multocida*, and *Streptobacillus moniliformis* (rat-bite fever).

5. Characterize the therapeutic index of penicillins.

The therapeutic index is high for these drugs, and they are, in general, considered very safe drugs.

6. Discuss the adverse effects of penicillins.

Adverse effects, in general, are low. However, all penicillins have the potential for causing interstitial nephritis (of allergic origin), and serious allergic reactions resulting in urticaria progressing to anaphylactic shock.

7. Describe allergic reactions to penicillin.

Common reactions are urticaria or skin rashes. Less common allergic reactions include severe reactions such as anaphylaxis and vasodilatation (anaphylactic shock).

245

8. Discuss the major cause of penicillin allergy.

The majority of allergic reactions are the result of sensitivity to the beta-lactam ring in the penicillin structure. The penicillin is metabolized to a penicilloyl moiety, which binds to plasma albumin. This combination triggers an immune reaction, resulting in massive histamine release.

9. What are the secondary (minor) causes of penicillin allergy?

Less common allergic reactions occur as a result of the side chain structures attached to the beta-lactam ring.

10. Explain the occurrence of pseudomembranous colitis with penicillin administration.

This condition is caused by the organism *Clostridium difficile*. Because this organism is less responsive than others to the actions of penicillin, it proliferates in the intestine as other populations of bacteria are killed by the drug. It thus gives rise to pseudomembranous colitis.

11. Discuss the changes in electrolyte balance seen with penicillin administration.

Penicillin is often administered as a sodium or potassium salt. The introduction of potentially large numbers on sodium or potassium ions along with the drug can result in changes in electrolyte balance. This is of particular occurrence with ticarcillin and carbenicillin salts.

12. Explain why penicillins are not administered as an IV bolus.

Penicillins are administered slowly to minimize shock to the system and decrease the potential for protein reactions (anaphylaxis).

13. How are penicillin G-K and penicillin G-Na administered?

These drugs are administered by slow intravenous route, either by intramuscular (IM) injection or by slow infusion (IV drip).

14. What adverse central nervous system (CNS) effect can be seen with high dose intravenous administration of penicillin G?

This drug may cause seizures if administered intravenously at high dose, particularly in the presence of renal failure.

15. Does penicillin G cross the blood-brain barrier?

Not in significant amounts, unless inflammation is present. High-dose administration can also result in entrance of the drug into the CNS.

16. Why does penicillin G cross into the CNS in a patient with meningitis but not in a patient with pneumonia.

Recall that penicillins exist bound to plasma albumin. In a patient with a systemic infection, the blood-brain barrier remains relatively intact, and does not allow the penicillin molecule or drug-protein complex to pass. In a patient with CNS inflammation (e.g., meningitis), however, the blood-brain barrier is compromised, and openings occur that are large enough for the drug to pass through.

17. Why are most penicillins not administered orally?

These drugs are rapidly degraded by gastric acid. Oral formulations of penicillin G are still marketed, but the dose is increased in order to compensate for the gastric acid degradation. Despite the increased dosage, therapeutic dosage is difficult to monitor because of individual variability in gastric acid production.

18. What are penicillin V and penicillin V potassium?

These are acid-resistant forms of penicillin, which are marketed as oral dosage forms.

19. Which bacteriocidal penicillin may be given orally to pediatric and geriatric patients?
Amoxicillin.

20. What is the effect of administering amoxicillin with drinks containing red dye (e.g., cherry "Kool-aid")?
Administration of amoxicillin with these drinks may reduce the potency of the drug because many red dyes chemically interact with the drug.

21. Which drugs are considered natural penicillins?
Penicillin G and Penicillin V.

22. Are first-generation penicillins bacteriostatic or bacteriocidal?
In general, these drugs are bacteriocidal.

23. Which penicillins are extended-spectrum drugs?
Amoxicillin, ampicillin, carbenicillin, mezlocillin, piperacillin, and ticarcillin.

24. What adverse effect occurs with the use of high-dose, extended-spectrum penicillins?
These drugs, particularly ticarcillin and carbenicillin, interfere with platelet function.

25. Which penicillins are resistant to bacterial penicillinases?
Cloxacillin, dicloxacillin, nafcillin, and oxacillin are penicillinase resistant.

26. Which penicillins are lipophilic in nature, with a high degree of efficacy against Staphylococcus?
Nafcillin and the isoxazolyl penicillins (oxacillin, cloxacillin, dicloxacillin).

27. How are the isoxazolyl penicillins eliminated?
These drugs are metabolized in the liver and excreted through the bile.

28. Why is methicillin of limited use?
This drug causes an unacceptably high rate of interstitial nephritis.

29. Discuss the use of piperacillin.
Piperacillin is a semisynthetic penicillin used in the therapy of serious gram-negative infections.

30. Describe the spectrum of action of piperacillin.
Piperacillin is considered to be an extended-spectrum penicillin. The gram-negative spectrum of piperacillin includes *Enterobacter* species, *E. coli*, *Klebsiella pneumoniae*, *Morganella morganii*, *Proteus mirabilis*, *Proteus vulgaris*, *Providencia*, *Serratia*, and *N. gonorrhoeae*. The anaerobic spectrum includes *Peptococcus* and *Peptostreptococcus*, *Clostridium perfringens*, *Clostridium tetani*, and *Bacteroides* (including many strains of *b. fragilis*).

31. Is piperacillin used in conjunction with aminoglycoside antibiotics?
Yes. Its actions are synergistic with those of aminoglycosides, and the combination is used in the therapy of systemic *Pseudomonas* infections.

32. Discuss penicillin resistance.
Resistance to penicillin can come about by several means. Normally, the organism evolves to produce an enzyme that can degrade the drug (penicillinase), or to produce a protective barrier on the cell wall (e.g., tuberculosis bacilli). An organism may also develop resistance through means of a plasmid, obtained from a resistant organism. The most common means of resistance is the production of penicillinase.

33. Why is penicillin G not effective against Staphylococcus (Staph) (e.g., *S. aureus*)?
Staphylococcus organisms produce a β-lactamase that is plasmid-mediated.

β-LACTAMASE INHIBITORS

34. Describe the mechanism of action of β-lactamase inhibitors.
These agents bind irreversibly to β-lactamase, inactivating the enzyme.

35. Describe the β-lactamase inhibitors currently in use.
Clavulanic acid, which may be used orally or intravenously, and the intravenous agents sulbactam and tazobactam.

36. What is clavulanic acid?
Clavulanic acid is a chemical similar in structure to penicillin, which acts as a substrate for penicillinase, thus inhibiting its action on penicillin. This agent is added to penicillin preparations to decrease the manifestation of bacterial resistance.

37. Describe the adverse effects of β-lactamase inhibitors.
These drugs cause nausea and vomiting, and can precipitate allergic reactions in penicillin-allergic patients.

38. Which organisms produce β-lactamases that are not affected by β-lactamase inhibitors?
These drugs do not reduce the activity of β-lactamases produced by *Enterobacter*, *Citrobacter*, *Serratia*, and *Pseudomonas* organisms.

39. Do β-lactamase inhibitors (e.g., clavulanic acid) increase penicillin efficacy against staph organisms?
No. The lactamase produced by *Staph* is not affected by these agents.

MISCELLANEOUS CELL WALL INHIBITORS

40. Discuss aztreonam.
This drug is a monobactam—possessing a β-lactam ring with a monocyclic structure. It possesses the major activity of penicillins and the susceptibility to β-lactamases.

41. Describe the cross-reactivity between penicillins and cephalosporins.
These drugs act with a similar mechanism—both are inhibitors of cell wall synthesis. The structures of both drug classes also possesses a β-lactam ring, which allows for cross-sensitivity between drugs.

42. Discuss the rationale behind the administration of cephalosporins to a penicillin-allergic patient.
Cephalosporins are an acceptable substitute for penicillin therapy. However, a patient allergic to penicillin can also be allergic to cephalosporins (depending on the portion of the penicillin molecule to which the patient has sensitivity). It is not wise to administer cephalosporins to a patient who has had an anaphylactic reaction to penicillins, because this presents a greater risk.

BIBLIOGRAPHY

1. Bertucci C, Barsotti MC, Raffaelli A, et al: Binding properties of human albumin modified by covalent binding of penicillin. Biochim Biophys Acta 1544(1–2):386–392, 2001.
2. Crichlow GV, Nukaga M, Doppalapudi VR, et al: Inhibition of class c beta-lactamases: Structure of a reaction intermediate with a cephem sulfone. Biochemistry 40(21):6233–6239, 2001.

3. Fogle-Hansson M, White P, Hermansson A, et al: Short-term penicillin-V prophylaxis did not prevent acute otitis media in infants. Int J Pediatr Otorhinolaryngol 59(2):119–123, 2001.
4. Hardman J, Limbird L, Gilman A: Goodman & Gilman's The Pharmacological Basis of Therapeutics, 10th ed. McGraw-Hill Publishers, 2001.
5. Hujer AM, Hujer KM, Bonomo RA: Mutagenesis of amino acid residues in the SHV-1 beta-lactamase: The premier role of Gly238Ser in penicillin and cephalosporin resistance. Biochim Biophys Acta 1547(1):37–50, 2001.
6. Jedrzejas MJ: Pneumococcal virulence factors: Structure and function. Microbiol Mol Biol Rev 65(2):187–207, 2001.
7. Katzung B: Basic and Clinical Pharmacology, 8th ed. Appleton & Lange, 2001.
8. Salkind AR, Cuddy PG, Foxworth JW: Is this patient allergic to penicillin? An evidence-based analysis of the likelihood of penicillin allergy [review]. JAMA 285(19):2498–2505, 2001.

40. CEPHALOSPORIN ANTIBIOTICS

1. What is a cephalosporin antibiotic?

Cephalosporin antibiotics are beta-lactam antibiotics, similar in structure and action to penicillin.

2. Describe the mechanism of action of cephalosporin antibiotics.

These agents bind to penicillin binding proteins. Like penicillins, they must enter the cell wall through porins and attach to penicillin-binding proteins (PBPs). The binding of the drug to these proteins mediates an inhibition of cell wall synthesis and leads to autolysis.

3. What is a cephamycin?

A beta-lactam-like antibiotic. These drugs are included in the cephalosporin classification but are not true cephalosporins. They are, however, similar in structure and mechanism.

4. List examples of cephamycin drugs.

Cefoxitin, cefotetan, and cefmetazole are cephamycins.

5. Why are cephalosporins not active against enterococcus?

Structural anomalies within the structure of the PBPs in these organisms results in decreased binding of the drug.

6. Are cephalosporins affected by β-lactamases?

Yes. The β-lactam ring is vulnerable to the enzyme, resulting in inaction of the drug. Organisms that secrete β-lactamases are resistant to cephalosporins.

7. Does the pH of surrounding tissues affect the activity of cephalosporins?

No. Cephalosporin activity is not affected by decreased tissue pH.

8. Describe the adverse effects of cephalosporins.

Hypersensitivity reactions occur, but otherwise the drugs are well tolerated.

9. In general, are cephalosporins metabolized?

No. With the exception of cephalothin, these drugs are secreted or filtered into the nephron and excreted unchanged.

10. Which cephalosporin has the longest half life?

Ceftriaxone.

11. Which cephalosporins require once-daily dosing?

Ceftriaxone, cefonicid, and cefotetan.

12. What was the first oral cephalosporin?

Cephalexin.

13. Which cephalosporins are considered to be first-generation drugs?

Cephalexin, cephazolin, and (possibly) cefaclor.

14. Describe the activity of the first-generation cephalosporins.

In general, first-generation cephalosporins possess excellent activity against gram-positive aerobic bacteria and poor activity against gram-negative organisms.

15. Are first-generation agents useful in the treatment of meningitis?
No. These agents do not penetrate the cerebrospinal fluid (CSF).

16. Describe the effect of cefoxitin on β-lactamases.
Cefoxitin is actually a potent inducer of this enzyme.

17. Are first-generation cephalosporins effective against *S. aureus*?
Yes, with the exception of methicillin-resistant strains.

18. How is cefazolin administered?
This drug is administered parenterally, because it is not well absorbed.

19. Is *b. fragilis* susceptible to cefazolin?
No.

20. Is cefazolin hepatically metabolized?
No. It is excreted unchanged into the urine.

21. Describe the degree of plasma protein binding seen with cefzolin.
Approximately 75–85% of circulating cefzolin is protein-bound.

22. Describe the spectrum of activity of cephalexin.
This agent is effective against gram-positive organisms. Activity against gram-negative organisms is limited to *E. coli*, *Klebsiella*, and *Proteus mirabilis*.

23. Is cephalexin useful in central nervous system (CNS) infections?
No. The drug does not reach therapeutic levels in the CSF.

24. Discuss the therapeutic uses of cefaclor.
Cefaclor is useful in the treatment of otitis media, sinusitis, and upper respiratory tract infection caused by *H. influenzae* that are resistant to ampicillin or amoxicillin.

25. Which drugs are "second-generation" cephalosporins?
Cefoxitin and cefamandole.

26. Against which class of organisms is cefoxitin active?
Gram-negative organisms and anaerobes.

27. Is cefamandole active against bowel anaerobes?
No.

28. Discuss the effect of cefamandole on coagulation.
Cefamandole can induce hypoprothrombinemia in predisposed individuals.

29. Compare cefuroxime and cefamandole.
Cefuroxime is equipotent to cefamandole in the killing of gram-negative organisms (including beta-lactamase strains of *H. influenzae*) but has a longer half-life and can be dosed less frequently. It does not produce hypoprothrombinemia.

30. Which drugs are classified as third-generation cephalosporins?
Cefoperazone, ceftizoxime, ceftriaxone, and ceftazidime.

31. Describe the activity of third-generation agents.
These agents are effective against gram-negative organisms.

32. How are cephaloridine and cephalothin administered?
These antibiotics are for intravenous use.

33. Does cefotetan cause hypoprothrombinemia?
Yes.

34. Which third-generation agent is effective against pseudomonas aeruginosa?
Ceftazidime.

35. Which parenteral cephalosporin is active against both gram-positive and gram-negative organisms?
Cefepime, a "fourth-generation" cephalosporin.

BIBLIOGRAPHY

1. Aguilar L, Garcia-Rey G, Gimenez MJ: Antibiotic pressure, development of resistance in Streptococcus pneumoniae and clinical failure: A not-so-vicious circle for some antibiotics. Rev Esp Quimioter 14(1):17–21, 2001.
2. Czeizel AE, Rockenbauer M, Sorensen HT, Olsen J: Use of cephalosporins during pregnancy and in the presence of congenital abnormalities: A population-based, case-control study. Am J Obstet Gynecol 184(6):1289–1296, 2001.
3. Fornas FL, Garcia FM, Salmeron JP, et al: Comparative study of treatment with pencillin, ceftriaxone, trovafloxacin, quinupristin-dalfopristin and vancomycin in experimental endocarditis due to pencicillin- and ceftriaxone-resistant Streptococcus pneumoniae. J Antimicrob Chemother 47(5):623–629, 2001.
4. Hardman J, Limbird L, Gilman A: Goodman & Gilman's The Pharmacological Basis of Therapeutics, 10th ed. McGraw-Hill Publishers, 2001.
5. Katzung B: Basic and Clinical Pharmacology, 8th ed. Appleton & Lange, 2001.
6. Kohda-Shimizu R, Li Y, Shitara Y, et al: Oral absorption of cephalosporins is quantitatively predicted from in vitro uptake into intestinal brush border membrane vesicles. Int J Pharm 4;220(1–2):119–128, 2001.
7. Paterson DL, Ko WC, Von Gottberg A, et al: Outcome of cephalosporin treatment for serious infections due to apparently susceptible organisms producing extended-spectrum beta-lactamases: Implications for the clinical microbiology laboratory. J Clin Microbiol 39(6):2206–2212, 2001.

41. MACROLIDE ANTIBIOTICS

1. What is the mechanism of action of macrolide antibiotics?
Macrolide antibiotics bind to the 50 S ribosomal subunit, inhibiting bacterial protein synthesis. This results in a decrease in bacterial cellular function and replication.

2. Are macrolides bacteriostatic or bacteriocidal?
These agents are bacteriostatic.

3. Describe the spectrum of activity of erythromycin.
Erythromycin is active against a wide range of microorganisms, but has superior activity against gram-positive organisms as compared to gram-negative activity.

4. Compare the spectrum of activity of azithromycin to that of erythromycin.
Azithromycin appears to have less gram-positive activity but greater gram-negative activity than erythromycin.

5. Which macrolide has potent activity against *chlamydiae*?
Azithromycin.

6. Contrast the bioavailability of the macrolide antibiotics.
Clarithromycin and azithromycin are more bioavailable than erythromycin.

7. Discuss the various forms of erythromycin.
Erythromycin lactobionate or gluceptate are used for parenteral administration, while erythromycin ethylsuccinate, estolate, stearate, and erythromycin base are administered orally.

8. Is erythromycin base absorbed well?
No.

9. Why is erythromycin dispensed as a coated tablet?
Erythromycin base is acid-labile and is degraded in the stomach. The majority of absorption takes place in the duodenum.

10. Is erythromycin highly plasma protein-bound?
Yes. The drug may be up to 81 percent protein-bound.

11. Describe the gastrointestinal (GI) effects of erythromycin.
This drug increases motility of the bowel.

12. Is azithromycin or erythromycin the best choice for treatment of a *Staphylococcus* (staph) infection?
Erythromycin is the best choice. Azithromycin is more active against gram-negative organisms but has less activity against streptococci and staphylococci than does erythromycin.

13. Why are clarithromycin and azithromycin useful in the treatment of AIDS-related Mycobacterium avium complex?
These drugs are concentrated within macrophages, and thus have increased activity against organisms that are taken up by macrophages.

14. Describe the half-life of azithromycin.
    This drug has a half-life of 11 to 14 hours, allowing once-daily dosing.

15. Discuss the protein binding of azithromycin.
    Protein binding varies with plasma concentration—the higher the plasma concentration, the lower the proportion of the drug is bound.

16. Does azithromycin penetrate well into the central nervous system?
    No. CNS penetration is poor with this drug.

17. What is the half-life of azithromycin?
    It is 68 hours.

18. What might account for the long serum half-life of azithromycin?
    Azithromycin has a high degree of tissue penetration and is sequestered by tissues. Thus, the drug leaches slowly out of tissue reservoirs, keeping plasma levels at therapeutic level. Enterohepatic recirculation may also play a role.

19. How is azithromycin eliminated?
    This drug is eliminated unchanged in the bile.

20. Which macrolide antibiotic has active metabolites?
    Clarithromycin.

21. Describe the use of clarithromycin in the therapy of ulcers.
    Clarithromycin is useful in the therapy of peptic ulcer as part of a combination regimen. It is also effective in the treatment of *H. pylori*-associated duodenal ulcer.

22. Is clarithromycin highly plasma protein-bound?
    No. Protein binding is low, and kinetics are approximately linear, in contrast to azithromycin.

23. Describe the role of plasma pH in the action of clarithromycin.
    Clarithromycin is ionized at physiological pH. Penetration of the drug into the bacterium is accomplished in the unionized state, and thus is facilitated by alkalinizing the plasma.

24. What effect does clarithromycin have on P-glycoprotein?
    This drug efflux pump is inhibited by clarithromycin.

25. Discuss the metabolites of clarithromycin.
    The major metabolite, 14-hydroxyclarithromycin, has antimicrobial activity up to twice that of the parent drug.

26. Discuss dirithromycin.
    Dirithromycin is a newly marketed macrolide antibiotic. It is similar in spectrum of action to erythromycin, but has an extremely long half-life, greater tissue penetration, and fewer interactions with other drugs metabolized by the cytochrome P_{450} system.

27. Does dirithromycin have active metabolites?
    Yes. The production of the active metabolite erythromycylamine is partly responsible for the long half-life of the drug.

28. What is the half-life of dirithromycin?
    The mean terminal half-life is approximately 44 hours. Plasma elimination half-life is approximately 8 hours, allowing once-daily dosage.

29. Describe the protein binding of dirithromycin.

Dirithromycin is primarily bound to alpha$_1$-acid glycoprotein. Protein binding is moderate— approximately 15–30 percent.

30. Rank the macrolide antibiotics with respect to their ability to cause gastrointestinal disturbances.

In general, erythromycin causes adverse GI effects in the highest number of patients (21 percent). Clarithromycin causes significantly less (10 percent of patients experience adverse GI effects), followed by azithromycin (5 percent of patients).

31. What serious adverse effect is caused by intravenous administration of erythromycin?

Erythromycin can produce ototoxicity, particularly if administered IV.

32. Discuss the activity of troleandomycin as compared to erythromycin.

Troleandomycin is significantly less efficacious than erythromycin, and is rarely prescribed.

BIBLIOGRAPHY

1. Guay DR, Gustavson LE, Devcich KJ, et al: Pharmacokinetics and tolerability of extended-release clarithromycin. Clin Ther 23(4):566–577, 2001.
2. Hardman J, Limbird L, Gilman A: Goodman & Gilman's The Pharmacological Basis of Therapeutics, 10th ed. McGraw-Hill Publishers, 2001.
3. Katzung B: Basic and Clinical Pharmacology, 8th ed. Appleton & Lange, 2001.
4. Prescott LM: Macrolides, azalides, and streptogrammins. J Int Assoc Physicians AIDS Care 2(4):35–37, 1996.
5. Prescott LM: Clarithromycin for MAC prevention offers additional benefits. Posit Aware 7(3):8, 1996.

42. FLUOROQUINOLONE ANTIBIOTICS

1. Discuss the mechanism of action of fluoroquinolone antibiotics.
These agents inhibit the actions of DNA gyrase (topoisomerase II), which is responsible for the supercoiling of bacterial DNA.

2. Do bacteria exhibit resistance to fluoroquinolones?
Bacterial resistance occurs rapidly to these agents.

3. Describe the mechanism of bacterial resistance to fluoroquinolones.
Two mechanisms have been delineated—the production of an altered gyrase by the bacteria, and the production of an altered permeability to the drug.

4. Describe the therapeutic use of norfloxacin.
Norfloxacin is primarily used for infections of the gut and urinary tract.

5. Does norfloxacin achieve adequate serum levels for the therapy of systemic infections?
No.

6. Which quinalones are used in the therapy of systemic infections?
Ciprofloxacin, ofloxacin, enoxacin, and lomefloxacin.

7. Describe the distribution of fluoroquinolones.
These drugs are widely distributed.

8. Describe the clearance of ofloxacin and lomefloxacin.
These drugs are excreted through the urine.

9. How are ciprofloxacin and enoxacin cleared?
These drugs are metabolized in the liver and cleared through the urine.

10. Which quinolone is hepatically metabolized and excreted through the bile?
Perfloxatin.

11. Describe the interaction of fluoroquinolones with antacids.
Divalent and trivalent ions (e.g., Ca^{++}, Mg^{++}, Al^{+++}) substantially reduce the absorption of fluoroquinolones.

12. Describe the adverse central nervous system effects seen with quinolones.
These drugs may cause insomnia, confusion, headaches, dizziness, and anxiety.

13. What is the most common adverse effect of quinolone administration?
Nausea and vomiting.

14. Describe the interactions of quinolones with theophylline.
Drugs of this class, especially those that undergo metabolism (e.g., norfloxacin, enoxacin and ciprofloxacin) can decrease the clearance of theophylline and significantly elevate plasma levels.

15. Describe the clinical effectiveness of fluoroquinolones.
These drugs are primarily effective against gram-negative rods.

16. Which quinolone is particularly effective against chlamydia?
Ofloxacin.

17. Which fluoroquinolone is most active against *P. aeruginosa*?
Ciprofloxacin.

18. Describe the postantibiotic effect of fluoroquinolones.
These agents have a significant postantibiotic effect.

19. Should patients on fluoroquinolone therapy be exposed to direct sunlight?
No. These drugs cause photosensitivity.

20. Describe the administration of quinolones to seizure patients.
Nadilicacid has been shown to cause seizures. Therefore, these drugs should be used with caution in seizure prone patients.

21. Are quinolones effective against stationary phase organisms?
Yes.

22. Which quinolone is appropriate for once-daily dosing?
Lomefloxacin, with a $T\frac{1}{2}$ of 8 hours.

BIBLIOGRAPHY

1. Appelbaum PC, Hunter PA: The fluoroquinolone antibacterials: Past, present and future perspectives. Int J Antimicrob Agents 16(1):5–15, 2000.
2. Bjornsson E, Olsson R, Remotti H: Norfloxacin-induced eosinophilic necrotizing granulomatous hepatitis. Am J Gastroenterol 95(12):3662–3664, 2000.
3. Fornas FL, Garcia FM, Salmeron JP, et al: Comparative study of treatment with penicillin, ceftriaxone, trovafloxacin, quinupristin-dalfopristin and vancomycin in experimental endocarditis due to penicillin- and ceftriaxone-resistant *Streptococcus pneumoniae*. J Antimicrob Chemother 47(5):623–629, 2001.
4. Hardman J, Limbird L, Gilman A: Goodman & Gilman's The Pharmacological Basis of Therapeutics, 10th ed. McGraw-Hill Publishers, 2001.
5. Katzung B: Basic and Clinical Pharmacology, 8th ed. Appleton & Lange, 2001.
6. Kundu AK: Norfloxacin-induced hallucination-an unusual CNS toxicity of 4-fluoroquinolones. J Assoc Physicians India 48(9):944, 2000.
7. Ohnishi K, Kimura K, Masuda G, et al: Oral administration of fluoroquinolones in the treatment of typhoid fever and paratyphoid fever in Japan. Intern Med 39(12):1044–1048, 2000.
8. Rizk M, Belal F, Ibrahim F, et al: Derivative spectrophotometric analysis of 4-quinolone antibacterials in formulations and spiked biological fluids by their Cu(II) complexes. J AOAC Int 84(2):368–375, 2001.
9. Shen LL: Quinolone interactions with DNA and DNA gyrase. Methods Mol Biol 95:171–184, 2001.
10. Smith A, Pennefather PM, Kaye SB, et al: Fluoroquinolones: Place in ocular therapy. Drugs 61(6): 747–761, 2001.

43. TETRACYCLINE ANTIBIOTICS

1. Discuss the mechanism of action of tetracyclines.
These drugs inhibit protein synthesis through the inhibition of peptidyl transferase activity.

2. Are tetracyclines bactericidal?
No. These drugs are bacteriostatic—only cellular function is disrupted.

3. Why should tetracyclines not be administered with food?
Tetracyclines form chelation complexes with divalent ions (e.g., Ca^{++}, Mg^{++}, Fe^{++}), which inhibit absorption of the drug.

4. Discuss the interaction of tetracyclines with antacids.
Antacids contain divalent or trivalent ions (e.g., Ca^{++}, Mg^{++}, Al^{+++}) which chelate the drug.

5. Describe the spectrum of action of tetracyclines.
These agents are considered broad spectrum, but are mainly active against gram-positive organisms.

6. Are tetracyclines protein-bound?
Yes. These drugs are highly protein-bound.

7. Do tetracyclines cross into the central nervous system (CNS)?
No.

8. Describe the major use of tetracyclines.
These drugs are useful in the therapy of Lyme disease and chlamydia infections. They are drugs of choice in rickettsial infections.

9. How are tetracyclines eliminated?
The majority of drugs are eliminated through the urine. Exceptions are the lipophilic drugs such as doxycycline and minocycline.

10. Which tetracyclines are drugs of choice for patients with compromised renal function?
Doxycycline and minocycline, because they are lipid-soluble and are not cleared by the kidney.

11. Which tetracyclines are long-acting?
Doxycycline and minocycline.

12. Why are doxycycline and minocycline long-acting?
These drugs are lipophilic and are excreted through the bile. They are thus subject to entero-hepatic recycling.

13. Which tetracycline is short-acting?
Tetracycline.

14. Describe the adverse effects of tetracyclines.
Tetracyclines can cause gastric irritation, particularly in large doses, and can also cause tooth discoloration in children. Hepatotoxicity may be seen with large doses (> 2g), as well as nephrotoxicity. Hypersensitivity reactions can also be seen.

15. Do tetracyclines cause superinfections?
Yes. These drugs have an increased potential for the development of superinfections.

16. Describe the contraindications of the exposure to sunlight with tetracycline therapy.
Tetracyclines cause photosensitivity and exposure to sunlight is thus contraindicated.

17. Are tetracyclines that have reached their expiration date still safe to use?
No. These drugs degrade into toxic products that may cause liver or kidney failure (the effects of these products cause a syndrome similar to Fanconi syndrome).

18. Why are tetracyclines contraindicated in pregnancy?
These drugs cross the fetal-placental barrier and can chelate calcium in developing bones, resulting in a decrease in bone integrity.

19. Does tetracycline administration affect human protein synthesis?
No. Human ribosomes and aminoacyl t-RNA are not affected.

20. Does the presence of the various divalent ions affect all tetracyclines equally?
No. Doxycycline appears to have a lower affinity for calcium and a higher affinity for iron than do the other agents.

21. Why are tetracyclines useful in the therapy of intracellular infections (e.g., rickettsia)?
These drugs are able to penetrate intracellularly and thus are drugs of choice for intracellular infections.

22. Which tetracycline drug is useful for meningococcal prophylaxis?
Minocycline, because it has a high degree of penetration of pulmonary secretions.

SULFA DRUGS

23. Describe the mechanism of action of sulfa drugs.
These drugs are similar in structure to paraaminobenzoic acid (PABA). Thus, they act as competitive antagonists in bacterial folic acid synthesis (see Figure).

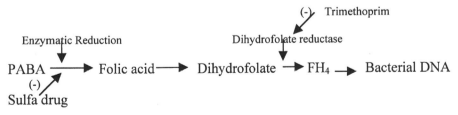

Diagrammatic representation of the steps in bacterial DNA synthesis and drug interference.

24. Discuss the elimination of sulfa drugs.
These drugs are acylated in the liver and excreted renally.

25. Why do sulfa drugs cause nephrotoxicity, particularly in the dehydrated patient?
The acylated drug forms crystals in the urine unless sufficient tubular fluid is present. The crystals can damage renal tubules.

26. Discuss the adverse effects of sulfa drugs.
These drugs can cause a rash and other allergic reactions. Blood dyscrasias (rare) and tubular necrosis may also be evident.

27. Which sulfa drugs are presently used clinically?

Sulfisoxazole, sulfamethoxazole, and sulfadine are used clinically.

28. Describe the pharmacokinetic parameters of clinically-used sulfa drugs.

These drugs are rapidly absorbed and excreted, and are widely distributed into fluids (e.g., synovial, peritoneal, pleural).

29. Discuss the synergistic action of sulfamethoxazole and trimethoprim.

Both of these drugs interfere with bacterial synthesis of folic acid and the production of nucleotides. Sulfamethoxazole decreases the enzymatic conversion of PABA, and trimethoprim decreases the activity of dihydrofolate reductase. Thus, the actions are synergistic (see Figure p 262).

BIBLIOGRAPHY

1. Baptist EC, Abdel-Rahman S: Recommendations for dosing antibiotics. Pediatr Infect Dis J 20(3):324–325, 2001.
2. Chopra I, Roberts M: Tetracycline antibiotics: Mode of action, applications, molecular biology, and epidemiology of bacterial resistance. Microbiol Mol Biol Rev 65(2):232–260, 2001.
3. Hardman J, Limbird L, Gilman A: Goodman & Gilman's The Pharmacological Basis of Therapeutics, 10th ed. McGraw-Hill Publishers, 2001.
4. Katzung B: Basic and Clinical Pharmacology, 8th ed. Appleton & Lange, 2001.
5. Savage PB: Multidrug-resistant bacteria: Overcoming antibiotic permeability barriers of gram-negative bacteria. Ann Med 33(3):167–171, 2001.
6. Salamah SD, Hossain MM, Ahmed T: Enquiry into the causes of misuse of antibiotics. Saudi Med J 21(10):986–987, 2000.

44. ANTIVIRAL AND ANTIFUNGAL DRUGS

1. Describe the mechanism of action of amphotericin B.

This drug binds to sterol groups in fungal cell membranes and forms channels though the fungal cell membrane. This results in increased permeability and cell death.

2. Describe the adverse effects of amphotericin B.

Reactions to this drug vary. However, patients can experience fever, chills, and rigor, accompanied by headache, joint and muscle pain, nausea, vomiting, and hypotension.

3. Describe the renal effects of amphotericin B.

This drug can cause renal toxicity that is the result of vasoconstriction and peritubular membrane damage.

4. Discuss the mechanism of action of the azole antifungal agents (e.g., ketoconazole, itraconazole).

These drugs interact with fungal cytochrome P_{450} enzymes (eg, 14α demethylase), which is involved in the synthesis of the fungal cell membrane.

5. Why must ketoconazole be administered orally?

The drug must undergo acid conversion in the stomach in order to be soluble in water. Thus, it is not administered parenterally.

6. Discuss the adverse reactions of ketoconazole.

Nausea and vomiting are frequently seen, and, rarely, hepatotoxicity.

7. Discuss the effects of ketoconazole on mammalian cholesterol synthesis.

Ketoconazole is a weak inhibitor of enzymatic conversion of lanosterol to cholesterol in humans.

8. Can ketoconazole have endocrine effects?

Yes, in high doses or with prolonged therapy. The decrease in cholesterol synthesis can affect the synthesis of steroid hormones. Additionally, the drug inhibits key enzymes in hormone biosynthesis, such as $14-\alpha$ demethylase and $11-\beta$ hydroxylase, resulting in lower levels of androgens.

9. Describe the drug interaction between ketoconazole and cyclosporine.

Ketoconazole decreases the clearance of cyclosporine, resulting in elevated serum levels. This can result in toxicity to normal cells.

10. Compare the actions of fluconazole and ketoconazole.

These drugs are similar in action. However, fluconazole is 100 times more specific for the fungal cytochrome P_{450} enzymes than the human enzymes. This leads to substantially less adverse effects.

11. Are itraconazole and fluconazole effective against candida?

No. Many strains of this organism are resistant to these drugs.

12. What is the major use of fluconazole?

This drug is effective against *Cryptococcus*. A major use of fluconazole has been in the therapy of cryptococcal meningitis seen with AIDS.

13. Describe flucytosine.

Flucytosine is a fluorinated pyrimidine antifungal agent.

14. Discuss the mechanism of action of flucytosine.

This drug is converted by fungal enzymes to 5-flouro-uracil (5-FU). This agent disrupts the actions of fungal DNA polymerase and RNA polymerase, disrupting DNA synthesis and protein synthesis.

15. Describe the specificity of flucytosine.

Flucytosine is only effective in organisms that posses the enzymes necessary for conversion of the drug to 5-FU.

16. Does flucytosine affect mammalian cells?

No. The necessary enzymes for conversion are lacking.

17. Describe the use of miconazole.

This agent is used topically for fungal infection (e.g., vaginal and scrotal infections and athlete's foot).

18. Is miconazole used for systemic fungal infections?

No, because it lacks water solubility and has potential adverse effects.

19. Describe the mechanism of action of imidazole antifungals (e.g., butoconazole, econazole).

These drugs inhibit the synthesis of ergosterol.

20. What is the use of griseofulvin?

Griseofulvin is used systemically in the therapy of fungal infections of the skin and nails.

21. Describe the mechanism of action of griseofulvin.

Griseofulvin disrupts microtubule assembly in the fungal cell. This results in lack of replication of actively reproducing cells.

22. Discuss the adverse effects of griseofulvin.

Headache is the most common adverse effect. This drug may also produce rashes (including erythema multiforme), hepatotoxicity, hematological disturbances, and gastrointestinal (GI) distress.

ANTIVIRAL AGENTS

23. Discuss the mechanism of action of vidarabine.

This drug is deaminated intracellularly and phosphorylated. The phosphorylated form (Ara-A) is similar to adenosine triphosphate (ATP), and, when incorporated into the viral DNA replication sequence, binds to DNA polymerase and inhibits DNA synthesis.

24. Against which viral infections is vidarabine particularly effective?

Those produced by herpes simplex virus (HSV).

25. Describe the adverse effects of vidarabine.

Minor effects include nausea and vomiting. More serious effects include encephalopathy associated with dizziness, headache, confusion, ataxia and tremors, progressing to coma.

26. Which patients are at risk for serious encephalopathy with vidarabine?

Those with renal insufficiency, because the drug is eliminated through the urine.

27. What blood and serum abnormalities occur with vidarabine therapy?
Decreased blood cell count (hematocrit), decreased hemoglobin, and elevated serum glutamic-oxaloacetic transaminase (SGOT).

28. Describe the mechanism of action of acyclovir and ganciclovir.
These drugs are synthetic acyclic guanine nucleosides. They are converted to triphosphate form by viral thymidine kinase and inhibit the action of DNA polymerase.

29. Describe the advantage of the use of acyclovir over vidarabine.
Acyclovir affects a greater diversity of viruses, as it inhibits the actions of viral thymidine kinase, which is ubiquitous among viruses.

30. Discuss the mechanism of action of azidothymidine (AZT).
This drug is useful in the treatment of AIDS. It is converted intracellularly into a triphosphate form, which is a competitive inhibitor of reverse transcriptase of HIV and other retroviruses.

31. Does azidothymidine affect human immune cells?
AZT can affect human cells, however, the retrovirus is exquisitely sensitive to the drug, resulting in therapeutic efficacy of the drug at concentrations too low to cause toxicity to host cells.

32. Describe the toxicity of AZT.
Because rapidly reproducing cells are most affected, blood dyscrasias and anemia are seen with this drug, over a period of weeks.

33. How is interferon effective as an antiviral agent?
This drug interferes at virtually all stages of viral replication—viral uncoating, RNA transcription, protein synthesis, and the assembly of new virions.

BIBLIOGRAPHY

1. Baker R: FDA approves oral ganciclovir as first drug to prevent CMV disease. Food and Drug Administration. BETA:8, 1995.
2. Carbone GM, Catapano CV, Fernandes DJ: Imbalanced DNA synthesis induced by cytosine arabinoside and fludarabine in human leukemia cells. Biochem Pharmacol 62(1):101–110, 2001.
3. Cook PP: Amphotericin B lipid complex for the treatment of recurrent blastomycosis of the brain in a patient previously treated with itraconazole. South Med J 94(5):548–549, 2001.
4. Cuenca-Estrella M, Mellado E, Diaz-Guerra TM, et al: Azasordarins: Susceptibility of fluconazole-susceptible and fluconazole-resistant clinical isolates of candida spp. to GW 471558. Antimicrob Agents Chemother 45(6):1905–1907, 2001.
5. de Bruijn P, Kehrer DF, Verweij J, et al: Liquid chromatographic determination of ketoconazole, a potent inhibitor of CYP 3A4-mediated metabolism. J Chromatogr B Biomed Sci Appl 753(2):395–400, 2001.
6. Fried MW, Sommadossi JP: Nucleoside analogues and other investigational modalities for the treatment of chronic hepatitis B. Antivir Ther 1(2):71–76, 1996.
7. Gilden D: Ganciclovir approved to prevent CMV. GMHC Treat Issues 9(11):3, 1995.
8. Gupta AK, Gregurek-Novak T: Efficacy of itraconazole, terbinafine, fluconazole, griseofulvin and ketoconazole in the treatment of Scopulariopsis brevicollis causing onychomycosis of the toes. Dermatology 202(3):235–238, 2001.
9. Gussak HM, Rahman S, Bastani B: Administration and clearance of amphotericin b during high-efficiency or high-efficiency/high-flux dialysis. Am J Kidney Dis 37(6):E45, 2001.
10. Hardman J, Limbird L, Gilman A: Goodman & Gilman's The Pharmacological Basis of Therapeutics, 10th ed. McGraw-Hill Publishers, 2001.
11. Herranz U, Rusca A, Assandri A: Emedastine-ketoconazole: Pharmacokinetic and pharmacodynamic interactions in healthy volunteers. Int J Clin Pharmacol Ther 39(3):102–109, 2001.
12. Josephson L, Rutkowski JV, Paul K, et al: Antiviral activity of a conjugate of adenine-9-beta-D-arabinofuranoside 5'-monophosphate and a 9 kDa fragment of arabinogalactan. Antivir Ther 1(3):147–156, 1996.

13. Katzung B: Basic and Clinical Pharmacology, 8th ed. Appleton & Lange, 2001.
14. Krupova Y, Mistrik M, Bojtarova E, et al: Liposomal nystatin (L-NYS) in therapy of pulmonary aspergillosis refractory to conventional amphotericin B in cancer patients. Support Care Cancer 9(3):209–210, 2001.
15. Millikan R, Baez L, Banerjee T, et al: Randomized phase 2 trial of ketoconazole and ketoconazole/doxorubicin in androgen independent prostate cancer: Urol Oncol 6(3):111–115, 2001.
16. Olivero OA, Reddy MK, Pietras SM, et al: Plasma drug levels compared with DNA incorporation of 3'-azido-3'-deoxythymidine (AZT) in adult cynomolgus (Macaca fascicularis) monkeys. Exp Biol Med (Maywood) 226(5):446–449, 2001.
17. Schouten JT: Oral ganciclovir. STEP Perspect 7(3):1, 11, 1995.
18. Scripture CD, Pieper JA: Clinical pharmacokinetics of fluvastatin. Clin Pharmacokinet 40(4):263–281, 2001.
19. Viudes A, Peman J, Canton E, et al: The activity of combinations of systemic antimycotic drugs. Rev Esp Quimioter 14(1):30–39, 2001.
20. White DJ, Habib AR, Vanthuyne A, et al: Combined topical flucytosine and amphotericin B for refractory vaginal Candida glabrata infections. Sex Transm Infect 77(3):212–213, 2001.
21. Woodward J: New developments in the delivery of ganciclovir for cytomegalovirus (CMV retinitis). STEP Perspect 7(2):2–4, 1994.

XI. Cancer Chemotherapy

Patricia K. Anthony, Ph.D., and Dal Yoo, M.D.

45. GENERAL CONCEPTS IN CANCER CHEMOTHERAPY

1. Describe the general premise behind cancer chemotherapeutics.

Most cancer chemotherapeutics work under the premise that metastatic cells grow and divide faster than normal cells. Thus, cancer drugs affect rapidly dividing cells more than normal cells.

2. List possible mechanisms of action of cancer chemotherapeutics.

These drugs may:
• Interfere with DNA synthesis by disrupting folic acid utilization
• Interfere with mitotic spindle formation
• Interfere with nucleic acid synthesis
• Interfere with protein synthesis

3. Do cancer chemotherapeutic agents affect normal cells?

Yes, particularly those that are rapidly dividing (e.g., bone marrow, hair follicles).

4. What adverse effects are usually seen with cancer chemotherapeutics?

Adverse effects are usually related to inhibition of the replication of cell populations that divide rapidly. Side effects include bone marrow suppression, immunosuppression, and alopecia. Nausea and vomiting are also seen, due to stimulation of the chemoreceptor trigger zone.

5. Do all types of cancer chemotherapeutics exhibit the same profile of adverse effects?

No. The profile of effects varies with the drug class and mechanism of action.

6. Why is combination therapy useful in the therapy of solid tumors?

These tumors contain heterogeneous cell populations, which may respond differently to differnt drugs.

7. What is tumor lysis syndrome?

This condition arises from the rapid death and subsequent lysis of tumor cells. It results from the rapid release of calcium, potassium, and phosphate by dying cells.

8. Describe the toxic effects of tumor lysis syndrome.

This condition is characterized by nephrotoxicity, which may arise shortly after the initiation of chemotherapy.

9. What is CHOP?

This drug regimen includes **c**yclophosphamide, epirubicin, vincristine (**O**ncovin), and **p**rednisone (the more potent epirubicin has replaced **h**ydroxydaunomycin). It is commonly used in the treatment of non-Hodgkin's lymphoma.

10. Why does the therapy of solid tumors often involve more than one agent?

Solid tumors often contain more than one cell population. These different cells may respond differently to a chemotherapeutic agent. For example, one cell population may be resistant to the drug whereas another is responsive, resulting in a single population of resistant cells.

11. Why might calcium channel blockers be useful in cancer chemotherapy?

Verapamil, in particular, has been shown to inhibit the membrane P170 glycoprotein, which is necessary for the expulsion of chemotherapeutic drugs from cancer cells. Thus, these drugs may augment traditional cancer chemotherapy.

12. What agents may be used in the therapy of bone marrow depression seen with cancer chemotherapeutics?

Whole blood transfusions may be administered. Alternatively, erythropoietin may be given to stimulate the production of erythrocytes.

13. Describe filgrastim.

Filgrastim is a granulocyte colony stimulating factor that may be administered to reduce depression of neutrophils (neutropenia) seen with cancer chemotherapeutics, particularly those used for acute nonlymphocytic leukemia.

14. Discuss the use of amifostine.

Amifostine is a cytoprotective agent that is used to protect normal cells from cancer chemotherapeutic agents.

15. A previously healthy HIV-negative 20-year-old man with recently diagnosed stage III Burkitt's lymphoma was admitted for fever, early satiety, and 20 lbs weight loss over 3 months. Chest exam was normal without respiratory stridor, but multiple enlarged lymph nodes and epigastric mass are palpable. Lab showed a moderate anemia (Hct 33%) and uric acid increased to 9.0 (normal is less than 8.0); otherwise, the remaining lab values are unremarkable. He was started on CHOP—cyclophosphamide, doxorubicin (hydroxydaunomycin), vincristine, and prednisone—chemotherapy, but was found dead in bed within 10 hours after chemotherapy. What would be the most likely cause of death in this patient's scenario?

Tumor lysis syndrome—resulting in hypercalcemia, hyperuricemia, and hyperphosphotemia, leading to sudden arrhythmia, and renal shutdown.

BIBLIOGRAPHY

1. Hardman J, Limbird L, Gilman A (eds): Goodman & Gilman's The Pharmacologic Basis of Therapeutics, 10th ed. New York, McGraw-Hill, 2001.
2. Katzung B: Basic and Clinical Pharmacology, 8th ed. New York, Appleton & Lange, 2001.
3. Zhou S, Paxton JW, Tingle MD, Kestell P: Identification of the human liver cytochrome P450 isoenzyme responsible for the 6-methylhydroxylation of the novel anticancer drug 5,6-dimethylxanthenone-4-acetic acid. Drug Metab Dispos 28:1449–1456, 2000.

46. ANTIMETABOLITE AGENTS

1. Describe the general mechanism of action of antimetabolite anticancer agents.
These drugs inhibit the synthesis of nucleotides. Classic cellular mechanisms include the inhibition of folic acid metabolism and pyrimidine antagonism.

PYRIMIDINE ANTAGONISTS

2. Describe the general mechanism of action of 5-fluorouracil (5-FU).
This drug is metabolized to 5-deoxyuridine monophosphate (5-dUMP), which binds to thymidylate synthase, inhibiting the interaction between the enzyme and its major cofactor. Thus, synthesis of thymidine is inhibited, causing cell death.

3. What are the adverse effects of 5-FU?
Bone marrow suppression and hand and foot syndrome.

4. How is 5-FU administered?
This drug may be administered orally or by infusion.

5. Describe the hand and foot syndrome seen with continuous administration of 5-FU.
This syndrome is characterized by a reddening of the palms and the soles of the feet. It is thought to be due to vascular endothelial damage caused by the drug.

6. Does administration of 5-FU by continuous infusion result in bone marrow suppression?
The incidence of bone marrow suppression with slow infusion is low—approximately 15%.

7. Describe the effect of large-dose 5-FU administration or administration by IV push.
The relatively large amounts of drug presented to the patient by these methods of administration result in suppression of bone marrow.

8. Compare the survival rates of patients treated with oral 5-FU versus continuous infusion.
Administration by continuous infusion results in decreased adverse effects. However, no difference in survival rate is apparent.

9. What pyrimidine antagonist can work like a central line of 5-FU?
Capecitabine.

10. Is capecitabine immediately active?
No. It is a prodrug. It is converted to the active form within the tumor cell.

11. Does capecitabine cause a high level of thrombocytopenia?
No. Because it is converted to an active form within the tumor cell, it has less effect on other rapidly proliferating cells (e.g., bone marrow).

12. List the adverse effects of capecitabine.
Diarrhea
Mucositis
Hand and foot syndrome

13. What are the advantages of capecitabine therapy compared with 5-FU?
Capecitabine does not require a central line, only vascular access. In addition, there is less bone marrow depression.

14. In what phase of the cell cycle is cytarabine active?
S phase.

15. Describe the action of cytarabine on DNA synthesis.
This drug is metabolized to arabinosylcytidine monophosphate (Ara-CMP), which is then converted to arabinosylcytidine triphosphate (Ara-CTP). This agent competitively inhibits DNA polymerase, resulting in decreased DNA synthesis.

16. Does cytarabine have direct effects on DNA and RNA?
Yes. The drug is incorporated into both RNA and DNA, resulting in altered chain elongation and altered ligation of Okazaki fragments.

PURINE ANTAGONISTS

17. Describe the mechanism of action of 6-mercaptopurine.
This drug is metabolized to 6-thioinosinic acid, which inhibits the purine nucleoside pathway.

18. What is the major use of fludarabine?
This drug is primarily used in lymphatic cancers.

19. Why does cladribine reach high intracellular concentrations?
This drug is resistant to adenosine deaminase.

FOLIC ACID INHIBITORS

20. Describe the mechanism of action of methotrexate.
This drug inhibits dihydrofolate reductase (DHFR) in mammalian cells. The conversion of folic acid to tetrahydrofolate is inhibited, resulting in decreased nucleotide synthesis. Thus, cellular replication and protein synthesis are inhibited.

21. What are the major adverse effects of methotrexate?
Bone marrow suppression, alopecia, and gastrointestinal tract ulceration.

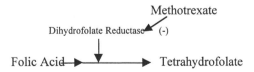

Schematic diagram of the competitive inhibition of DHFR by methotrexate.

22. Describe the mechanisms of tumor cell resistance to methotrexate.
Altered DHFR may confer resistance, or the cell may produce abnormally high levels of the enzyme. Decreased drug transport into the tumor cell may also be a factor.

23. A previously healthy 50-year-old woman with a recently diagnosed metastatic colon cancer accompanying multiple unresectable liver metastases underwent her first weekly IV bolus of standard dose 5-FU (Fluorouracil) chemotherapy without incident. She developed

severe side effects, including nausea, vomiting, complete hair loss, prolonged neutropenia, and watery diarrhea, but these adverse effects slowly improved in 3–4 weeks with supportive care only. Why is she reacting so unusually?

She is deficient in dihydropyrimidine dehydrogenease (DPD deficiency).

BIBLIOGRAPHY

1. Berghammer P, Pohnl R, Baur M, Dittrich C: Docetaxel extravasation. Support Care Cancer 9:131–141, 2001.
2. Hardman J, Limbird L, Gilman A (eds): Goodman & Gilman's The Pharmacologic Basis of Therapeutics, 10th ed. New York, McGraw-Hill, 2001.
3. Katzung B: Basic and Clinical Pharmacology, 8th ed. New York, Appleton & Lange, 2000.
4. Moon C, Verschraegen CF, Bevers M, et al: Use of docetaxel (Taxotere) in patients with paclitaxel (Taxol) hypersensitivity. Anticancer Drugs 11:565–568, 2000.
5. Shin DM, Khuri FR, Glisson BS, et al: Phase II study of paclitaxel, ifosfamide, and carboplatin in patients with recurrent or metastatic head and neck squamous cell carcinoma. Cancer 91:1316–1323, 2001.

47. ALKYLATING AGENTS AND RELATED DRUGS

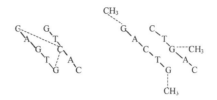

Schematic representation of the actions of alkylating agents. The drug (---) may be bifunctional, resulting in DNA cross-links (*left*) or monofunctional, resulting in guanine alkylation (*right*).

1. Discuss the various cellular mechanisms of drugs described as alkylating agents.

Classically, these drugs alkylate nucleotides, resulting in subsequent errors in RNA translation, DNA transcription, and DNA replication. Alkylation may be monofunctional (affecting one strand) or bifunctional (cross-linking two strands) depending on the agent. Other drugs included in this class cause DNA cission, also resulting in aberrant cellular replication.

2. Describe the mechanism of action of alkylating agents in cancer chemotherapy.

Classic alkylating agents add an alkyl group to nucleosides in DNA (primarily guanine). This results in DNA cross-linking or strand cission.

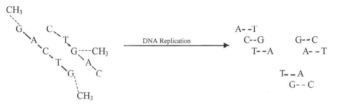

Schematic representation of the disruption of DNA replication by monofunctional alkylating agents. Cross-linked DNA arising from the actions of bifunctional agents would not be available for replication.

3. Which drugs are considered nonclassic alkylating agents?

Procarbazine, dacarbazine, and altretamine.

4. Are alkylating agents useful in the therapy of slow-growing tumors?

Because these agents interfere with DNA replication, they are less useful in slow-growing tumors.

5. Discuss the adverse effects of alkylating agents.

Adverse effects are related to effects of the drug on rapidly growing cells. These include bone marrow suppression, alopecia, and emesis.

6. Which alkylating agents are prodrugs?

Decarbazine, procarbazine, altretamine, ifosfamide, cyclophosphamide, and the nitrosureas all require activation

7. Which alkylating agent does not cause myelosuppression?

Cisplatin.

8. Which agents cause delayed hematopoietic effects?

The nitrogen mustards, carmustine and lomustine. Myelosuppression may not be evident for several weeks after initial therapy.

9. Name two agents that cause hemorrhagic cystitis.

Cyclophosphamide and ifosfamide.

10. Adverse effects due to alkylating agents are commonly seen on which organs?

Adverse effects on the lung and gonads are common.

11. What side effects of procarbazine may contribute to drug interactions?

Procarbazine can cause a disulfiram-like reaction and is a monoamine oxidase inhibitor. Thus, ingestion of alcohol, foods containing tyramine (e.g., cheese), drugs that increase sympathetic activity, and MAOI-type antidepressants (e.g., tranylcypromine) should be avoided.

12. Describe the mechanism of action of cisplatin.

Cisplatin is a bifunctional alkylating agent. By attaching alkyl groups to opposing guanine residues, the drug cross-links DNA strands, causing inhibition of DNA replication and transcription.

13. What are the major adverse effects of cisplatin?

Nephrotoxicity
Emesis
Peripheral neuropathy
Ototoxicity

14. Contrast the mechanisms of action of cisplatin and carboplatin.

These drugs share the same mechanism of action, but cross-links formed by carboplatin persist longer than those formed by cisplatin. However, cisplatin cross-links are formed more quickly (6–8 hours after administration) than those of carboplatin (18 hours after administration).

15. Describe the cellular activation of carboplatin.

These drugs must enter the cell before they are activated. Once inside the cell, the ring structure of the drug is hydroxylated to form the active moiety, which effectively cross-links the strands of DNA and RNA, functionally inactivating these nucleic acids.

16. Compare the adverse effects of cisplatin and carboplatin.

Carboplatin has a much more favorable adverse effect profile than cisplatin; however, it does exhibit myelosuppression.

17. How is carboplatin eliminated?

Elimination is biphasic, through the urine.

18. Can carboplatin be used concurrently with radiation therapy?

No. This drug sensitizes tissue to radiation, and severe myelosuppression may result.

19. Describe the effects of carboplatin on the ear.

This drug may cause ototoxicity, particularly in children receiving high-dose therapy. Effects on adults are rare.

20. Does carboplatin cause peripheral neuropathy?

Yes. The elderly are particularly at risk.

21. Discuss the secondary malignancies seen with cisplatin and carboplatin.

Platinum-based therapy has been associated with an increased risk of secondary malignancy, primarily acute myelogenous leukemia, myelodysplastic syndromes, acute lymphocytic leukemia, and chronic myelogenous leukemia. The risk of secondary malignancy increases with cumulative carboplatin doses > 2000 mg.

22. Discuss the major clinical use of cisplatin and carboplatin.

These drugs are used primarily in the therapy of reproductive organ cancers (e.g., ovarian cancer).

23. Describe the clinical use of busulfan.

Busulfan is no longer used clinically as an antineoplastic agent. It is now used to destroy the myeloid cell line prior to an allogeneic bone marrow transplant for leukemia.

24. What is the clinical use of procarbazine?

This drug is effective in Hodgkin's lymphoma.

25. Describe the clinical use of dacarbazine.

This drug is used in the therapy of melanoma. It is not curative.

26. Describe the clinical use of streptozotocin.

Because of its unique toxicity against beta cells of the pancreas, streptozotocin is used almost exclusively to treat islet cell carcinoma of the pancreas. Its use is rare.

27. Discuss mitomycin as a cancer chemotherapeutic agent.

Mitomycin is a broad-spectrum antibiotic that also functions effectively as a monofunctional or bifunctional alkylating agent for mammalian DNA. Its activity is not considered cell-cycle specific, but maximum cytotoxic effects occur in cells in late G_1 and S phases.

BIBLIOGRAPHY

1. Hardman J, Limbird L, Gilman A (eds): Goodman & Gilman's The Pharmacologic Basis of Therapeutics, 10th ed. New York, McGraw-Hill, 2001.
2. Hsu CH, Chen J, Wu CY, et al: Combination chemotherapy of cisplatin, methotrexate, vinblastine, and high-dose tamoxifen for transitional cell carcinoma. Anticancer Res 21(1B):711–715, 2001.
3. Katzung B: Basic and Clinical Pharmacology, 8th ed. New York, Appleton & Lange, 2001.
4. Kaiser U, Uebelacker I, Havemann K: Non-Hodgkin's lymphoma protocols in the treatment of patients with Burkitt's lymphoma and lymphoblastic lymphoma: A report on 58 patients. Leuk Lymphoma 36(1–2):101–108, 1999.
5. Shin DM, Khuri FR, Glisson BA, et al: Phase II study of paclitaxel, ifosfamide, and carboplatin in patients with recurrent or metastatic head and neck squamous cell carcinoma. Cancer 91:1316–1323, 2001.

48. ANTIBIOTICS AND MITOTIC SPINDLE INHIBITORS

ANTIBIOTICS

1. Which drugs are classified as anthracycline antibiotics?

Daunorubicin, doxorubicin, epirubicin, and idarubicin are examples of anthracycline antibiotic agents. These agents are used as antineoplastic agents.

2. Describe the mechanism of action of anthracycline antineoplastics (e.g., daunorubicin).

These drugs combine with DNA by intercalating DNA base pairs, causing altered configuration of the DNA helix.

3. What is the cellular effect of anthracycline antineoplastics?

The conformational change produced by these drugs results in altered strand elongation and interferes with DNA polymerase activity. Protein synthesis is also inhibited because of the effects on RNA polymerase.

4. Are the actions of anthracyclines cell cycle phase specific?

These drugs are not considered to be specific for a single phase of the cell cycle.

5. In which phases of the cell cycle do anthracyclines have antineoplastic effects?

The majority of effects occur in the S phase of the cell cycle. However, cells exposed to the drug in G_1 also will be affected.

6. Do anthracycline antineoplastics interfere with nucleoside uptake?

Yes. These drugs inhibit the uptake of thymidine into cancer cells and fibroblasts.

7. Describe the effects of anthracycline antineoplastics on topoisomerase II.

These drugs inhibit topoisomerase II, resulting in decreased or altered DNA repair.

8. Describe the interactions of anthracyclines with divalent ions.

These drugs may form complexes with divalent ions, such as iron or copper.

9. What are the effects of anthracyclines on the heart?

These drugs are cardiotoxic.

10. How do anthracycline antibiotics affect mitochondria?

As the drug enters a cell, it forms superoxide anions. These free radicals (e.g., hydrogen peroxide) normally are destroyed by glutathione peroxidase; however, this enzyme, and the required glutathione, is of limited concentration in cardiac cells. Thus, the radicals complex with available Fe^{++} ions, forming highly reactive radicals that rapidly cause lipid peroxidation and extensive mitochondrial destruction.

11. Discuss the cellular mechanisms of anthracycline-induced cardiac failure.

In addition to mitochondrial damage, the superoxide radicals formed from these drugs cross into the cardiac myocytes and inhibit ATPase. This results in a decreased ability of cardiac cells to store and release intracellular calcium (e.g., sarcoplasmic reticulum).

12. List the various forms of neoplastic drug resistance to anthracyclines.
- Multidrug resistance mechanisms mediated by an overexpression of P170-glycoprotein.
- Changes in topoisomerase II conformation or activity
- Changes in glutathione levels or activity

13. Describe the role of P170-glycoprotein in multidrug resistance.
This protein functions as an energy-dependent membrane pump, which actively pumps the antineoplastic drug out of the cancerous cell.

14. Is there a pharmacologic remedy to multidrug resistance?
Yes. Calcium channel blockers, such as verapamil, may block this process and reduce resistance. Cyclosporine and its analogs also may be effective.

15. Discuss the pharmacokinetics of anthracyclines.
These drugs are bound extensively to DNA and are 75% protein bound. They are eliminated through hepatic metabolism and glucuronidation. Metabolites are excreted primarily through the bile, with some elimination through the urine. These drugs tend to have long half-lives and are administered intravenously.

16. Is the cardiotoxicity of doxorubicin due to the parent drug or the metabolite?
Cardiotoxicity primarily is due to the effects of the parent drug, but the primary metabolite, doxorubicinol, is also cardiotoxic.

17. Describe the therapeutic uses of doxorubicin.
This drug is useful in the therapy of a variety of tumor types and is effective against most solid tumors. It is part of standard regimens for breast, lung, gastric, and ovarian cancers, Hodgkin's disease, non-Hodgkin's lymphoma, sarcoma, myeloma, and acute lymphocytic leukemia.

18. What is the primary therapeutic use of daunorubicin?
Daunorubicin is used primarily in the treatment of acute leukemias.

19. Contrast the cardiotoxicity seen with doxorubicin and daunorubicin.
Daunorubicin has a lower incidence of cardiotoxicity than doxorubicin.

20. Is daunorubicin effective against solid tumors?
Yes, particularly neuroblastoma.

21. What is idarubicin?
Idarubicin is an analog of daunorubicin. It is indicated for use in combination with cytarabine (Ara-C) for induction therapy of acute myelogenous leukemia (AML).

22. Compare doxorubicin and idarubicin.
Idarubicin is less lipophillic and therefore has less cardiotoxicity than doxorubicin (or daunorubicin). It has a greater affinity for DNA and increased DNA binding compared with doxorubicin and is more readily taken up into target cells.

23. Contrast the potency of idarubicin and other anthracyclines.
Idarubicin inhibits the uptake of thymidine into cancer cells at lower concentrations. It, therefore, may be considered more potent.

24. For which neoplastic conditions is idarubicin designated an orphan drug?
Idarubicin has orphan drug designation for AML, acute lymphoblastic leukemia in pediatrics, chronic myelogenous leukemia, and myelodysplastic syndrome.

25. Is idarubicin susceptible to multidrug resistance?
Yes, but to a substantially lower degree than other drugs of the class.

26. In which phase of the cell cycle are etoposide and teniposide active?
These agents are specific for G_2.

27. Describe the mechanism of action of etoposide and teniposide.
Etoposide is an inhibitor of topoisomerase II. Unlike the anthracyclines, the drug does not bind directly to the enzyme but stabilizes the complex formed by the enzyme and DNA. When DNA and topoisomerase II are bound together, further progression in the cell cycle is halted. DNA strand breaks develop, and the cell dies.

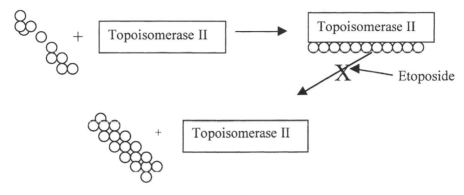

Schematic representation of the actions of etoposide.

28. Does etoposide cross the blood–brain barrier?
Yes, but only to a small degree (approximately 5%).

29. Do fluoroquinolone antibiotics affect neoplastic cells?
No. These agents are specific for bacterial topoisomerases.

30. What is plicamycin?
Plicamycin is a parenteral cell cycle-phase nonspecific antineoplastic agent.

31. Describe the use of plicamycin in antineoplastic therapy.
This drug is used primarily in refractory cases of embryonal-type testicular cancer.

32. Describe the mechanism of action of plicamycin.
This drug intercalates DNA base pairs, causing the helix to uncoil and thereby inhibiting the synthesis of DNA and transcriptional synthesis of RNA.

33. How is plicamycin administered?
Intravenously.

34. Describe the distribution of plicamycin.
This drug is most concentrated in renal tubular cells, hepatocytes, and bone—particularly areas of active bone resorption.

35. Does plicamycin cross the blood–brain barrier?
Yes. The serum and cerebrospinal fluid (CSF) concentrations of the drug are approximately equal.

36. Which drugs are included in the camptothecin class of antineoplastics?
Topotecan and iridotecan.

37. What is topotecan?
Topotecan is a cytotoxic plant alkaloid isolated from the Chinese tree *Camptotheca acuminata*. It is used as an intravenous antineoplastic agent.

38. Are camptothecins cell-cycle phase specific?
Yes. These agents are highly S-phase specific.

39. Describe the mechanism of action of topotecan and iridotecan.
These drugs inhibit topoisomerase I, resulting in DNA strand fragmentation upon replication and deficient RNA synthesis.

40. What are the therapeutic uses of topotecan?
This drug is used as first-line therapy for ovarian cancer and is effective as second-line therapy in the treatment of small cell lung cancer.

41. Can camptothecins be used in conjunction with radiation therapy?
No. Topoisomerase I inhibitors appear to inhibit initial DNA repairs including sealing of broken strands and repair of base damage following radiation therapy.

42. Discuss the mechanism of action of bleomycin.
This drug is converted to a heme complex, which binds to DNA and results in strand breakage during DNA cleavage. It is G_2 specific.

43. Is bleomycin therapy detrimental to bone marrow?
No. Bone marrow contains high levels of bleomycin hydrolase, which converts the drug to an inactive form.

44. Is bleomycin susceptible to multidrug resistance?
No. It is not affected by P-glycoproteins.

45. How is bleomycin administered?
Because of its poor absorption, the drug must be administered parenterally.

46. Describe the distribution of bleomycin.
Bleomycin distributes mainly into the tissues of the skin, lungs, kidneys, peritoneum, and lymph.

47. Is bleomycin highly protein bound?
No. Less than 10% of the drug is bound to plasma proteins.

48. List the primary sites of bleomycin toxicity.
Primary toxicity occurs in lung and skin tissue.

VINCA ALKALOIDS AND SPINDLE INHIBITORS

49. Are vinca alkaloids cell-cycle specific?
Yes. They are S-phase specific.

50. List the two major vinca alkaloids used as antineoplastic agents.
Vincristine and vinblastine.

51. Describe the mechanism of action of vinca alkaloids.
These drugs bind to tubulin at low-affinity sites, resulting in splitting of tubules into spiral aggregates or protofilaments and spindle disintegration. Cells are thus arrested in metaphase.

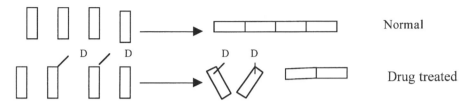

Schematic representation of the actions of mitotic spindle inhibitors on tubulin assembly. The drug binds to tubulin in S_1 and disrupts the assembly of microtubules.

52. Do vinca alkaloids affect intracellular transport and cell migration?
Yes. These and other actions requiring microtubule formation are disrupted.

53. List the mechanisms for resistance to vinca alkaloids.
• Multidrug resistance
• Alteration in the alpha and beta subunits of tubulin, which would affect drug binding

54. What adverse effects may be mediated by vinca alkaloids?
These agents decrease the transport of amino acids into cells and mediate inhibition of purine synthesis; inhibition of RNA, DNA, and protein synthesis; disruption of lipid metabolism; inhibition of glycolysis; changes in antidiuretic hormone release; and disruption of cell membrane integrity and membrane function.

55. How is vinblastine administered?
Parenterally.

56. Describe the actions of vinblastine on blood.
This drug binds readily to platelets and leukocytes because of their high content of tubulin.

57. Does vinblastine cross the blood–brain barrier?
No.

58. Which vinca alkaloid has the shortest half-life?
Vinblastine has the shortest terminal half-life and highest clearance of all available vinca alkaloids.

59. How is vinblastine metabolized?
This drug is metabolized by the cytochrome P3A4 isoenzyme of cytochrome P450.

60. Does vinblastine produce active metabolites?
Yes.

61. Why does vincristine have greater potency with bolus dosing than vinblastine?
Vincristine has more cellular retention than vinblastine.

62. Is vincristine effective in the therapy of brain tumors?
Yes.

63. Describe the adverse central nervous system (CNS) effects of vincristine.
Because of its ability to cross into the CNS and its long half-life, vincristine causes an increased incidence of neurotoxicity.

64. Describe vinorelbine.

Vinorelbine is a vinca alkaloid that may be administered orally. The spectrum of activity is similar to that of vincristine and vinblastine.

65. Compare the neurotoxic effects of vincristine and vinorelbine.

Vinorelbine produces substantially less neurotoxicity than vincristine.

66. Is vinorelbine highly protein bound?

Yes. Vinorelbine is 80–91% bound to both albumin and α_1 acid glycoprotein.

67. Does vinorelbine have active metabolites?

Yes.

68. Describe the use of asparaginase in cancer chemotherapy.

This enzyme depletes cells of asparagine, an amino acid crucial to the manufacture of cellular proteins used in growth and metabolism. This depletion results in inhibition of protein synthesis and cell death.

69. For which type of tumor is asparaginase useful?

This enzyme has been shown to be useful in the therapy of lymphomas.

BIBLIOGRAPHY

1. Hardman J, Limbird L, Gilman A (eds): Goodman & Gilman's The Pharmacologic Basis of Therapeutics, 10th ed. New York, McGraw-Hill, 2001.
2. Katzung B: Basic and Clinical Pharmacology, 8th ed. New York, Appleton & Lange, 2001.
3. Laack E, Mende T, Benk J, et al: Gemcitabine and vinorelbine as first-line chemotherapy for advanced non-small cell lung cancer: A phase II trial. Eur J Cancer 37:583–590, 2001.
4. Liu YY, Han TY, Giuliano AE, Cabot MC: Ceramide glycosylation potentiates cellular multidrug resistance. FASEB J 15:719–730, 2001.
5. Liu JH, Yang MH, Fan FS, et al: Tamoxifen and colchicine-modulated vinblastine followed by 5-fluorouracil in advanced renal cell carcinoma: A phase II study. Urology 57:650–654, 2001.
6. Mi Q, Cui B, Silva GL, et al: A novel tropane alkaloid that reverses the multidrug-resistance phenotype. Cancer Res 61:4030–4037, 2001.
7. Sersa G, Krzic M, Sentjurc M, et al: Reduced tumor oxygenation by treatment with vinblastine. Cancer Res 61:4266–4271, 2001.
8. Tesch H, Sieber M, Diehl V: Treatment of advanced stage Hodgkin's disease. Oncology 60:101–109, 2001.

XII. Herbal and Over-the-Counter Preparations and Toxicology

Patricia K. Anthony, Ph.D., and Donald Kautz, Ph.D.

49. HERBAL MEDICATIONS AND OVER-THE-COUNTER DRUGS

HERBAL PREPARATIONS

1. Define and discuss ginkgo biloba.
This herb is a vasodilator that has activity in the cerebral cortex. It is reputed to enhance memory and cognition.

2. Discuss the effects of ginkgo biloba on the blood.
This drug has significant antithrombotic activity and thus may potentiate the effects of anticoagulants or other antithrombotics.

3. What are the reputed therapeutic uses of alfalfa?
Alfalfa is used to alleviate inflammation of the bladder, bloating or water retention, indigestion, constipation, and halitosis.

4. Describe the adverse effects of alfalfa in pregnancy.
Alfalfa, particularly the seeds, contains stachydrine and homostachydrine, which promote menstruation and in some cases can lead to miscarriage.

5. Discuss the effects of alfalfa on the blood.
In moderate doses, alfalfa is beneficial because of the large quantities of iron and vitamins it contains. However, the seeds contain relatively high levels of the toxic amino acid canavanine, which may promote pancytopenia with routine ingestion of large quantities of seeds.

6. Describe the effects of dong quai.
This herb is used to control bleeding. Its primary use is in herbal therapy of irregular or painful menstruation.

7. What are the contraindications of dong quai?
It should be avoided in the first trimester of pregnancy.

8. What are the active chemical compounds found in echinacea?
1. Echinacoside, an ingredient that may have antibiotic effects
2. Echinacein, which may block viral and bacterial invasion

9. Describe the external use of echinacea.
This herb may be used as a topical anti-infective on burns, boils, and minor wounds. It is also used as a topical agent in the therapy of skin disorders such as eczema.

10. Discuss the two therapeutically useful portions of aloe.
The therapeutically useful portions of the aloe plant are the green gel and the yellowish layer (latex) just beneath the skin of the leaves.

11. What are the uses of the green gel portion of the aloe plant?
This portion is soothing and is used to heal burns. It is also useful in digestive disorders, gastritis, and stomach ulcers.

12. Describe the mechanism of action of aloe in the relief of burns.
Components of the aloe gel are thought to function by inhibiting bradykinin.

13. Does aloe have an anti-inflammatory effect?
Yes. In addition to anti-inflammatory compounds, the leaves are believed to contain magnesium lactate, an effective antihistamine.

14. Describe the use of the latex portion of the aloe plant.
The latex portion is a powerful laxative and is used in the therapy of constipation.

15. What are the adverse effects of ingested aloe?
Intestinal cramps and irritated bowel.

16. What is butcher's broom?
This herb is an astringent, which may be used as a laxative or diuretic.

17. What are the active components of butcher's broom?
Two steroidal components have been identified: ruscogenin and neuroscogenin.

18. Describe the vascular effects of butcher's broom.
The astringent action causes minor irritation and narrowing of blood vessels. Therefore, it may be used as a therapeutic agent for varicose veins and hemorrhoids.

19. What are the uses of chamomile?
This herb is useful in alleviating digestive disorders, menstrual cramping, and insomnia.

20. Describe the topical uses of chamomile.
Applied topically, the extract may be useful in decreasing swelling and pain in the joints, skin inflammation, sunburn, cuts and scrapes, teething pain, varicose veins, hemorrhoids, and sore or inflamed eyes.

21. Does chamomile cause allergic reactions?
Yes. Those patients allergic to ragweed, chrysanthemums, or other plants of the same family may have allergic reactions ranging from contact dermatitis to anaphylaxis.

22. What are the major uses of evening primrose oil?
This oil may be used to decrease the inflammation of arthritis and to treat premenstrual syndrome (PMS). It also has reputed activity in the therapy of arthritis, dry eyes, hyperactivity in children, high blood pressure, and eczema.

23. What is the primary component of primrose oil?
Gamma linoleic acid, which may facilitate production of prostanoids.

24. Describe the use of garlic as an antifungal agent.
Garlic has been used topically in the therapy of various fungal and parasitic infections, including hookworm, roundworm, ringworm, and athlete's foot.

25. Discuss the actions of ginger on the digestive system.

Ginger root contains gingerols, which soothe the digestive tract and relieve excess gas.

26. Describe the effects of ginger on the cardiovascular system.

Ginger is shown to have an antithrombotic action, reducing clotting and the risk of stroke and vessel infarct. It also has been shown to decrease blood pressure.

27. Describe the actions of parsley oil on the cardiovascular system.

Parsley oil lowers serum cholesterol and decreases blood pressure. It may also be of benefit in congestive heart failure.

28. Discuss the therapeutic effects of uva ursi.

The leaves of this plant are used as a diuretic. It is also useful as a urinary antiseptic.

29. What are the major components of uva ursi?

The leaves contain arbutin, which is converted in the urinary tract to the antiseptic hydroquinone. Also present are tannin, an astringent useful in treating wounds, and allantoin, which soothes and accelerates wound healing.

30. Is the use of uva ursi recommended in pregnancy?

No. The active components of the herb stimulate uterine contraction.

31. What is the active component of St. John's wort?

Hypericin. This compound has germicidal, antidepressant, and anti-inflammatory properties.

32. To which class of prescription drugs is the mechanism of St. John's wort similar?

This drug is a monoamine oxidase (MAO) inhibitor. It appears to affect both MAOA and MAOB.

33. What things should be avoided when taking St. John's wort?
- Foods containing tyramine (e.g., wine, cheese) and amino acids such as tyrosine and tryptophan
- Sympathetic agonists, such as isoproterenol, phenylephrine, amphetamines, phenylpropanolamine, and amphetamines

34. Why are rose hips a good source of vitamin C?

Rose hips contain flavonoids, which increase the body's utilization of vitamin C.

35. How does processing affect vitamin C?

Vitamin C is heat labile, and up to 90% of the vitamin may be lost in processing.

OVER-THE-COUNTER DRUG PRODUCTS

36. What is phenolphthalein?

This drug is an irritant to the intestinal mucosa. It is used as a laxative (e.g., Ex-Lax).

37. How do stool softeners work?

These products are usually oils (e.g., glycerin, mineral oil, docusate) intended to become incorporated into the stool and cause it to be soft and "slippery."

38. Why is phenylephrine used in hemorrhoid preparations?

Phenylephrine stimulates alpha receptors on vessels, resulting in shrinkage of swollen tissue.

39. Describe the interactions of phenylpropanolamine and antihypertensive agents.

Cold medications or diet aids containing phenylpropanolamine can interfere with the action of antihypertensive agents. Phenylpropanolamine increases circulating levels of catecholamines, which can result in increased cardiac output and vascular tension.

40. What products contain pyrantel pamoate?

Pyrantel pamoate is used in products that treat pinworm infections.

41. Describe the problems with aerosol inhalers (e.g., isoproterenol) for asthma.

These drugs may have systemic effects (e.g., tachycardia, insomnia, headache, hypertension) if the drug is applied to the buccal tissue or mixed with saliva. Isoproterenol, in particular, is well absorbed from the lung.

42. What is pamabrom?

This drug is a thiazide class diuretic sold over the counter in preparations for menstrual bloating.

43. Describe the use of magnesium salicylate.

This agent is used as a calming agent in the over-the-counter therapy of PMS.

BIBLIOGRAPHY

 1. Duke JA: The Green Pharmacy. Ephrata, PA, Rodale Press, 1997.
 2. Elvin-Lewis M: Should we be concerned about herbal remedies? J Ethnopharmacol 75(2–3):141–164, 2001.
 3. Jacobson JS, Troxel AB, Evans J, et al: Randomized trial of black cohosh for the treatment of hot flashes among women with a history of breast cancer. J Clin Oncol 19:2739–2745, 2001.
 4. Parker V, Wong AH, Boon HS, Seeman MV: Adverse reactions to St. John's wort. Can J Psychiatry 46:77–79, 2001.
 5. Pinn G: Herbs and metabolic/endocrine disease. From past to present. Aust Fam Physician 30:146–150, 2001.
 6. Pinn G: Herbs used in obstetrics and gynaecology. Aust Fam Physician 30:351–356, 2001.
 7. Ryan EA, Pick ME, Marceau C: Use of alternative medicines in diabetes mellitus. Diabet Med 18:242–245, 2001.
 8. Spirling LI, Daniels IR: Botanical perspectives on health: Peppermint: More than just an after-dinner mint. J R Soc Health 121(1):62–63, 2001.
 9. Townsend RR: Common questions and answers in the management of hypertension: Everyday practice in hypertension: Herbal remedies for high blood pressure. J Clin Hypertens (Greenwich) 2:54–55, 2000.
10. Tyler VE: Herbal medicine: From the past to the future. Public Health Nutr 3(4A):447–452, 2000.

50. TOXICOLOGY

1. Define *toxicity*.
Toxicity is the ability of an agent to cause injury.

2. Define *hazard*.
Hazard is a measure of the probability that a given agent will cause injury.

3. What is *acute exposure*?
Acute exposure occurs when an individual is exposed to an agent only once or is exposed infrequently over a period of 1–2 days.

4. Define *chronic exposure*.
Regular exposure over a long period of time.

5. Describe the effects of exposure to multiple agents.
Multiple exposures may be described as **additive** exposure, **synergistic** exposure, or **antagonistic** exposure.

6. Describe the ways in which a toxin may enter the body.
Toxins may enter through cutaneous absorption, injection, ingestion, or exposure to mucous membranes (e.g., mouth, rectum). They also may be inhaled or enter through the membranes of the eye or lacrimal ducts. If cuts or abrasions are present, toxic substances may enter directly into the bloodstream.

7. How are toxins eliminated from the body?
Drugs and toxins may be metabolized and eliminated through the bile, feces, or urine. They also may be eliminated through the lung, skin, and bodily secretions.

8. Describe the ramifications of protein binding with respect to drug overdose.
Drugs that are highly protein bound, whether to plasma or tissue proteins, will not be removed easily by hemodialysis, because proteins are not filtered. This may result in increased potential for toxicity with overdose.

9. Discuss the potential toxicity of small amounts of ingested cyanide.
Cyanide is buffered by deoxygenated hemoglobin (methemoglobin) within red blood cells. A patient with a normal red cell count and normal methemoglobin concentration is able to buffer approximately 175 µg of cyanide ion per kilogram of body weight.

10. Discuss the potential toxic physiologic effects of caffeine consumption.
Caffeine consumption appears to have adverse cardiovascular effects including enhanced sympathetic nerve activity and increased pulse pressure and systolic pressure.

11. Describe the potential health hazards involved with the administration of gamma butyrolactone (GBL), gamma hydroxybutyric acid (GHB), and 1,4-butanediol (BD).
These agents are sold over the counter as body-building supplements. Ingestion of these agents may cause severe respiratory depression. They also may produce unconsciousness or coma, vomiting, seizures, bradycardia, and death.

12. What toxic effects may be seen with troglitazone?
Severe hepatotoxicity.

13. Why should albumin solution not be diluted with sterile water?

If water is used as the diluent in place of an isotonic solution such as D_5W or saline, hemolysis may result.

14. Why are diuretics useful in the therapy of fluoride or bromide poisoning?

Halogens such as bromine, fluorine, and iodide are all reabsorbed in the thick ascending limb of the loop of Henle, using the sodium/potassium/2-chloride cotransporter. Thus, inhibition of this transport system by loop diuretics would result in these ions remaining in the urine and an increased rate of elimination.

15. Discuss the use of mannitol in the therapy of drug overdose.

Mannitol may be used alone or in combination with other diuretic agents to promote urinary excretion of toxins such as salicylates, barbiturates, lithium, and bromides.

16. Explain the rationale for the use of citric acid as an adjunct in the therapy of erythromycin overdose.

Drugs that are basic in nature, such as erythromycin, ionize in an acid environment. Acidification of the plasma by the administration of a weak acid would result in ionization of the drug an an increase in renal elimination. Concurrently, acidification of the urine will increase the rate of elimination of the drug by decreasing reabsorption.

17. Discuss the treatment of organophosphate poisoning.

If treatment is administered early, bound acetylcholinesterase may be reactivated with the use of pralidoxime. Otherwise, the patient must be managed with supportive care.

18. Discuss the mechanism of action of pralidoxime in organophosphate poisoning.

This drug is a substrate for organophosphates. Organophosphates have an increased affinity for pralidoxime compared to acetylcholinesterase. The weakly bound organophosphate may be removed from the enzyme by the pralidoxime, thus reactivating the enzyme.

19. Should ipecac be administered to a patient with a sedative overdose?

No. If the patient lost consciousness before vomiting, chemical pneumonia or suffocation could result.

20. What are the ramifications of excessive use of sodium bicarbonate antacids?

These drugs may cause systemic alkalosis, because sodium bicarbonate is absorbed quickly.

BIBLIOGRAPHY

1. Bond JA, Medinsky MA: Insights into the toxicokinetics and toxicodynamics of 1,3-butadiene. Chem Biol Interact 135–136:599–614, 2001.
2. Clarke JJ, Sokal DC, Cancel AM, et al: Re-evaluation of the mutagenic potential of quinacrine dihydrochloride dihydrate. Mutat Res 494(1–2):41–53, 2001.
3. Gill SS, Pulido OM: Glutamate receptors in peripheral tissues: Current knowledge, future research, and implications for toxicology. Toxicol Pathol 29:208–223, 2001.
4. Isbister G, Whyte I, Dawson A: Pediatric acetaminophen poisoning. Arch Pediatr Adolesc Med 155:417–419, 2001.
5. Katzung B: Basic and Clinical Pharmacology, 8th ed. New York, Appleton & Lange, 2001.
6. Melum MF: Emergency. Organophosphate toxicity. Am J Nurs 101:57–58, 2001.
7. Rosenheck R, Kosten T: Buprenorphine for opiate addiction: Potential economic impact. Drug Alcohol Depend 63:253–262, 2001.
8. Yang JM: Toxicology and drugs of abuse testing at the point of care. Clin Lab Med 21:363–374, 2001.

APPENDIX
Physiology Review: Selected Systems

THE AUTONOMIC NERVOUS SYSTEM

The autonomic nervous system (ANS) consists of parasympathetic and sympathetic neurons. The transmitter for the parasympathetic system is acetylcholine (ACh), which acts on muscarinic and nicotinic cholinergic receptors. Muscarinic receptors are located on effector organs and mediate typical parasympathetic responses, such as *s*alivation, *l*acrimation, *u*rination, and *d*efecation (SLUD), as well as various cardiovascular responses. Prototypical muscarinic actions are:

- **Negative chronotropic and dromotropic effects**. ACh acts to decrease the rate of spontaneous depolarization of the cells of the SA node, decreasing heart rate. It also acts to decrease the rate of conduction through the atrioventricular (AV) node, through changes in sodium and calcium conductance.
- **Decreased inotropic effect**. ACh decreases the force of contraction of cardiac muscle, resulting in decreased ejection fraction and decreased cardiac output.
- **Miosis**. Ach constricts the circular muscle of the iris, resulting in reduced pupillary diameter.
- **Increased secretion rate**. This includes secretion of gastric acid, mucous secretions, and saliva.

The major transmitter involved in the sympathetic system is norepinephrine. Receptors stimulated by norepinephrine are:

- The α_1 receptor, which mediates vasoconstriction and venoconstriction
- The α_2 receptor, which is autoregulatory, mediating a decrease in noradrenergic outflow
- the β_1 receptor, which increases cardiac inotropic, chronotropic, and dromotropic action. It also stimulates renin secretion, glycogenolysis, and gluconeogenesis
- The β_2 receptor, which mediates vasodilatation and bronchodilatation, as well as insulin synthesis

The two factions of the ANS work as opposing forces to maintain homeostasis. There is a yin/yang effect, with the parasympathetic system (i.e., resting state) being dominant. It is important to realize that both systems are constantly present and active, so if the effects of the parasympathetic system are blocked, the sympathetic effects will predominate.

THE PHYSIOLOGIC EFFECTS UNDERLYING HYPERTENSION

The following are the primary determinants of hypertension:

- Arteriolar diameter
- Cardiac output
    - i. Preload (venous tone)
    - ii. Afterload (arterial tone)
    - iii. Heart rate
    - iv. Myocardial contractility
- Blood (fluid) volume

Hypertension results from an increase in transmural pressure across the vessel wall. The primary determinants of vascular tension are the more muscular arterioles, which are able to change diameter and thus change resistance. Thus, total peripheral resistance (TPR) is the primary determinant of hypertension. The amount of fluid within the vessels is also a determinant. Therefore, cardiac output and blood (fluid) volume are also determinants. Recall also that cardiac output = heart rate × force of contraction and is influenced by preload (venous tone) and afterload (arterial tone).

THE CARDIAC ACTION POTENTIAL

The major determinants of cardiac action are sodium, potassium, and calcium. The equilibrium potentials are: sodium = +60, potassium = –90, calcium = +50

More channels open as the membrane potential approaches the ionic equilibrium potential. However, the reversal potential is never reached because the membrane potential is due to a combination of ionic potentials; no one channel type is open during a particular phase of the action potential.

The shape of the action potential is determined by the rapidity of influx or efflux of ions with time. Therefore, if calcium channels are blocked, phase 2 will be elongated, and blockade of potassium channels will result in elongation of phase 2 and prolonged or skewed phase 2.

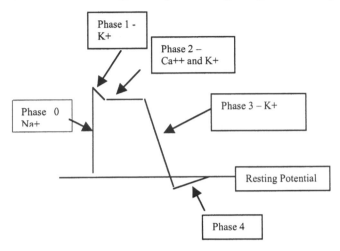

Normal cardiac action potential.

THE ETIOLOGY AND TYPES OF CARDIAC ARRHYTHMIAS

Arrhythmias arise from ectopic foci in the cardiac tissue. Recall that all cardiac myocytes have the potential for spontaneous depolarization because of their smooth muscle–like properties and the close proximity of the cell membrane to depolarization threshold. Normally, these foci are eliminated by the powerful depolarization of the SA nodal cells. Unopposed, these foci generate depolarizations that cause small premature contractions and inhibit full contraction of cardiac muscle in response to the normal SA nodal depolarization. This is of primary importance in ventricular tissue.

Supraventricular Arrhythmias

Supraventricular arrhythmias arise from atrial or accessory pathways. They are not life threatening unless the arrhythmia is communicated to ventricular pathways. Atrial arrhythmias include atrial flutter and atrial fibrillation.

Supraventricular arrhythmias arising from accessory conduction pathways include Wolff-Parkinson-White syndrome (re-entrant arrhythmias). In this case, a depolarization and conduction occur in an accessory pathway, which circumvents the upper portion of the AV node and weakly depolarizes AV nodal tissue. Then, because the tissue is quickly repolarized, it is able to rapidly depolarize the upper portion of the AV node after depolarization of myocardial tissue, causing a re-entrant "loop" or circus rhythm. (The nodal tissue is normally refractory to stimulus, and thus serves as the termination stimulus for ventricular conduction.) The therapy of supraventricular arrhythmias involves partial blockade of the AV node.

Ventricular Arrhythmias

Ventricular arrhythmias arise most often from cells in the bundle of His and Purkinje's fibers. These ectopic foci can cause premature contraction of ventricular cells, resulting in no beneficial physiologic effect but leaving the cells of the conduction pathway hypopolarized, causing a conduction blockade or a small depolarization and subsequent contraction. These arrhythmias can be life threatening.

Therapy of ventricular arrhythmias involves depression of the excitability of cells in the bundle of His and Purkinje's fibers, leaving the AV nodal conduction pathways relatively unopposed.

PROSTANOID SYNTHESIS AND FUNCTION

Prostanoid synthesis begins with the release of arachidonic acid from cellular membranes by phospholipase A_2. Arachidonic acid is cleaved by cyclooxygenase, resulting in the generation of subsequent precursors, which enter the various pathways to become prostaglandins (PGA, B, C, D, or F), prostacyclin (PGI_2), or thromboxane A (e.g., TxA series). These mediators act on smooth muscle to promote constriction or dilation; on neurons (e.g., pain fibers) to promote excitation; or as mediators released from endogenous cells (e.g., leukocytes), which act on brain structures (e.g., the hypothalamus). Inhibition of the first step of the prostaglandin synthesis cascade (e.g., cyclooxygenase) results in dose-dependent inhibition of the various pathways that follow. Products of the 5-lipoxygenase pathway (e.g., leukotrienes and lipoxins) are not affected by cyclooxygenase inhibitors.

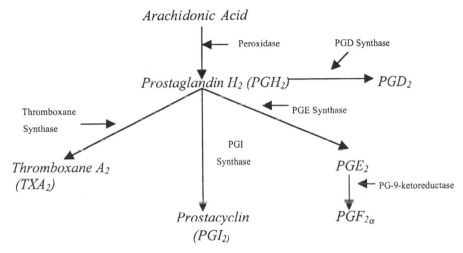

Schematic diagram of prostanoid synthesis.

INDEX

Page numbers in **boldface type** indicate complete chapters.